Clinical Cases in
Orofacial Pain

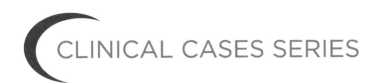

CLINICAL CASES SERIES

Clinical Cases in
Orofacial Pain

Edited by

Malin Ernberg

Karolinska Institutet
Department of Dental Medicine
Section for Orofacial Pain and Jaw Function
Scandinavian Center for Orofacial Neurosciences (SCON)
Huddinge
Sweden

Per Alstergren

Malmö University
Faculty of Odontology
Department of Orofacial Pain and Jaw Function
Scandinavian Center for Orofacial Neurosciences (SCON)
Malmö
Sweden

Skåne's University Hospital
Specialized Pain Rehabilitiation
Lund
Sweden

WILEY Blackwell

This edition first published 2017
© 2017 John Wiley and Sons

The right of Malin Ernberg and Per Alstergren to be identified as the Editors of the editorial material in this work has been asserted in accordance with law.

Registered Offices
John Wiley & Sons, Inc., 111 River Street, Hoboken, NJ 07030, USA
John Wiley & Sons Ltd, The Atrium, Southern Gate, Chichester, West Sussex, PO19 8SQ, UK

Editorial Office
9600 Garsington Road, Oxford, OX4 2DQ, UK
For details of our global editorial offices, customer services, and more information about Wiley products visit us at www.wiley.com.
Wiley also publishes its books in a variety of electronic formats and by print-on-demand. Some content that appears in standard print versions of this book may not be available in other formats.

Limit of Liability/Disclaimer of Warranty
The contents of this work are intended to further general scientific research, understanding, and discussion only and are not intended and should not be relied upon as recommending or promoting scientific method, diagnosis, or treatment by physicians for any particular patient. The publisher and the authors make no representations or warranties with respect to the accuracy and completeness of the contents of this work and specifically disclaim all warranties, including without limitation any implied warranties of fitness for a particular purpose. In view of ongoing research, equipment modifications, changes in governmental regulations, and the constant flow of information relating to the use of medicines, equipment, and devices, the reader is urged to review and evaluate the information provided in the package insert or instructions for each medicine, equipment, or device for, among other things, any changes in the instructions or indication of usage and for added warnings and precautions. Readers should consult with a specialist where appropriate. The fact that an organization or website is referred to in this work as a citation and/or potential source of further information does not mean that the author or the publisher endorses the information the organization or website may provide or recommendations it may make. Further, readers should be aware that websites listed in this work may have changed or disappeared between when this works was written and when it is read. No warranty may be created or extended by any promotional statements for this work. Neither the publisher nor the author shall be liable for any damages arising herefrom.

Library of Congress Cataloging-in-Publication Data

Names: Ernberg, Malin, editor. | Alstergren, Per, editor.
Title: Clinical cases in orofacial pain / edited by Prof. Malin Ernberg,
    Prof. Per Alstergren.
Other titles: Clinical cases (Ames, Iowa)
Description: 1 edition. | Hoboken, NJ : John Wiley & Sons, Inc., [2017] |
    Series: Wiley-Blackwell's clinical cases series | Includes bibliographical
    references and index.
Identifiers: LCCN 2016055411 (print) | LCCN 2016057074 (ebook) | ISBN
    9781119194798 (pbk.) | ISBN 9781119194804 (pdf) | ISBN 9781119194828 (epub)
Subjects: | MESH: Facial Pain–diagnosis | Temporomandibular Joint
    Disorders–diagnosis | Case Reports
Classification: LCC RK322 (print) | LCC RK322 (ebook) | NLM WU 141 | DDC
    617.5/2–dc23
LC record available at https://lccn.loc.gov/2016055411

The contents of this work are intended to further general scientific research, understanding, and discussion only and are not intended and should not be relied upon as recommending or promoting scientific method, diagnosis, or treatment by physicians for any particular patient. The publisher and the authors make no representations or warranties with respect to the accuracy and completeness of the contents of this work and specifically disclaim all warranties, including without limitation any implied warranties of fitness for a particular purpose. In view of ongoing research, equipment modifications, changes in governmental regulations, and the constant flow of information relating to the use of medicines, equipment, and devices, the reader is urged to review and evaluate the information provided in the package insert or instructions for each medicine, equipment, or device for, among other things, any changes in the instructions or indication of usage and for added warnings and precautions. Readers should consult with a specialist where appropriate. The fact that an organization or website is referred to in this work as a citation and/or potential source of further information does not mean that the author or the publisher endorses the information the organization or website may provide or recommendations it may make. Further, readers should be aware that websites listed in this work may have changed or disappeared between when this works was written and when it is read. No warranty may be created or extended by any promotional statements for this work. Neither the publisher nor the author shall be liable for any damages arising herefrom.

Cover image: Per Alstergren
Cover design: Wiley

Set in 10/13pt, UniversLTStd by SPi Global, Chennai, India
Printed and bound in Singapore by Markono Print Media Pte Ltd

10 9 8 7 6 5 4 3 2 1

This book is dedicated to our patients, you are the greatest source to our understanding of orofacial pain

CONTENTS

List of Contributors

Editors

Malin Ernberg DDS, PhD
Professor and Head
Section of Orofacial Pain and Jaw Function
Department of Dental Medicine
Karolinska Institutet
Scandinavian Center for Orofacial Neurosciences (SCON)
Huddinge
Sweden

Per Alstergren DDS, PhD
Professor and Head
Department of Orofacial Pain and Jaw Function
Faculty of Odontology
Malmö University
Scandinavian Center for Orofacial Neurosciences (SCON)
Malmö
Sweden
Skåne's University Hospital
Specialized Pain Rehabilitiation
Lund
Sweden

Contributors

Sowmya Ananthan BDS, DMD, MSD
Division of Orofacial Pain
Rutgers School of Dental Medicine
Newark
USA

Peter Abrahamsson DDS
Senior Consultant
Käkkirurgiska kliniken
Region Halland
Halmstad
Sweden

Lene Baad-Hansen DDS, PhD
Associate Professor
Section of Orofacial Pain and Jaw Function
Department of Odontology
Aarhus University
Scandinavian Center for Orofacial Neurosciences
  (SCON)
Aarhus
Denmark

Merete Bakke DDS, PhD, Dr Odont
Associate Professor
Department of Odontology
Faculty of Health and Medical Sciences
Copenhagen University
Copenhagen
Denmark

Karina Bendixen DDS, PhD
Associate Professor
Section of Orofacial Pain and Jaw Function
Department of Odontology
Aarhus University
Scandinavian Center for Orofacial Neurosciences
  (SCON)
Aarhus
Denmark

Rafael Benoliel BDS
Professor
Division of Orofacial Pain
Rutgers University School of Dental Medicine
Newark
USA

Tore Bjørnland DDS, Dr Odont
Professor
Department of Oral Surgery and Oral Medicine
Institute of Clinical Dentistry
Faculty of Dentistry
University of Oslo
Oslo
Norway

Paulo César R Conti DDS, PhD
Professor
Department of Prosthodontics
Bauru School of Dentistry
University of São Paulo
Bauru
Brazil

Randy Q Cron MD, PhD
Division of Pediatric Rheumatology
University of Alabama
Children's Park Place
Birmingham
USA

Lars Eriksson DDS, PhD
Professor
Department of Oral and Maxillofacial Surgery
Faculty of Odontology
Malmö University
Malmö
Sweden

Natasha M Flake DDS, MSc, PhD
Associate Professor
University of Washington Medical Center
Seattle
USA

Dorothy Foigelman-Holland PT, DPT
Ken-Ton Physical Therapy
Kenmore
USA

Daniela AG Gonçalves DDS, PhD
Professor
Department of Dental Materials and Prosthodontics
UNESP–Universidad Estadual Paulista
São Paulo
Brazil

Jean-Paul Goulet DDS, MSD, FRCD
Professor
Section of Stomatology
Faculty of Dentistry
Laval University
Montreal
Canada

Britt Hedenberg-Magnusson DDS, PhD
Associate Professor
Section of Orofacial Pain and Jaw Function
Department of Dental Medicine
Karolinska Institutet
Scandinavian Center for Orofacial Neurosciences
    (SCON)
Huddinge
Department of Orofacial Pain and Jaw Function
Eastman Institute
Stockholm
Sweden

Gary M Heir DMD
Professor
Center for Temporomandibular Disorders and
    Orofacial Pain
Rutgers University School of Dental Medicine
Newark
USA

Fredrik Hallmer DDS
Department of Oral and Maxillofacial Surgery
Skåne University Hospital
Lund
Sweden

Birgitta Häggman-Henriksson DDS, PhD
Associate Professor
Department of Orofacial Pain and Jaw Function
Faculty of Odontology
Malmö University
Scandinavian Center for Orofacial Neurosciences
    (SCON)
Malmö
Sweden

Stanimira I Kalaykova DDS, PhD
Associate Professor
Department of Oral Function and Prosthetic Dentistry
College of Dental Science
Radboud University Medical Center
Nijmegen
The Netherlands

Junad Khan BDS, MSD, PhD
Division of Orofacial Pain
Rutgers University School of Dental Medicine
Newark
USA

Eiro Kubota DDS, PhD
Professor
Department of Oral and Maxillofacial Surgery
Kanagawa Dental College
Kanagawa
Japan

Thomas List DDS, PhD
Professor
Department of Orofacial Pain and Jaw Function
Faculty of Odontology
Malmö University
Scandinavian Center for Orofacial Neurosciences
    (SCON)
Malmö
Sweden

Daniele Manfredini DDS
Professor
Temporomandibular Disorders Clinic and School of
    Dentistry
Department of Neurosciences
University of Padova
Padova
Italy

Ambra Michelotti BDS, DDS
Professor
Section of Orthodontics
Department of Neuroscience
Section of Temporomandibular Disorders and
    Orofacial Pain
University of Naples "Federico II"
Naples
Italy

Egild Møller DDS, PhD
Professor
Department of Odontology
Faculty of Health and Medical Sciences
University of Copenhagen
Copenhagen
Denmark

Christine Nadeau DMD, MSc
Laval University
Québec
Canada

Richard Ohrbach DDS, PhD
Professor
University at Buffalo
Buffalo
USA

Maria Pigg DDS, PhD
Assistant Professor
Department of Endodontics
Faculty of Odontology
Malmö University
Scandinavian Center for Orofacial Neurosciences
    (SCON)
Malmö
Sweden

Massimiliano Politi DDS
Department of Biomedical, Surgical and Dental
    Sciences
Section of Orthodontics
IRCCS Galeazzi Orthopaedic Institute
University of Milan
Milan
Italy

Bachar Reda DDS
Department of Orthodontics and Gnathology
University of Trieste
Trieste
Italy

Claudia Restrepo DDS
Professor
CES-LPH Research Group
Faculty of Dentistry
Universidad CES
Medellín
Colombia

Annemiek Rollman PT, PhD
Department of Oral Kinesiology
Academic Centre for Dentistry Amsterdam (ACTA)
Amsterdam
The Netherlands

Juliana Stuginski-Barbosa DDS, MSc, PhD
Department of Prosthodontics
Bauru School of Dentistry
University of São Paulo
Bauru
Brazil

Peter Svensson DDS, PhD, Dr Odont
Professor
Section of Orofacial Pain and Jaw Function
Department of Odontology
Aarhus University
Scandinavian Center for Orofacial Neurosciences
   (SCON)
Aarhus
Denmark
Department of Dental Medicine
Karolinska Institutet
Huddinge
Sweden

Peter Wetselaar DDS, PhD
Department of Oral Kinesiology
Academic Centre for Dentistry Amsterdam (ACTA)
Amsterdam
The Netherlands

**Joanna Zakrewska BDS, MB BChir, MD, FDSRCS,
   FFDRCSI, FFPM RCA, FHEA**
Professor
Eastman Dental Hospital
UCLH NHS Foundation Trust
London
UK

Vincent B Ziccardi DDS, MD, FACS
Assistant Dean of Hospital Affairs
Chief of Service
University Hospital
Division of Oral and Maxillofacial Surgery
Newark
USA

Preface

Chronic pain is an excessive burden for those affected and leads to severe consequences and reduced quality of life for the patient as well as their closest family. It also has a great impact on society in terms of costs for health care, sick leave and early retirement. The most common type of chronic pain in the orofacial region is temporomandibular disorders (TMDs) pain, but chronic orofacial pain may also be caused by, for example, nerve lesions in the trigeminal system, diseases, or being a part of a generalized pain condition. The knowledge about chronic pain has evolved considerably during the last 20 years. Chronic pain is nowadays considered not as a symptom but rather recognized by the World Health Organization as a disease in itself. Likewise, medical education, including dentistry and orofacial pain, has also evolved to include case-based teaching to better reinforce this more holistic approach. Traditional textbooks are an excellent resource but by necessity present information in artificially constrained topic groupings. For orofacial pain conditions, not only the physical symptoms and signs, but also psychosocial issues and health status need to be addressed simultaneously to properly assess the patient and manage the care. A case-based approach to education allows students to use foundational knowledge obtained from reference texts and didactic courses to learn strategies for providing patient-centered care.

The clinical cases included in this book were conceived to provide case studies for a wide array of learning situations, but the cases are primarily aimed at undergraduate and postgraduate teaching. For undergraduate students the cases may provide a more clinically oriented complement to text books about orofacial pain. Residents can use these cases as they prepare for case-based exams during their training and board certification. The cases can also be used as a quick introduction to orofacial pain, and as a study guide for case-based curricula and exams for students at all educational levels; for example, undergraduate, postgraduate, and doctoral students as well as residents. This book will also be a useful tool for educators, who will now have a ready collection of clinical cases, covering the essentials of orofacial pain, to discuss with their students.

Each case emphasizes a particular diagnosis, but any particular patient case may have other diagnoses as well. The case presentation is accompanied by pink boxes within the text containing background information, diagnostic criteria, and fundamental points. The background may include a more in-depth presentation of the particular knowledge about, for example, etiology, epidemiology, diagnostics, and treatment for the particular diagnosis that the case represents. The Diagnostic Criteria for TMD (DC/TMD) are primarily used as these criteria are validated. For orofacial pain diagnoses not included in the DC/TMD the criteria proposed in the expanded taxonomy for DC/TMD are used, or other recommended criteria (e.g., the criteria for headache by the International Headache Society). Fundamental points address issues that are of importance to the diagnosis, treatment plan, and management of the case.

Even if the book can be used as a "dictionary" to retrieve information about specific diagnoses, it is strongly recommended that the reader also read the first chapter. This chapter gives thorough information about diagnostics in chronic orofacial pain, including the DC/TMD classification as a basis for diagnostics. The reader could then read the information provided on patient presentation and history, to determine what additional diagnostic information is necessary and how it would be best obtained. A differential diagnosis and problem list could then be compiled and used for comparison with that provided in the case. Following this, a treatment plan can be proposed which should then also be compared with that listed in the text. At the end of each chapter a number of study questions with answers are provided that can be used to review the key elements of the topic or as a study guide for self-evaluation in preparation exams.

Although each clinical case in this book was designed to focus on a particular diagnosis, we also wanted it to be possible to only read about single cases. Therefore, there will be some repetition from case to case. The editors have tried to minimize this as much as possible by referring to other cases, but it will be evident particularly regarding management, as this does not differ very much across diagnoses.

We have selected highly competent contributors with an international perspective to make the content universally relevant. However, for consistency we have chosen to use the FDI nomenclature.

The structure of the book is based on the diagnostic list in the proposed Expanded taxonomy for DC/TMD and the cases have been selected to represent the essentials of orofacial pain. However, some diagnoses are very rare and have therefore been excluded, or excluded due to other reasons. Other diagnoses have been added, as they are not included in the Expanded DC/TMD taxonomy (e.g., neuropathic and dental pains).

It was also beyond the scope of this type of book to provide comprehensive citations, so for each chapter only a few key references are listed.

We hope that students, educators, and clinicians will find this book a useful resource as we advance and broaden the scope of orofacial pain for the benefit of our patients.

Acknowledgments

We, the Editors, would like to express our gratitude to those who have contributed in compiling all these excellent cases and thus made this book project possible. There are more than 35 co-authors from Europe, Asia, USA, and South America that have contributed with writing of cases. Without your help sharing your cases there would have been no book. Thank you!

We would also like to thank Catriona Cooper, Mary Aswinee Anton, Tanya McMullin, and Jessica Evans at Wiley-Blackwell for excellent guidance and editorial assistance throughout the process.

Finally, we would like to thank all the patients that have consented to appear in this book.

Abbreviations

Abbreviation	Term
AAOP	American Academy for Orofacial Pain
ACPA	Anti-citrullinated peptide antibody
CBCT	Cone-beam computerized tomography
CBT	Cognitive behavioural therapy
CRP	C-reactive protein
CT	Computerized tomography
DC/TMD	Diagnostic Criteria for Temporomandibular Disorders
ENT	Ear, Nose, and Throat
EPT	Electric Pain Threshold
ESR	Erythrocyte sedimentation rate
GAD-7	Generalized Anxiety Disorder-7 questionnaire (anxiety)
GCPS	Graded Chronic Pain Scale
ICHD-3 beta	International Classification of Headache Disorders version 3 beta
IHS	International Headache Society
MRI	Magnetic resonance imaging
NRS	Numerical rating scale
NSAID	Nonsteroidal anti-inflammatory drug
OBCL	Oral Behavior Checklist
PCS	Patient Catastrophizing Scale
PHQ-9	Patient Health Questionnaire-9 (depression)
PHQ-15	Patient Health Questionnaire-15 (physical symptoms)
PSQI	Pittsburgh Sleep Quality Index questionnaire
PSS-10	Perceived Stress Scale-10
RDC/TMD	Research Diagnostic Criteria for Temporomandibular Disorders
RF	Rheumatoid factor
SNRI	Serotonin and noradrenaline reuptake inhibitor
SSRI	Selective serotonin reuptake inhibitor
TCA	Tricyclic antidepressant
TMD	Temporomandibular disorder
TMJ	Temporomandibular joint
VAS	Visual analog scale

1

Diagnostics of Orofacial Pain and Temporomandibular Disorders

Thomas List and Richard Ohrbach

Temporomandibular disorders (TMDs) and orofacial pain occur in about 5–12% of the adult population and in approximately 4–7% of youth and adolescents (Drangsholt, 1999; Nilsson *et al.*, 2005; NIDCR, 2014). About half of the individuals with TMD and orofacial pain perceive a need for treatment and seek consultation (Nilsson *et al.*, 2009; NIDCR, 2014). The consequences of TMD and orofacial pain for the patient are often a limitation in daily activities, lower quality of life, and personal suffering; the consequences for society include high economic costs for treatment and loss of productivity (NIDCR, 2014).

Although several professional groups routinely encounter patients with TMD and orofacial pain, it is the general practicing dentist who will initially manage the care of these patients. One problem is that general dentists are often unsure about diagnosing patients with TMD and orofacial pain (Tegelberg *et al.*, 2001). Thus, there is great need for a simplified and reliable diagnostic classification with clear instructions on how to conduct the clinical examination and which questions to ask in the history to get an overall picture of the patient's difficulties and choose suitable therapy. In addition to determining diagnoses through the examination of subjective symptoms and clinical findings, it is important to assess the patient's psychosocial status, including the consequences of chronic pain, in order to reveal an overall picture of the patient. The clinical condition (Axis I) and the psychosocial assessment (Axis II) together provide the information necessary for planning and executing suitable therapy with an optimal prognosis.

Diagnostic Classifications

There are many diagnostic systems for TMD and orofacial pain (Dworkin and LeResche, 1992; de Leeuw and Klasser, 2013; Headache Classification Committee of the International Headache Society (IHS), 2013; Peck *et al.*, 2014; Schiffman *et al.*, 2014). Of these, the Research Diagnostic Criteria for Temporomandibular Disorders (RDC/TMD) and the American Academy of Orofacial Pain (AAOP) diagnostic criteria for TMD-related masticatory disorders have been the ones most used internationally (Dworkin and LeResche, 1992; de Leeuw and Klasser, 2013). The RDC/TMD standardized assessment of the most common TMD diagnoses and the AAOP criteria, while not as strictly defined, covered a larger range of conditions.

The RDC/TMD has been translated into more than 20 languages, and the publication that introduced it is one of the most cited in the dental literature (Dworkin and LeResche, 1992; List and Greene, 2010). After identification of some limitations of the system, the RDC/TMD was revised and the new classification system Diagnostic Criteria for Temporomandibular Disorders (DC/TMD) (Schiffman *et al.*, 2014) was developed, which was also incorporated into the newest edition of the AAOP guidelines (de Leeuw and Klasser, 2013), thereby bringing research and clinical practice together.

Clinical Cases in Orofacial Pain, First Edition. Edited by Malin Ernberg and Per Alstergren.
© 2017 John Wiley & Sons Ltd. Published 2017 by John Wiley & Sons Ltd.

The most common temporomandibular disorders

The DC/TMD is based both on extensive multicenter clinical studies, including studies funded by the National Institutes of Health in the USA, and on international consensus conferences (Schiffman et al., 2014). It is important to point out here that the DC/TMD only covers the most commonly occurring TMD conditions. The DC/TMD is comprised of two domains: a physical Axis I and a psychosocial Axis II.

The strength of the DC/TMD Axis I protocol includes reliable and valid diagnostic criteria for the common pain-related disorders and for the intraarticular disorders. The Axis I protocol provides standardized evaluation of subjective symptoms, contains clearly defined examination methods, and utilizes specific diagnostic criteria based on the clinical findings. The Axis II protocol, a psychosocial assessment, is simplified compared with the RDC/TMD version and has two options: a brief assessment and a comprehensive set of instruments for expanded assessment. The AAOP guidelines, in parallel, include the 12 common DC/TMD diagnoses.

Less common temporomandibular disorders: the expanded taxonomy

The DC/TMD covers the most common TMD conditions for which data were readily available. This created a need to expand the taxonomy to cover less common but still clinically relevant conditions. The expanded taxonomy (Peck et al., 2014) is a consolidation of the common disorders in the DC/TMD and the less common disorders described in the fourth edition of the AAOP guidelines for TMD (De Leeuw, 2008). The expanded taxonomy defines the diagnostic criteria for

Table 1.1 Expanded taxonomy of the DC/TMD

I TMJ DISORDERS
  1. Joint pain
     A. **Arthralgia***
     B. Arthritis
  2. Joint disorders
     A. **Disc disorders***
        1. **Disc displacement with reduction***
        2. **Disc displacement with reduction with intermittent locking***
        3. **Disc displacement without reduction with limited opening***
        4. **Disc displacement without reduction without limited opening***
     B. Hypomobility disorders other than disc disorders
        1. Adhesions/adherence
        2. Ankylosis
           a. Fibrous
           b. Osseous
     C. Hypermobility disorders
        1. Dislocations
           a. **Subluxation***
           b. Luxation
  3. Joint diseases
     A. **Degenerative joint disease***
        1. Osteoarthrosis
        2. Osteoarthritis
     B. Systemic arthritides
     C. Condylysis/idiopathic condylar resorption
     D. Osteochondritis dissecans
     E. Osteonecrosis
     F. Neoplasm
     G. Synovial chondromatosis
  4. Fractures

Table 1.1 (*Continued*)

1. Congenital/developmental disorders
   A. Aplasia
   B. Hypoplasia
   C. Hyperplasia
II MASTICATORY MUSCLE DISORDERS
   1. Muscle pain
      A. ***Myalgia****
         1. Local myalgia
         2. Myofascial pain
         3. ***Myofascial pain with referral****
      B. Tendonitis
      C. Myositis
      D. Spasm
   2. Contracture
   3. Hypertrophy
   4. Neoplasm
   5. Movement disorders
      A. Orofacial dyskinesia
      B. Oromandibular dystonia
   6. Masticatory muscle pain attributed to systemic/central pain disorders
      A. Fibromyalgia/widespread pain
III HEADACHE
   1. ***Headache attributed to TMD****
IV ASSOCIATED STRUCTURES
   1. Coronoid hyperplasia

*DC/TMD with sensitivity and specificity.

the less common TMD conditions and includes a total of 37 disorders; for example, temporomandibular joint (TMJ) arthritis in cases of systemic inflammatory diseases, local TMJ arthritis, ankylosis, myositis, and orofacial dyskinesia (Peck *et al.*, 2014) (Table 1.1). Note that while the diagnostic criteria for the less common disorders are clearly stated such that each disorder is defined without overlap, the criteria have not yet been operationalized; in addition, there is at present no information regarding the sensitivity, specificity, reliability, or validity of the diagnoses for these less common conditions (Peck *et al.*, 2014).

Other orofacial pain conditions

Other orofacial pain conditions – such as trigeminal neuropathic pain, persistent idiopathic orofacial pain, and burning mouth syndrome – are not included in the expanded taxonomy because they are considered to be orofacial pain conditions, not TMDs. Other classification systems should be consulted in order to diagnose these conditions.

Trigeminal neuropathic pain is caused by injury or diseases of the peripheral or central somatosensory nervous system. The pain is usually constant with variations in intensity over several days, but, in rare cases, it may also occur intermittently throughout the day. Pain from normally nonpainful stimuli (such as touch, pressure, or cooling) can be a significant part of suffering in trigeminal neuropathic pain.

Treede and colleagues have published a frequently used diagnostic algorithm for neuropathic pain, proposing three levels of pain (Treede *et al.*, 2008; Geber *et al.*, 2009).

Possible neuropathic pain

This requires both of the following:

(i) Pain distribution is neuroanatomically plausible.

(ii) History suggests lesion or disease of the somatosensory system.

Possible neuropathic pain indicates that the condition is not confirmed and requires further investigation.

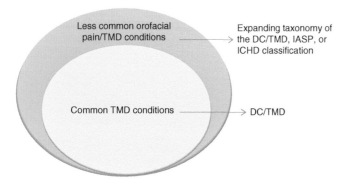

Figure 1.1 Orofacial pain and TMD conditions and the application of different diagnostic classifications.

Probable neuropathic pain

Requires (i) and (ii) with one of the following two clinical confirmatory tests being positive:

(iii) Negative or positive sensory signs confined to the innervation territory of the lesioned nervous structure (according to qualitative or quantitative sensory tests).

(iv) Diagnostic tests confirming lesion or disease explaining neuropathic pain (imaging, biopsy, neurophysiological, or laboratory tests).

Definite neuropathic pain

Requires (i) and (ii) with both clinical confirmatory tests (iii) and (iv) positive.

If a patient does not meet the criteria for any of these three levels, it is unlikely that the patient has neuropathic pain.

Figure 1.1 provides recommendations for which classification to use for orofacial pain/TMD. In summary, it is best to use the DC/TMD for the most common types of TMDs. For less common TMDs, use the expanded taxonomy of the DC/TMD. And finally, for other orofacial pain conditions, consult the classifications published by the International Association for the Study of Pain or the International Headache Society (Headache Classification Committee of the International Headache Society (IHS), 2013).

Clinical Assessment for the Most Common Temporomandibular Disorders/Orofacial Pain Conditions

It is necessary to conduct an interview to collect a comprehensive history in order to guide the clinician to make a relevant and accurate examination and provide a diagnosis, prognosis, and treatment plan for the patient. The following three steps have been recommended to simplify the clinical assessment of patients:

(i) screening of all patients at general dental clinics or by other care providers to identify patients with possible orofacial pain/TMD, (ii) a brief and focused examination by the general dentist of patients identified in the screening, and (iii) a comprehensive examination by a specialist.

Since the following chapters in this book are based on diagnoses within the expanded taxonomy of DC/TMD, the focus of this chapter is to help explain the steps leading to a diagnosis. It will provide an overview of how to establish an Axis I diagnosis (physical diagnosis) and an Axis II evaluation of psychosocial distress in orofacial pain/TMD patients.

Readers who seek more detailed information on history data collection, clinical procedures, and laboratory tests in the examination of orofacial pain patients should refer to the Schiffman *et al.* (2014), Svensson *et al.* (2014), Goulet *et al.* (2014), and Ohrbach *et al.* (2014, 2015).

Screening

Screening instruments can help simplify identification of patients with TMD and orofacial pain (Nilsson *et al.*, 2006; Gonzalez *et al.*, 2011; Zhao *et al.*, 2011). One of these instruments consists of a questionnaire with a long version (six items) and a shorter version (three items) to detect individuals with TMD pain (Gonzalez *et al.*, 2011) (Table 1.2). The long version of this instrument is also integrated into the Symptom Questionnaire of the DC/TMD. All the screening instruments demonstrate good reliability and validity (Nilsson *et al.*, 2006; Gonzalez *et al.*, 2011; Zhao *et al.*, 2011), and have been used in epidemiological studies (Nilsson *et al.*, 2006).

There are several screening instruments developed to detect neuropathic pain (Mathieson *et al.*, 2015). They are most likely useful for trigeminal neuropathic pains, but none have been validated for these conditions yet.

Screening questionnaires are an important first step in detecting patients with TMD pain in the general practice, but they do not replace the need for a physical examination.

Clinical examination

Axis I diagnostics require a patient history including questionnaires and a structured clinical examination that is described below. Assessment of the patient's psychosocial situation and pain consequences are based on validated instruments (questionnaires), which are

Table 1.2 Screening questions for TMD

1. In the last 30 days, on average, how long did any pain in your jaw or temple area on either side last?
   a. No pain
   b. From very brief to more than a week, but it does stop
   c. Continuous
2. In the last 30 days, have you had pain or stiffness in your jaw on awakening?
   a. No
   b. Yes
3. In the last 30 days, did the following activities change any pain (i.e., make it better or make it worse) in your jaw or temple area on either side?
   A. Chewing hard or tough food
      a. No
      b. Yes
   B. Opening your mouth or moving your jaw forward or to the side
      a. No
      b. Yes
   C. Jaw habits such as holding teeth together, clenching, grinding, or chewing gum
      a. No
      b. Yes
   D. Other jaw activities such as talking, kissing, or yawning
      a. No
      b. Yes

A positive score of 2 or more indicates a high probability of pain-related TMD.

described under Axis II below. The DC/TMD distinguishes two levels of inquiry in assessing the patient. The first level is designed for the general practitioner using a brief questionnaire, and the second, more advanced, level uses a more comprehensive questionnaire and is designed for the specialist. At either level it is important to evaluate both clinical status and psychosocial factors in order to get as complete a picture of the patient, given the level of assessment, when making a diagnosis, determining the best therapy, or deciding upon possible referral. Table 1.3 illustrates this through two cases. Since most patients presenting in a dental setting with a facial pain complaint will have a common TMD, we will explain the standardized protocol leading to a diagnosis and psychosocial assessment of the patient with a TMD (DC/TMD).

Clinical conditions (Axis I)

History questionnaire

The instrument called the "DC/TMD symptom questionnaire," together with data from the clinical examination, is the basis for diagnosis of clinical conditions in the DC/TMD. This questionnaire solicits information relevant for Axis I diagnoses; that is, pain, joint sounds, ability to open the mouth wide, and headache. The 14-item questionnaire, together with the clinical findings, provides enough information to diagnose the most common TMD conditions.

Clinical examination

The clinical examination consists of precise verbal instructions that the care giver gives to the patient and a detailed description of the clinical measurements to be made. One example of a verbal instruction is "Open your mouth as wide as you can without feeling any pain, or without increasing any pain you may have right now." The aim of these instructions is high reliability for examinations, as studies evaluating their use have demonstrated (Schiffman *et al.*, 2014).

The DC/TMD is built on two central concepts that must be defined for the patient before the examination: (i) pain is a personal experience and responses to whether pain is present are "yes" or "no," and (ii) familiar pain is pain that the patient recognizes; that is, pain that is similar to pain that the patient may have had in the same area sometime in the last 30 days.

That the pain experienced in the clinical examination is familiar to the patient has proved to be very important for excluding irrelevant pain. Likewise, the timeframe "in the last 30 days" emphasizes a more clinically relevant pain that is both important to the individual and a part of why the patient is seeking care. These concepts are used in the provocation of pain – for example, through jaw movements and palpation – as criteria to minimize false-positive findings.

Clinical assessments evaluate pain localization, jaw movement limitations (lateral, protruding, and mouth opening), movement pain, TMJ noises, and pain upon palpation of the masticatory muscles and TMJ. The DC/TMD requires only extraoral palpation of the *musculus temporalis*, the *musculus masseter*, and the TMJ. The palpation of other regions is unreliable (Turp and Minagi, 2001) and does not increase the sensitivity or specificity of the diagnosis. Palpation of the TMJ has been expanded to include not only the lateral pole but also the area around it to increase the scope of assessment for arthralgia. The examination protocol is standardized and recommends a palpation pressure of

Table 1.3

	Anna	Cecilia
Case history	Anna is a 19-year-old girl with frequent headaches and pain in the jaw and ear region. The pain is recurrent and greater in the morning. She has been examined by her physician and her ENT status is normal. Her physician asked her to be examined by her dentist to see if the pain could be related to orofacial pain.	Cecilia is 51 years old and has had pain for 8 years in the face, head, neck, back and arms. The average pain intensity is NRS 5. The pain started after a neck trauma. She previously received several treatments (e.g., occlusal appliance, instructions in jaw exercises, and occlusal grinding) with limited improvement. She is listless and appears to be slightly depressed.
Diagnosis (Axis I)	Myalgia Arthralgia	Myalgia Arthralgia
Pain drawing		
Characteristic pain intensity	6	5
Pain-related interference	2	8
GCPS (Axis II)	I	IV
PHQ-9	Mild	Severe
GAD-7	Mild	Severe
Treatment plan	Information and education in behavioral changes Jaw exercises Occlusal appliances	Information and education in behavioral changes Antidepressant Referral to multidisciplinary pain treatment (CBT, physical therapy)

CBT: cognitive behavioral therapy; ENT: Ear, Nose, and Throat; GCPS: Graded Chronic Pain Scale; PHQ: Patient Health Questionnaire; GAD: Generalized Anxiety Disorder.

1.0 kg for the masseter muscle, temporalis muscle, and around the lateral pole of the TMJ, and 0.5 kg for direct palpation of the lateral pole. An additional test is to examine whether the patient experiences the pain provoked by pressure only under the finger or somewhere else (referred pain), which is a sign of central sensitization.

The reader who is interested in details of the examination may download written, illustrated instructions and an instructional video at http://www.rdc-tmdinternational.org.

The DC/TMD clinical examination comprises only those measurements necessary to provide a DC/TMD diagnosis. Supplemental examinations – such as neck examination, sensory examination, cranial nerve status, occlusal measurement, or intraoral palpation of the *pterygoideus lateralis* and/or the attachment of the temporalis muscle – may be necessary for differential diagnostics, but are not part of the DC/TMD diagnoses.

Expanded Taxonomy of the Diagnostic Criteria for Temporomandibular Disorders (Axis I)

I. Temporomandibular joint disorders

Joint pain

TMJ pain (arthralgia) is defined as pain from the TMJ that is affected by jaw movements, jaw function, or jaw parafunction (Figure 1.2a). The pain should be reproducible upon provocation of the TMJ via jaw movements or palpation of the joint. Arthralgia often occurs together with a diagnosis of myalgia; only in rare cases (about 2%) is arthralgia the only diagnosis (Schiffman *et al.*, 2010). Arthritis, in contrast, is pain originating in the TMJ with clinical characteristics of inflammation over the affected joint: edema, erythema, and/or increased temperature.

Joint disorders

Disc displacement is a biomechanical disorder involving the condyle-disc complex. Clinical studies report its prevalence at 10% for healthy youths and adolescents and around 30% for healthy adults, while in clinical patients approximately 20% of youths and 40% of adults have disc displacement with reduction (List and Dworkin, 1996; List *et al.*, 1999; Anastassaki Köhler *et al.*, 2012). For the majority of individuals who experience joint sounds, the sounds are harmless, as long as there is no pain and no functional limitation due to a catch in the jaw movement.

Disc displacement with reduction and with intermittent locking includes not only clicking but also locking and catching (temporary locking) of the jaw. Patients often experience pain during locking. This group has a considerably higher risk of permanent disk displacement than the group that does not experience pain.

In disc displacement without reduction, the disc is permanently displaced. The sensitivity and specificity for a diagnosis of disc displacement without reduction and with limited mouth opening are good, while they are poor for disc displacement without reduction and without limited mouth opening. These diagnoses can be confirmed with magnetic resonance imaging (MRI), when necessary. For a definite diagnosis, MRI is required.

Hypomobility disorders other than disc disorders include intraarticular fibrous adhesion/adherence and ankylosis. These are characterized by restricted mandibular movement with deflection to the affected side on opening. They may occur as a long-term sequel of trauma, and in turn can lead to contracture of the soft tissues.

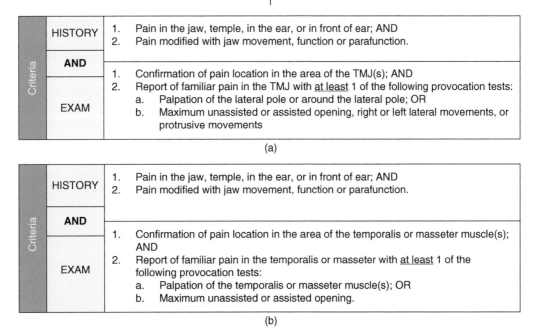

(a)

(b)

Figure 1.2 Diagnostic criteria for TMD (a) arthralgia (sensitivity, 0.91; specificity, 0.96) and (b) myalgia (sensitivity, 0.84; specificity, 0.95).

Hypermobility disorders involve a TMJ dislocation in which the condyle is positioned anterior to the articular eminence and is unable to return to a closed position without a specific maneuver by the patient or the clinician.

Joint diseases

Arthrosis/osteoarthrosis is a degenerative joint disease (DJD) characterized by loss of cartilage and bone with concurrent remodeling of underlying bone tissue. Diagnostic criteria include patient reports of crepitation from the TMJ during jaw movements and clinical findings that confirm this. Arthrotic changes, combined with a positive finding for arthralgia, indicate osteoarthritis. Sensitivity and specificity are reasonably high for the clinical diagnosis of DJD. Computed tomography of the TMJ detecting sclerosis, subchondral cyst(s), osteophytes, flattening, and space reduction between joint surfaces confirms the clinical diagnosis (Ahmad *et al.*, 2009).

Systemic arthritis is when the TMJ inflammation resulting in pain or structural changes is caused by a generalized systemic inflammatory disease, such as rheumatoid arthritis or juvenile idiopathic arthritis. Clinical signs and symptoms of ongoing chronic TMJ inflammation vary between patients, and often in the same patient over time.

There are several other rare joint diseases, such as condylysis/idiopathic condylar resorption, osteochondritis dissecans, osteonecrosis, neoplasm, and synovial chondromatosis that lead to structural changes in the TMJ. More detailed descriptions will follow in their respective chapters.

Fractures and congenital/developmental disorders

Subcondylar fracture is most common and may result in malocclusion and impaired opening. Congenital developmental disorders are characterized by incomplete or overdeveloped cranial bones or mandibles. They are often associated with mandibular or facial asymmetries and malocclusions.

II. Masticatory muscle disorders
Muscle pain

Muscle pain – that is, myalgia – is the most common TMD diagnosis and occurs in about 80% of patients with TMD (List and Dworkin, 1996; Schiffman *et al.*, 2010). Myalgia is defined as pain that occurs in the masticatory muscles; changes with jaw movements, jaw function, or parafunction; and can be reproduced by provocation. Provocation tests consist of opening the mouth wide and palpitating the temporalis and/or the masseter (Figure 1.2b). During provocation, patients must also indicate that they recognize the pain, that the pain is familiar to them. Myofascial pain with referral is defined as myalgia plus referred pain beyond the boundary of the masticatory muscles being palpated, such as in the ear, teeth, or eye.

Other masticatory muscle disorders

Other masticatory muscle disorders, such as tendonitis, myositis spasm, contracture, hypertrophy, and neoplasm, are rare. A detailed description will follow in their respective chapters.

Movement disorders

Movement disorders include patients with involuntary movements that mainly involve the face, lips, tongue, and/or the jaw. The movements can be mainly choreatic (dance-like) or involve excessive sustained contractions. A detailed description will follow in the respective chapter.

Masticatory muscle pain attributed to systemic/central pain disorders

Masticatory muscle pain with concurrent widespread pain is found in patients with conditions such as fibromyalgia.

III. Headache
Headache attributed to temporomandibular disorder

Headache is common, both in adults and in youths and adolescents (Lipton *et al.*, 2007; Stovner *et al.*, 2007). Tension-type headache and TMD have overlapping symptoms. Both conditions involve the trigeminus system and are characterized by pain and tenderness upon palpation of the head and/or face (Ciancaglini and Radaelli, 2001; Ballegaard *et al.*, 2008). However, this does not mean that the pathophysiology of the pain is identical (Svensson, 2007).

Headache attributed to TMD is defined as headache that occurs in the temple region secondary to a pain-related TMD and that is affected by jaw movement, jaw function, or parafunction. The headache should be reproducible upon provocation of the masticatory system. A prerequisite for the diagnosis is eliminating other possible headache diagnoses. Sensitivity and specificity are high for the diagnosis. This new diagnosis simplifies communication between dentists, neurologists, and headache specialists. The primary utility of this diagnosis, in contrast to a primary diagnosis (commonly, tension-type headache or migraine without aura), is that it points to TMD treatment as the therapeutic approach.

IV. Associated structures

Conditions such as coronoid hyperplasia are characterized by progressive enlargement of the coronoid process, which impedes mandibular opening when it is obstructed by the zygomatic process of the maxilla.

Psychosocial Evaluation (Axis II)

Chronic pain affects the patient's cognitive, emotional, sensory, and behavioral reactions. These can, in turn, aggravate and maintain pain. For example, a patient with chronic pain may exhibit difficulties concentrating, impaired memory function, anxiety, feelings of mild depression, dizziness, numbness, increased pain sensitivity, decreased motor functions (such as difficulties chewing and opening wide), social isolation, and absence from work due to sickness. Thus, it is very important to assess the patient's psychosocial situation when experiencing chronic pain and consider it during treatment planning and prognosis evaluation. To assess the psychosocial burden for each patient, there are instruments with structured questions and validated interpretation guidelines. Use of these instruments in treatment planning and for prognosis assessment has great patient benefit (Dworkin et al., 2002a,b).

The DC/TMD Axis II includes new instruments for assessing pain behavior, jaw function, and psychosocial functioning and distress (Schiffman et al., 2014). Table 1.4 shows the instruments recommended for the

Table 1.4 Recommended Axis II assessment protocol

Domain	Instrument	Brief	Comprehensive
Pain location	Pain drawing	✓	✓
Physical function	GCPS	✓	✓
Limitation	JFLS–8	✓	
	JFLS–20		✓
Distress	PHQ–4	✓	
Depression	PHQ–9		✓
Anxiety	GAD–7		✓
Physical symptoms	PHQ–15		✓
Parafunctions	OBCL	✓	✓

JFLS: Jaw Function Limitation Scale; OBCL: Oral Behaviors Checklist.

general practitioner (brief), and for the orofacial pain specialist (comprehensive).

Pain and daily activities

The GCPS assesses pain intensity and the degree that pain affects daily activities. The scale has been used to evaluate a range of pain conditions, and not only for the orofacial area (von Korff et al., 1992).

The GCPS records pain intensity on a 0–10 scale from three perspectives: the worst pain experienced, average pain, and current pain. The average of these values determines characteristic pain intensity, where a mean >5.0 is considered "high intensity." The GCPS also assesses the effect of pain on daily activities based on the number of days that pain interferes with daily activities and the degree to which it limits social interaction, work, or common daily activities, each rated on a 0–10 scale. High pain and a high degree of limitation of daily activities indicate a considerably worse prognosis and warrant further investigation and possibly a referral to a specialist.

The GCPS has been shown to be extremely helpful during treatment planning and prognosis evaluation in which patients with low levels of daily limitation (simple patient cases) can be treated with simpler methods while persons with greater limitations in their daily life (complex patient cases) receive more multidisciplinary treatment (Kotiranta et al., 2015).

Jaw function

The masticatory system performs many tasks, including functional use (e.g., chewing, swallowing, eating, yawning) as well as emotional expression and communication (e.g., smiling, laughing, shouting, kissing). The JFLS measures global jaw function by describing limitations in opening and chewing abilities as well as communication abilities. The scale can also be used to document changes over time (Ohrbach et al., 2008a).

Depression, anxiety, and physical symptoms

Many studies have shown that psychological distress (such as depression, anxiety) is usual in chronic TMD pain (List and Dworkin, 1996; Schiffman et al. 2010). Since pain and psychosocial distress occur together and affect each other, it is important that the overall assessment of a patient considers depression and anxiety (Schiffman et al., 2014). The following instruments are in widespread use across the world and have been translated into many languages.

The PHQ-4 is a short and sufficiently reliable instrument. It contains two questions on depression and two questions on anxiety. The instrument can indicate the presence of moderate or severe distress. For interpretation of the PHQ-4, more than 3 points indicates possible distress, while a total of more than 6 points indicates moderate distress, and a total of 9 points indicates severe distress (Kroenke et al., 2009).

For a more reliable assessment of depressive symptoms, the PHQ-9 assesses the core diagnostic areas underlying clinical depression. Data indicate that depression is more often a consequence than a cause of chronic pain. The presence of depression can substantially undermine a patient's attempts at self-management as well as contribute to impaired pain modulation. Scoring is simple with cut-offs of 5, 10, 15, and 20 representing, respectively, mild, moderate, moderately severe and severe levels of depression (Kroenke et al., 2001).

Anxiety symptoms, also represented on the PHQ-4, can be more reliably assessed with the slight longer GAD-7. The central processes associated with anxiety increase vigilance to the body and symptoms, increase body scanning and catastrophizing interpretations, and activate tension states in the body. All of these are detrimental towards improving pain. Scoring is simple, and the GAD-7 relies on cut-offs of 5, 10 and 15 representing, respectively, mild, moderate and severe levels of anxiety (Löwe et al., 2008).

The PHQ-4, PHQ-9, and GAD-7 contain a final item regarding the amount of difficulty the person has encountered due to the marked symptoms, and this response from the patient serves as an excellent starting point for discussion of the reported symptoms, by focusing on their impact on functioning.

Physical symptoms representing pain or functional problems remain one of the core methods for assessing presence of disorders that are likely comorbid with the TMD; such problems contribute greatly to chronicity, to pain facilitation, and to overall suffering (Fillingim et al., 2011). The PHQ-15 is a simple checklist for the more common functional and pain disorders. Scoring is based on cut-offs of 5, 10, and 15 representing, respectively, low, medium, and high somatic symptom severity (Kroenke et al., 2002).

Note that use of these instruments that assess mood, anxiety, and physical symptoms does not provide any psychiatric diagnoses. Instead, they give an indication of the degree of psychological distress and symptom dysregulation. This information, in turn, is very important for treatment planning and prognosis evaluation. It can also indicate a need to refer the patient to a doctor or recommend that the patient seeks care from a psychologist for psychosocial distress.

Parafunctions

Many studies have found that bruxism or other parafunctions are associated with TMD and orofacial pain (Manfredini and Lobbezoo, 2010). Most likely, certain types of bruxism or parafunctions lead to overloading in the jaw system and thereby trigger or maintain TMD and orofacial pain. Observation by the patients themselves or by friends and family is the most common method of identifying bruxism and parafunction and it is generally more reliable than a clinical assessment, except in cases of severe abrasions and muscle hypertrophy.

The OBCL gives an overview of parafunctions that occur during sleep and those that occur during the waking hours (Ohrbach et al., 2008b; Manfredini and Lobbezoo, 2010). This indicates whether treatment should target parafunction during sleep (e.g., with an occlusal splint) or during the waking period (e.g., through behavior modification). The use of a self-report instrument for the assessment of behaviors that often occur outside of normal conscious awareness often leads to the patient testing each behavior while completing the instrument in order to assess whether the behavior is familiar or not; this leads to substantially better assessment for the presence or absence of these behaviors. Reports on the OBCL, like any self-report instrument, should be followed up with further clinical interview and, as necessary, field observation for confirmation and linking to symptom patterns.

The pain drawing

The pain drawing gives a good picture of the extent and localization of the patient's pain. The pain drawing covers the entire body in order to capture all pain conditions besides TMD and orofacial pain. The most common comorbid pain conditions are headache and neck and back pain. Co-occurrence of other pain conditions is common and indicates a higher risk of developing TMD and orofacial pain (Lim et al., 2010; Marklund et al., 2010; Nilsson et al., 2013). Another important point is that widespread pain may indicate a need for medical assessment to investigate, for example, systemic diseases or central pain conditions.

We do not clearly understand why chronic orofacial pain often occurs together with other pain conditions, but it is clear that comorbid pain conditions maintain chronic orofacial pain (Rammelsberg et al., 2003;

LeResche *et al.*, 2007; Lim *et al.*, 2010; Velly *et al.*, 2010), probably via central sensitization, while reducing treatment effects and making diagnosis extremely difficult (Velly end Fricton, Velly and Fricton, 2011).

Learn About Doing These Procedures

Download the instructional video, the documentation and the questionnaires from http://www.rdc-tmdinternational. org.

1. Use the screening questions to identify patients with TMD and orofacial pain (Table 1.1).
2. Use the DC/TMD – both Axis I and Axis II – with those patients who you identified from the screening questions.

References

Ahmad M, Hollender L, Anderson Q, *et al.* (2009) Research diagnostic criteria for temporomandibular disorders (RDC/TMD): development of image analysis criteria and examiner reliability for image analysis. *Oral Surg Oral Med Oral Pathol Oral Radiol Endod* **107**:844–860.

Anastassaki Köhler A, Hugoson A, Magnusson T (2012) Prevalence of symptoms indicative of temporomandibular disorders in adults: cross-sectional epidemiological investigations covering two decades. *Acta Odontol Scand* **70**:213–223.

Ballegaard V, Thede-Schmidt-Hansen P, Svensson P, Jensen R (2008) Are headache and temporomandibular disorders related? A blinded study. *Cephalalgia* **28**:832–841.

Ciancaglini R, Radaelli G (2001) The relationship between headache and symptoms of temporomandibular disorder in the general population. *J Dent Res* **29**:93–98.

De Leeuw R (2008) *The American Academy of Orofacial Pain. Orofacial pain. Guidelines for assessment, diagnosis, and management*. Chicago, IL: Quintessence.

De Leeuw R, Klasser GD (eds) (2013) *Orofacial pain: Guidelines for assessment, diagnosis, and management*, 5 edn. Hanover Park, IL: Quintessence Publishing.

Drangsholt M (1999) Temporomandibular pain. In: Crombie I, Croft P, Linton S, *et al.* (eds), *Epidemiology of pain*. Seattle, WA: IASP Press; pp 203–234.

Dworkin SF, LeResche L (1992) Research Diagnostic Criteria for Temporomandibular Disorders: review, criteria, examinations and specifications, critique. *J Craniomandib Disord* **6**:301–355.

Dworkin SF, Huggins KH, Wilson L, *et al.* (2002a) A randomized clinical trial using research Diagnostic Criteria for Temporomandibular Disorders–Axis II to target clinic cases for a tailored self-care TMD treatment program. *J Orofac Pain* **16**:48–63.

Dworkin SF, Turner JA, Mancl L, *et al.* (2002b) A randomized clinical trial of a tailored comprehensive care treatment program for temporomandibular disorders. *J Orofac Pain* **16**:259–276.

Fillingim RB, Ohrbach R, Greenspan JD, *et al.* (2011) Potential psychosocial risk factors for chronic TMD: descriptive data

and empirically identified domains from the OPPERA case–control study. *J Pain* **12**:T46–T60.

Geber C, Baumgartner U, Schwab R, *et al.* (2009) Revised definition of neuropathic pain and its grading system: an open case series illustrating its use in clinical practice. *Am J Med* **122**:S3–S12.

Gonzalez YM, Schiffman E, Gordon SM, *et al.* (2011) Development of a brief and effective temporomandibular disorder pain screening questionnaire: reliability and validity. *J Am Dent Assoc* **142**:1183–1191.

Goulet JP, Schiffman E, Manfredini D (2014) Clinical examination and adjunctive laboratory tests for physical diagnosis. In: Sessle BJ (ed), *Orofacial pain: Recent advances in assessment, management, and understanding of mechanisms*. Washington, DC: IASP Press; pp 99–120.

Headache Classification Committee of the International Headache Society (IHS) (2013) The international classification of headache disorders, 3rd edition (beta version). *Cephalalgia* **33**:629–808.

Kotiranta U, Suvinen T, Kauko T, *et al.* (2015) Subtyping patients with temporomandibular disorders in a primary health care setting on the basis of the research diagnostic criteria for temporomandibular disorders Axis II pain-related disability: a step toward tailored treatment planning? *J Oral Facial Pain Headache* **29**:126–134.

Kroenke K, Spitzer RL, Williams JB (2001) The PHQ-9: validity of a brief depression severity measure. *J Gen Intern Med* **16**:606–613.

Kroenke K, Spitzer RL, Williams JB (2002) The PHQ-15: validity of a new measure for evaluating the severity of somatic symptoms. *Psychosom Med* **64**:258–266.

Kroenke K, Spitzer RL, Williams JB, Löwe B (2009) An ultra-brief screening scale for anxiety and depression: the PHQ-4. *Psychosomatics* **50**:613–621.

LeResche L, Mancl LA, Drangsholt MT, *et al.* (2007) Predictors of onset of facial pain and temporomandibular disorders in early adolescence. *Pain* **129**:269–278.

Lim PF, Smith S, Bhalang K, *et al.* (2010) Development of temporomandibular disorders is associated with greater bodily pain experience. *Clin J Pain* **26**:116–120.

Lipton RB, Bigal ME, Diamond M, *et al.* (2007) Migraine prevalence, disease burden, and the need for preventive therapy. *Neurology* **68**:343–349.

List T, Dworkin SF (1996) Comparing TMD diagnoses and clinical findings at Swedish and US TMD centers using research diagnostic criteria for temporomandibular disorders. *J Orofac Pain* **10**:240–253.

List T, Greene CS (2010) Moving forward with the RDC/TMD. *J Oral Rehabil* **37**:731–733.

List T, Wahlund K, Wenneberg B, Dworkin SF. (1999) TMD in children and adolescents: prevalence of pain, gender differences, and perceived treatment need. *J Orofac Pain* **13**:9–20.

Löwe B, Decker O, Müller S, *et al.* (2008) Validation and standardization of the Generalized Anxiety Disorder Screener (GAD-7) in the general population. *Med Care* **46**:266–274.

Manfredini D, Lobbezoo F (2010) Relationship between bruxism and temporomandibular disorders: a systematic review of literature from 1998 to 2008. *Oral Surg Oral Med Oral Pathol Oral Radiol Endod* **109**:e26–e50.

Marklund S, Wiesinger B, Wanman A (2010) Reciprocal influence on the incidence of symptoms in trigeminally and spinally innervated areas. *Eur J Pain* **14**:366–371.

Mathieson S, Maher CG, Terwee CB, *et al.* (2015) Neuropathic pain screening questionnaires have limited measurement properties. A systematic review. *J Clin Epidemiol* **68**:957–966.

NIDCR (2014) *Facial pain.* National Institute of Dental and Craniofacial Research. http://www.nidcr.nih.gov/ DataStatistics/FindDataByTopic/FacialPain/ (accessed November 3, 2016).

Nilsson IM, List T, Drangsholt M (2005) Prevalence of temporomandibular pain and subsequent dental treatment in Swedish adolescents. *J Orofac Pain* **19**:144–150.

Nilsson IM, List T, Drangsholt M (2006) The reliability and validity of self-reported temporomandibular disorder pain in adolescents. *J Orofac Pain* **20**:138–144.

Nilsson IM, Drangsholt M, List T (2009) Impact of temporomandibular disorder pain in adolescents: differences by age and gender. *J Orofac Pain* **23**:115–122.

Nilsson IM, List T, Drangsholt M (2013) Headache and co-morbid pains associated with TMD pain in adolescents. *J Dent Res* **92**:802–807

Ohrbach R, Larsson P, List T (2008a) The jaw functional limitation scale: development, reliability, and validity of 8-item and 20-item versions. *J Orofac Pain* **22**:219–230.

Ohrbach R, Markiewicz MR, McCall WD, Jr, (2008b) Waking-state oral parafunctional behaviors: specificity and validity as assessed by electromyography. *Eur J Oral Sci* **116**:438–444.

Ohrbach R, Durham J, Fillingim RB (2014) Self-report assessment of orofacial pain and psychosocial status. In: Sessle BJ (ed), *Orofacial pain: Recent advances in assessment, management, and understanding of mechanisms.* Washington, DC: IASP Press; pp 121–141.

Ohrbach R, Blasberg B, Greenberg MS (2015) Temporomandibular disorders. In: Glick M (ed), *Burket's oral medicine*, 12th edn. Shelton, CT:PMPH-USA, Ltd; pp 263–308.

Peck CC, Goulet JP, Lobbezoo F, *et al.* (2014) Expanding the taxonomy of the diagnostic criteria for temporomandibular disorders. *J Oral Rehabil* **41**:2–23.

Rammelsberg P, LeResche L, Dworkin S, Mancl L (2003) Longitudinal outcome of temporomandibular disorders: a 5-year epidemiologic study of muscle disorders defined by research diagnostic criteria for temporomandibular disorders. *J Orofac Pain* **17**:9–20.

Schiffman EL, Truelove EL, Ohrbach R, *et al.* (2010) The Research Diagnostic Criteria for Temporomandibular Disorders. I: overview and methodology for assessment of validity. *J Orofac Pain* **24**:7–24.

Schiffman E, Ohrbach R, Truelove E, *et al.* (2014) Diagnostic Criteria for Temporomandibular Disorders (DC/TMD) for clinical and research applications: recommendations of the International RDC/TMD Consortium Network and Orofacial Pain Special Interest Group. *J Oral Facial Pain Headache* **28**:6–27.

Stovner L, Hagen K, Jensen R, *et al.* (2007) The global burden of headache: a documentation of headache prevalence and disability worldwide. *Cephalalgia* **27**:193–210.

Svensson P (2007) Muscle pain in the head: overlap between temporomandibular disorders and tension-type headaches. *Curr Opin Neurol* **20**:320–325.

Svensson P, Baad-Hansen L, Drangsholt M, Jaaskelainen SK (2014) Neurosensory testing for assessment, diagnosis, and prediction of orofacial pain. In: Sessle BJ (ed), *Orofacial pain: Recent advances in assessment, management, and understanding of mechanisms.* Washington, DC: IASP Press; pp 143–164.

Tegelberg A, List T, Wahlund K, Wenneberg B (2001) Temporomandibular disorders in children and adolescents: a survey of dentists' attitudes, routine and experience. *Swed Dent J* **25**:119–127.

Treede RD, Jensen TS, Campbell JN, *et al.* (2008) Neuropathic pain: redefinition and a grading system for clinical and research purposes. *Neurology* **70**:1630–1635.

Turp JC, Minagi S (2001) Palpation of the lateral pterygoid region in TMD – where is the evidence? *J Dent Res* **29**:475–483.

Velly AM, Fricton J (2011) The impact of comorbid conditions on treatment of temporomandibular disorders. *J Am Dent Assoc* **142**:170–172.

Velly AM, Look JO, Schiffman E, *et al.* (2010) The effect of fibromyalgia and widespread pain on the clinically significant temporomandibular muscle and joint pain disorders – a prospective 18-month cohort study. *J Pain* **11**:1155–1164.

Von Korff M, Ormel J, Keefe FJ, Dworkin SF (1992) Grading the severity of chronic pain. *Pain* **50**:133–149.

Zhao NN, Evans RW, Byth K, *et al.* (2011) Development and validation of a screening checklist for temporomandibular disorders. *J Orofac Pain* **25**:210–222.

2

Temporomandibular Joint Disorders

Clinical Cases in Orofacial Pain, First Edition. Edited by Malin Ernberg and Per Alstergren.
© 2017 John Wiley & Sons Ltd. Published 2017 by John Wiley & Sons Ltd.

A: Joint Pain

Case 2.1

Arthralgia

Per Alstergren

A. Demographic Data and Reason for Contact

- Caucasian woman (Figure 2.1), 29 years old, referred to orofacial pain specialist from ENT specialist for pain in front of and in ear left side. ENT examination found no reason to suspect ear pathology.

B. Symptom History

- Today: sharp pain in front of left ear at some occasions on mouth opening. Sometimes minor pain on chewing. No resting pain and pain fades away quickly after each occurrence. Pain occurs more frequently in the mornings but may occur throughout the day.
- Large mouth opening (yawning, singing) elicits pain but the patient does not know any factor that can relieve the pain.
- Pain intensity varies between 0 (at rest) and 7 (on mouth opening) on a 0–10 numerical rating scale (NRS). No headache. No neck pain. No occlusal changes.
- Characteristic pain intensity 16 (NRS 0–100), current pain intensity 0 (0–10 NRS), pain-related disability 30 (NRS 0–100; GCPS).
- JFLS reveals limitation in mouth opening and singing. Infrequent daytime parafunctions (chewing gum, clenching) according OBCL.
- Debut 4 months ago for unknown reason. The pain condition has increased somewhat since the debut; occurs more often today. Ten years ago a history of clicking in the left jaw, but this went away about 2 years ago. Trauma to right cheek and head after fall from horse 3 years ago. Initial pain and decreased mouth opening, the trauma thereafter resolved by itself in 1 week; no medical attention was sought.

C. Medical History

- Hypothyreosis, stable with Levaxin® medication.
- No allergies.

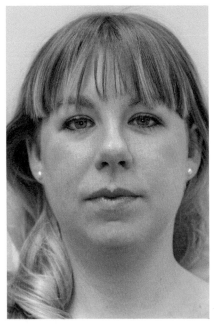

Figure 2.1 A 29-year-old Caucasian woman presenting with pain in her left TMJ on mouth opening and chewing.

D. Psychosocial History

- Unmarried, lives together with boyfriend, no children. Happy with home situation.
- Sings in a choir two times a week.
- Works as an administrative secretary in a computer game company. Very satisfied with work situation, although often stressful work tasks in periods. Frequent computer work.
- Exercises regularly at a gym.
- Describes herself as a calm person with good stress management. Normal scores for depression (PHQ-9), no anxiety (GAD-7). No physical symptoms (PHQ-15) and moderate level of stress (Perceived Stress Scale (PSS)-10). Good sleep quality (Pittsburgh Sleep Quality Index (PSQI)).
- GCPS grade I; that is, low intensity, low disability.
- No smoking, little alcohol consumption.

E. Previous Consultations and Treatments

- General practitioner (dentist) tried nonsteroidal anti-inflammatory drug (NSAID) for 2 weeks. So far unclear indication; basically no effect. Referral to ENT for ear pain.
- ENT specialist excluded ENT condition. Referral to orofacial pain specialist.

F. Extraoral Status
Asymmetries
- None.

Swelling or redness
- None.

Somatosensory abnormalities
- Maxillary branch on left side shows hyperesthesia for touch and cold. Pinprick: normal findings (compared with the right side).
- Normal findings for the other two branches of the trigeminal nerve on the left side (compared with the right side) regarding touch, cold, and pinprick.

Temporomandibular joint
- No palpation pain.
- Brief familiar pain in left TMJ on maximum mouth opening (48 mm).

Masticatory muscles
- Familiar palpation pain in masseter muscle and temporalis insertion, left side.

Jaw movement capacity
- Maximum unassisted mouth opening 48 mm, laterotrusion to the right 9 mm and to the left 14 mm, protrusion 11 mm.
- Lower jaw deviates to the left on maximum mouth opening and protrusion.

Neck
- Normal movement capacity; no pain on movement or palpation.

G. Intraoral Status
Hard tissues and dentition
- Complete dentition with few and minor fillings.

Occlusion
- Stable with bilateral contacts on molars and premolars.

H. Additional Examinations and Findings
- None needed at this point.

I. Diagnosis/Diagnoses
DC/TMD
- Arthralgia in the left TMJ.
- Myalgia of the masticatory muscles.

J. Case Assessment
- Intermittent and rather intense pain on mouth opening in the left TMJ. Painful mouth opening does not elicit prolonged TMJ pain or pain at rest. Muscular palpation pain on the same side is interpreted as local sensitization; no other indications of a muscle tension problem.
- Anamnestic information gives rise to a suspicion of disc displacement without reduction in the left TMJ, but it is so far unclear to what extent that a possible disc displacement contributes to the current pain. In summary, most likely a mechanically induced nociceptive pain in the left TMJ, possibly related to a disc displacement without reduction and perhaps also the trauma to the right side of the face (implies trauma to left TMJ). No specific clinical signs of arthritis (prolonged pain, pain at rest, pain on movement, pain on loading, occlusal changes, swelling, etc.).
- Very little psychosocial distress.

K. Evidence-based Treatment Plan including Aims
- Counselling and patient education. Aims: to increase knowledge and understanding, to reduce anxiety and to correct expectations.
- Jaw exercises. Aims: increase physical activity in the masticatory system to reduce pain-eliciting factors, improve coordination, reduce arthralgia and myalgia.
- Stabilization appliance. Aim: reduce morning time increase in pain frequency by unloading the joint and by altering the sensory input during sleep.

L. Prognosis and Discussion
- The prognosis is good, both due to a rather short duration of the pain problem and due to the low characteristic pain intensity, pain-related disability, and psychological distress.

Background Information
- Arthralgia means "pain in a joint" and can be part of nociceptive pain during overextension,

overloading or mechanical impingement, part of inflammation in articular tissues, i.e. arthritis, or a sensitization of the articular and adjacent tissues (Peck *et al.*, 2014).

- There are only a few patients presenting with solely "arthralgia" of the TMJ. Only about 1.9–2.3% of patients referred to an orofacial pain clinic will have "arthralgia" and not "myalgia" as well. It is much more common, as in this case, that the patients have both "arthralgia" and "myalgia" (Schiffman *et al.*, 2010).
- TMJ effusions lack adequate specificity for identifying TMJ arthralgia and were not associated with pain (Shaefer *et al.*, 2001).

Diagnostic Criteria

DC/TMD criteria for **Arthralgia** (Schiffman *et al.*, 2014). Sensitivity of 0.89 and specificity 0.98.

TMJ arthralgia definition: pain of joint origin that is affected by jaw movement, function, or parafunction, and replication of this pain occurs with provocation testing of the TMJ.

History.   Positive for both of the following:

1. Pain in the jaw, temple, in front of the ear, or in the ear.
   AND
2. Pain modified with jaw movement, function or parafunction.

Examination.   Positive for both of the following:

1. Confirmation of pain location in the area of the TMJ(s).
   AND
2. Report of familiar pain in the TMJ with at least one of the following provocation tests:
   (a) Palpation of the lateral pole or around the lateral pole.
   OR
   (b) Maximum unassisted or assisted opening, right or left lateral movements, or protrusive movements.

Note: The pain is not better accounted for by another pain diagnosis.

Criteria for DC/TMD **Myalgia** (Schiffman *et al.*, 2014), see Case 3.3.

Fundamental Points

- The diagnosis "arthralgia" is highly unspecific and does not give any indication of the cause (Peck *et al.*, 2014).
- Since treatment success depends on the underlying cause of the arthralgia, it is important to try to figure that out in addition to setting the diagnosis. The reason behind the arthralgia should be used to indicate which treatment modalities and treatment goals to use.
- Arthralgia in the TMJ can severely influence daily activities and life quality, at least if the arthralgia is due to systemic inflammatory disease affecting the TMJ (Voog *et al.*, 2003; Ahmad *et al.*, 2015).

Self-study Questions

1. What underlying mechanisms may cause "arthralgia"?
2. What is the difference between "arthralgia" and "arthritis"?
3. How common is it that a patient presents with solely TMJ arthralgia?
4. Can MRI be used to confirm TMJ arthralgia?

References

Ahmed N, Mustafa HM, Catrina AI, Alstergren P (2013) Impact of temporomandibular joint pain in rheumatoid arthritis. *Mediators Inflamm* **2013**:597419.

Peck CC, Goulet JP, Lobbezoo F, *et al.* (2014) Expanding the taxonomy of the diagnostic criteria for temporomandibular disorders. *J Oral Rehabil* **41**(1):2–23.

Shaefer JR, Jackson DL, Schiffman EL, Anderson QN (2001) Pressure-pain thresholds and MRI effusions in TMJ arthralgia. *J Dent Res* **80**(10):1935–1939.

Schiffman EL, Ohrbach R, Truelove EL, *et al.* (2010) The Research Diagnostic Criteria for Temporomandibular Disorders. V: methods used to establish and validate revised Axis I diagnostic algorithms. *J Orofac Pain* **24**(1):63–78.

Schiffman E, Ohrbach R, Truelove E, *et al.* (2014) Diagnostic Criteria for Temporomandibular Disorders (DC/TMD) for Clinical and Research Applications: recommendations of the International RDC/TMD Consortium Network and Orofacial Pain Special Interest Group. *J Oral Facial Pain Headache* **28**(1):6–27.

Voog U, Alstergren P, Leibur E, *et al.* (2003) Impact of temporomandibular joint pain on activities of daily living in patients with rheumatoid arthritis. *Acta Odontol Scand* **61**(5):278–282.

Answers to Self-study Questions

1. Arthritis, overstretching, overloading, impingement, regional sensitization.

2. Arthritis is inflammation of articular tissues. One symptom of arthritis may be arthralgia, but there are examples of ongoing arthritis of the TMJ without pain. A common example is TMJ arthritis in children due to juvenile idiopathic arthritis, which in younger years is usually not associated with pain. At the same time, there could be an inflammatory degradation of cartilage and bone tissue in the joint.

   Arthralgia means just "pain in a joint" and may be due to other problems than arthritis. See question 1.

3. About 1.9–2.3% of the patients referred to an orofacial pain specialist clinic will have solely TMJ arthralgia (Schiffman *et al.*, 2010).

4. No, at least not in an accurate or reliable manner (Shaefer *et al.*, 2001).

Case 2.2

Arthritis

Per Alstergren

A. Demographic Data and Reason for Contact

- Male, 34 years of age (Figure 2.2).
- Born in Sweden of Swedish parents.
- Referred to orofacial pain specialist from general practitioner due to TMJ pain and chewing difficulties.

B. Symptom History

- Today the pain is from the right TMJ at rest, movement, and chewing. When the pain intensity increases, a spread of the pain area occurs with pain in the ear, eye, upper molars, and temple, all on the right side. Difficulties opening mouth wide as before.
- Chewing, mouth opening, and talking worsens the pain. Rest and ibuprofen may decrease the pain. Otherwise, no apparent fluctuation of pain intensity during the day or night.
- Pain intensity varies between 3 at rest and 8 on mouth opening (NRS 0–10).
- Characteristic pain intensity 40 (NRS 0–100), current pain intensity 3 (0–10 NRS), pain-related disability 62 (NRS 0–100; GCPS).
- JFLS reveals limitation in mouth opening and chewing. Few and infrequent daytime parafunctions according to OBCL.
- No headache. No neck pain.
- Grating sounds from both TMJs.
- Debut (pain) 9 months ago after falling at a party. Trauma to the left side of the face but with only very minor soft tissue injury. The next day severe pain and difficulties opening the mouth. Pain and movement difficulties subsided, but not fully, during the first 3 weeks (self-medication with paracetamol and ibuprofen). Since 1 month later, increasing pain and opening difficulties.
- Six months ago the patient noticed difficulties chewing food due to occlusal changes. Since then a gradual loss of occlusal contacts, especially in the front. Today, no contacts in the front and harder contacts on the right side (molar and premolar area) resulting in gradually increasing chewing difficulties.

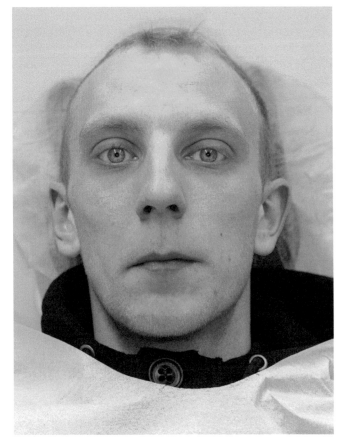

Figure 2.2 A 34-year-old Swedish man with bilateral TMJ arthritis and referred to orofacial pain specialist from general practitioner due to TMJ pain and chewing difficulties.

C. Medical History

- Healthy, no medications.

D. Psychosocial History

- Married, one child (4 years of age).
- Works in a truck garage shop, enjoys his work very much. Few sick-leave days in general, two last months sick-leave for about 10 days in total due to the orofacial pain.
- In his spare time: gym, family, friends, and parachuting.

- Describes himself as a stable person normally but with limited stress management. Moderate scores for depression (PHQ-9) and anxiety (GAD-7). Some physical symptoms (PHQ-15; 11 p) but high level of stress (PSS-10). Poor sleep quality (PSQI).
- GCPS grade III; that is, high and moderately limiting disability.
- No smoking, moderate alcohol consumption.

E. Previous Consultations and Treatments

- General practitioner who suspected arthralgia and myalgia of the masticatory system. The dentist made an attempt to treat the arthralgia with a stabilization splint for 4 months with no effect on the TMJ pain.
- Increasing occlusal changes, also on the splint, during the treatment period prompted the referral.

F. Extraoral Status
Asymmetries

- No apparent swelling or other facial asymmetries. No redness. No increased skin temperature over either TMJ.

Somatosensory abnormalities

- Mandibular branch on right side shows hyperesthesia for touch and cold and hyperalgesia to pinprick compared with the contralateral side.
- Normal findings for the other two branches of the trigeminal nerve on the left side (compared with the right side) regarding touch, cold, and pinprick.

TMJ

- No familiar palpation pain on either side. Reduced translatory movement on the right side. Pain from the right TMJ on mouth opening, laterotrusion to the left, and on protrusion.
- Palpable crepitus from both TMJs.

Masticatory muscles

- Familiar palpation pain in right and left masseter muscles and in the temporal muscle insertion on the right side. No referred pain.

Jaw movement capacity

- Maximum mouth opening without pain is 22 mm, maximum unassisted opening is 30 mm with familiar pain in right TMJ, and maximum assisted mouth opening is 42 mm with familiar pain in the right TMJ. Right laterotrusion 10 mm (no familiar pain), left laterotrusion 5 mm with familiar pain in the right TMJ and masseter muscle, and protrusion 6 mm with familiar pain in the right TMJ.

Neck examination

- Normal range of motion; no familiar neck pain on movement or palpation.

G. Intraoral Status
Soft tissues

- Normal findings.

Hard tissues and dentition

- Complete dentition with few and minor fillings.

Occlusion

- Dentition: 17–24, 26, 27, 37–45, 47. Hard occlusion shows contacts on the following teeth in the upper jaw: 17, 24, 27 (Figures 2.3, 2.4, and 2.5).

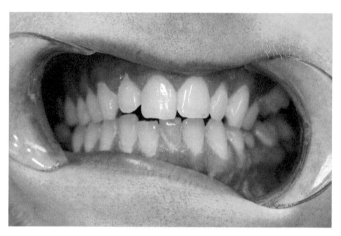

Figure 2.3 Frontal view of occlusion on hard biting. Loss of anterior contacts.

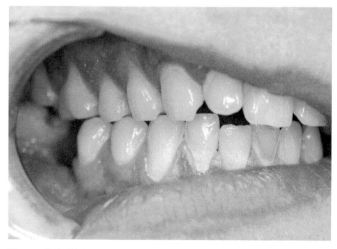

Figure 2.4 Right side view of occlusion on hard biting. Loss of anterior contacts, only contact between 17 and 47.

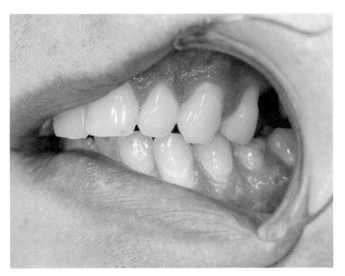

Figure 2.5 Left side view of occlusion on hard biting. Loss of anterior contacts, only contact between 24–34 and 27–37.

H. Additional Examinations and Findings

- The occlusal changes motivate a radiographic examination, especially regarding the left TMJ. The purpose would be to identify structural changes due to an inflammatory process in both TMJs that may explain the anterior open bite and help deciding if treatment would be required of none, one or both TMJs.
- The radiographic examination was performed by a radiologist using a bilateral cone-beam computerized tomography (CBCT) of both TMJs. This examination showed substantial structural changes in both TMJs with signs of condylar erosions and loss of compact bone on both condyles, bilateral condyle bone loss, condylar and temporal flattening as well as bilateral osteophytes (Figure 2.6).

I. Diagnosis/Diagnoses
Expanded DC/TMD taxonomy

- Right TMJ arthritis.

DC/TMD

- Arthralgia in the right TMJ.
- Bilateral TMJ degenerative joint disease.
- Myalgia of the masticatory muscles.

Other

- Left TMJ arthritis.

J. Case Assessment

- Many factors point to a bilateral TMJ arthritis as the main problem: continuous and sometimes intense pain on mouth opening and chewing in the right TMJ as well as pain on all mandibular movements (opening, laterotrusion. and protrusion) in the right TMJ. In addition, bilateral TMJ crepitus, bilateral radiographic signs of structural changes in accordance with inflammation and with signs of probable ongoing inflammatory activity (erosions, loss of compact bone). The anamnesis points to a trauma that very well may have induced a traumatic arthritis that now has become chronic with both pain and structural changes, resulting in occlusal changes, as a consequence.
- The patient also had myalgia and degenerative joint disease in the right TMJ. The myalgia is probably to a substantial part a consequence of a local sensitization since there are no other indications of a muscle tension problem.
- The diagnosis degenerative joint disease in DC/TMD is based on the presence of crepitus. The crepitus in this particular patient is most likely a consequence of inflammatory damage to articular cartilage and bone tissue (i.e., part of the arthritis).
- There were somatosensory abnormalities in the right trigeminal branch III that have to be interpreted as consequences of the TMJ arthritis on the same side that comprised pain. No neuropathic-type pain can be suspected.

K. Evidence-based Treatment Plan including Aims

- The main problem seems to be a traumatic bilateral TMJ arthritis that has become chronic. The initial treatment should therefore be anti-inflammatory with the goal to stop the inflammatory activity in both TMJs. It is, however, very important to supplement the pharmacological anti-inflammatory treatment with a treatment modality that has the possibility to reduce the risk of a relapse of the arthritis. For example, jaw exercise.
- When the inflammatory activity is substantially reduced and under control, the reduced chewing ability, probably in part due to the occlusal changes, should be addressed. The aim for this part should be adequate chewing ability and stable, comfortable occlusion.
- Initial treatment: anti-inflammatory treatment of both TMJs. Treatment options range from intraarticular corticosteroids, NSAIDs per os, de-loading of the joint (splint) and jaw exercise (Kopp and Wennerberg, 1981; Nicolakis *et al.*, 2002; Ta and Dionne, 2004; Conti *et al.*, 2006; Fredriksson *et al.*, 2006).

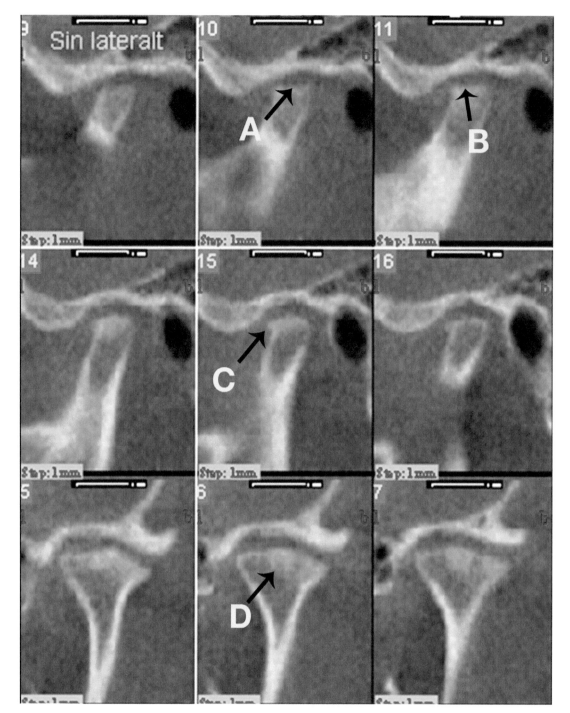

Figure 2.6 CBCT of both TMJs showing substantial structural changes in both TMJs with signs of condylar erosions and loss of compact bone on both condyles and bilateral condyle bone loss (A), condylar and temporal flattening (B), bilateral osteophytes (C), and sclerosis (D).

- When the inflammatory activity in both TMJs is under control, the reduced chewing ability due to the occlusal changes should be addressed. Treatment options range from no treatment and natural normalization of the occlusion, via occlusal adjustment, prosthodontic therapy, orthodontic therapy, surgery, or combinations of these. The goal here must be increased or normalized chewing capacity. Also, the treatment should be minimal, since there is an increased risk of future arthritic episodes that may have the possibility to further change the occlusion.

L. Prognosis and Discussion

- The prognosis is very much dependent on how well it will be possible to stop the inflammatory activity. The supposedly long duration of arthritis, including pain and later occlusal changes due to the bone tissue destruction, is a negative prognostic factor. The short-term prognosis for treatment of arthritis must be considered as good, especially if intraarticular corticosteroids are used. However, the long-term prognosis is unclear and depends on how well the inflammation will be controlled, also over time.

Background Information

- Arthritis (i.e., inflammation in articular tissues) in the TMJ is a disorder due to either local factors like micro- or macrotrauma, secondary to disc displacement or degenerative joint disease or infection or part of a systemic inflammatory disorder such as rheumatic diseases or reactive arthritis.
- Inflammation is a complex, rapid, first-line and highly unspecific immune system response with the purpose to locate and eliminate pathogens and injured tissue as well as to promote tissue healing. This reaction has a clear and important biologic purpose in the acute phase but may transfer into a chronic state with very unclear, if any, biologic purpose. The unspecific nature means that, regardless of cause, the reaction to a great extent involves the same cells, mediators, enzymes, and so on. In addition, autoantibodies and autoinflammation may contribute to initiate and maintain the chronic inflammation (Doria et al., 2012).
- Signs and symptoms of arthritis can lie on a continuum from no signs/symptoms to a combination of pain, swelling/exudate, tissue degradation and/or growth disturbance. The presentation at any time point may include none or one or more of these signs and symptoms. On the other hand, TMJ arthritis may cause arthralgia, but arthralgia could also be due to other factors that trigger articular nociceptors (e.g., noxious mechanical stimuli), referred pain, and general/central sensitization. However, pain is likely the most common clinical finding in TMJ arthritis (Peck et al., 2014).
- There are no established diagnostic criteria for TMJ arthritis. The Expanded DC/TMD suggests swelling, redness, increased temperature, and pain as a starting point for research into diagnosis. However, swelling, redness, and increased temperature are extremely rare findings in TMJ arthritis. Also, there can be arthritis without pain but with disease progression occurring, causing tissue degradation and/or growth disturbance. Therefore, the use of cardinal signs of inflammation as the only basis for clinical diagnosis of TMJ arthritis may lack clinical utility (Peck et al., 2014).

Diagnostic Criteria

Expanded DC/TMD criteria for **Arthritis** (Peck et al., 2014). Sensitivity and specificity have not been established.

Pain of joint origin with clinical characteristics of inflammation or infection over the affected joint: edema, erythema, and/or increased temperature. Associated symptoms can include dental occlusal changes (e.g., ipsilateral posterior open bite if intraarticular swelling or effusion is present unilaterally). This disorder is also referred to as synovitis or capsulitis, although these terms limit the sites of nociception. This is a localized condition; there should be no history of systemic inflammatory disease.

History. Positive for both of the following:
1. Arthralgia as defined in DC/TMD.
AND
2. Swelling, redness, and/or increased temperature in front of the ear OR dental occlusal changes resulting from articular inflammatory exudate or swelling (e.g., posterior open bite).

Examination. Positive for both of the following:
1. Arthralgia as defined in DC/TMD.
AND
2. Presence of edema, erythema, and/or increased temperature over the joint OR reduction in dental occlusal contacts noted between two consecutive measurements (unilateral/ bilateral posterior open bite), and not attributable to other causes

Rheumatologic consultation when needed:
1. Negative for rheumatologic disease.

Note: The pain is not better accounted for by another pain diagnosis.

DC/TMD criteria for **Arthralgia**, see Case 2.1, for **Degenerative joint disease**, see Case 2.10, and for **Myalgia**, see Case 3.3 (Schiffman *et al.*, 2014).

Fundamental Points

- Inflammation of the articular tissues in the TMJ may result in pain as well as cartilage and bone tissue destruction (Alstergren *et al.*, 2008). In adolescents, it may also result in growth disturbances and micrognathia since the growth site of the mandible is the condyles.

- The inflammatory process is rapid and highly unspecific, but when chronic the signs and symptoms of arthritis can lie on a continuum from no signs/symptoms to a combination of pain, swelling/exudate, tissue degradation, and/or growth disturbance. The presentation at any time point may include none or one or more of these signs and symptoms (Peck *et al.*, 2014). This means that some patients have pain but no tissue destruction, whereas others may show severe tissue destruction but no pain. This makes the diagnostic process more difficult.

- In systemic arthritides, as well as monoarthritic conditions, TMJ pain on jaw movements has been found to be strongly related to an inflammatory intraarticular milieu (Alstergren and Kopp, 1997; Alstergren *et al.*, 2008). TMJ pain on jaw movement may thus in the future be proven as a useful clinical symptom or sign when attempting to diagnose TMJ arthritis.

- Intraarticular corticosteroid treatment has been found to be efficient and safe for treatment of various arthritic conditions, including osteoarthritis, leading to significant pain relief and functional improvement for months up to 1 year. (Cheng and Abdi, 2007; Cheng *et al.*, 2012).

Self-study Questions

1. What is the difference between arthritis and arthralgia?
2. In most other joints than the TMJ, swelling and palpation pain are important clinical findings pointing to arthritis. Why is that not the case for the TMJ?
3. TMJ arthritis may cause two (adults) or three (children, adolescents) specific problems in the masticatory system. Which?
4. When should you consider occlusal therapy in a patient with TMJ arthritis and recent occlusal changes?

References

Alstergren P, Kopp S (1997) Pain and synovial fluid concentration of serotonin in arthritic temporomandibular joints. *Pain* **72**(1–2):137–143.

Alstergren P, Fredriksson L, Kopp S (2008) Temporomandibular joint pressure pain threshold is systemically modulated in rheumatoid arthritis. *J Orofac Pain* **22**(3):231–238.

Conti PC, dos Santos CN, Kogawa EM, *et al.* (2006) The treatment of painful temporomandibular joint clicking with oral splints: a randomized clinical trial. *J Am Dent Assoc* **137**(8):1108–1114.

Cheng J, Abdi S (2007) Complications of joint, tendon, and muscle injections. *Tech Reg Anesth Pain Manag* **11**(3):141–147.

Cheng OT, Souzdalnitski D, Vrooman B, Cheng J (2012) Evidence-based knee injections for the management of arthritis. *Pain Med* **13**(6):740–753.

Doria A, Zen M, Bettio S, *et al.* (2012) Autoinflammation and autoimmunity: bridging the divide. *Autoimmun Rev* **12**(1):22–30.

Fredriksson L, Alstergren P, Kopp S (2006) Tumor necrosis factor-alpha in temporomandibular joint synovial fluid predicts treatment effects on pain by intra-articular glucocorticoid treatment. *Mediators Inflamm* **2006**(6):59425.

Kopp S, Wenneberg B (1981) Effects of occlusal treatment and intraarticular injections on temporomandibular joint pain and dysfunction. *Acta Odontol Scand* **39**(2):87–96.

Nicolakis P, Erdogmus CB, Kollmitzer J, *et al.* (2002) Long-term outcome after treatment of temporomandibular joint osteoarthritis with exercise and manual therapy. *Cranio* **20**(1):23–27.

Peck CC, Goulet JP, Lobbezoo F, *et al.* (2014) Expanding the taxonomy of the diagnostic criteria for temporomandibular disorders. *J Oral Rehabil* **41**(1):2–23.

Schiffman E, Ohrbach R, Truelove E, *et al.* (2014) International RDC/TMD Consortium Network, International Association for Dental Research; Orofacial Pain Special Interest Group, International Association for the Study of Pain. Diagnostic Criteria for Temporomandibular Disorders (DC/TMD) for Clinical and Research Applications: recommendations of the International RDC/TMD Consortium Network and Orofacial Pain Special Interest Group. *J Oral Facial Pain Headache* **28**(1):6–27.

Ta LE, Dionne RA (2004) Treatment of painful temporomandibular joints with a cyclooxygenase-2 inhibitor: a randomized placebo-controlled comparison of celecoxib to naproxen. *Pain* **111**(1–2):13–21.

Answers to Self-study Questions

1. Arthritis can cause arthralgia but there may be other reasons for arthralgia (overstretching, mechanical impingement, and sensitization). Also, TMJ arthritis may not cause pain but there is still an ongoing inflammatory process causing cartilage and bone tissue destruction.

2. TMJ swelling is very rare. TMJ palpation pain is mainly modulated by systemic factors and does not usually reflect an intraarticular inflammatory milieu.

3. Pain, cartilage and tissue destruction, and growth disturbance (in children/adolescents)

4. If ever, you must make sure that the inflammatory activity in the TMJ has been eliminated before attempting to make any irreversible treatments in order to restore occlusal stability and function.

B: Disc Disorders

Case 2.3

Disc Displacement with Reduction

Bachar Reda and Daniele Manfredini

A. Demographic Data and Reason for Contact

- Caucasian male, 20 years old. Joint sounds and abrasion of lower front incisors.

B. Symptom History

- Popping sounds, left side, during jaw movements.

C. Medical History

- Review of systems is negative.
- No known allergies.
- No routine medications or drug administration.
- No previous hospitalizations or emergency-room visits.

D. Psychosocial History

- First-year mechanical engineering university student.
- Light athletics practitioner.
- Very good relationship with parents.
- Normal socioeconomic status.
- GCPS grade 0; that is, no pain and no pain-related disability.

E. Previous Consultations and Treatments

- No consultation necessary.
- Third molars extractions; fixed orthodontic treatment.

F. Extraoral Examination

- No noticeable asymmetry or redness (Figure 2.7a).
- Maximum unassisted mouth opening: 45 mm. No pain on mandibular movement.
- During opening movements, the jaw deviates to the left and then recovers the middle sagittal line (Figure 2.7b–d).
- Facial profile: slightly hyperdivergent.
- Reciprocal click in the left joint.
- No palpation pain of the temporomandibular joints or the masticatory muscles.

G. Intraoral Examination

- Marginal gingivitis and presence of plaque.
- Class I molar and canine relationship on the right side and class II on the left side, with asymmetrical incisor midline.

H. Additional Examinations and Findings

- Panoramic radiograph: normal findings (Figure 2.8). MRI confirmed the clinical diagnosis of left TMJ disc displacement with reduction, with the disc located ahead of the condyle in the closed mouth position (Figure 2.9a) and physiologically positioned over the condyle, showing a "butterfly" form, in the opened mouth position (Figure 2.9b). No effusion could be detected (Figure 2.9c). The right side showed a disc in normal position in both the closed (Figure 2.9d) and opened mouth position (Figure 2.9e).

I. Diagnosis/Diagnoses
DC/TMD

- Disc displacement with reduction (left side).

J. Case Assessment

- Patient with a nonpainful disc displacement in the left TMJ. No functional interference. In the case presented here there was no need to get deeper into the psychosocial assessment for prognostic purposes owing to the absence of pain and, consequently, pain-related disability.

K. Evidence-based Treatment Plan including Aims

- Counselling and reassurance. However, the patient may be worried by the click sounds or misinformed about their relevance. That is why it is fundamental to spend enough time to reassure patients during the first appointment to increase the patient's knowledge, correct the expectations and to lower any anxiety. This includes showing a drawing of the TMJ and the

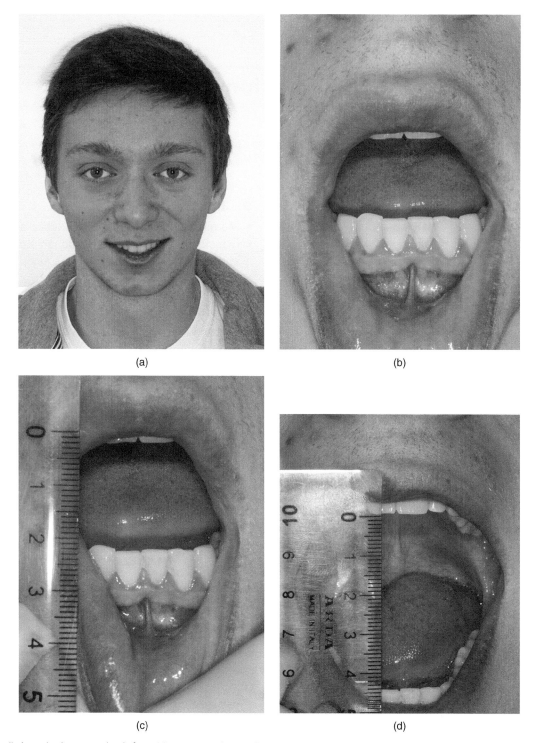

(a)

(b)

(c)

(d)

Figure 2.7 (a–d) Jaw deviates to the left at 23 mm opening and then centers again on maximum mouth opening (45 mm).

jaw muscles, explaining how the TMJ works and what a disc displacement is. This should also include information that this is a benign condition that may very well fluctuate over time.

L. Prognosis and Discussion

- Absence of pain and pain-related disability (GCPS grade 0) strongly indicate an observational approach.

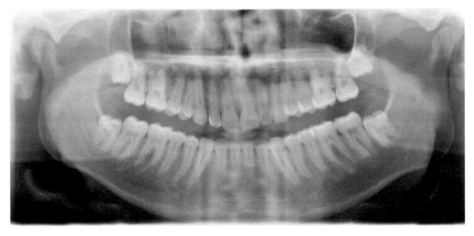

Figure 2.8 Panoramic radiograph showing an absence of gross morphological changes of the TMJ condyles.

- The prognosis regarding escalating symptoms is good. There is no increased risk of developing a disc displacement without reduction in this case, compared with a normal joint case.

Background Information
- Disc displacement with reduction is an intracapsular biomechanical disorder involving the condyle–disc complex. In the closed mouth position the disc is in an anterior position relative to the condylar head and the disc reduces upon opening of the mouth. Displacements can be anterior, medial, lateral, and posterior, with the antero-medial one being the most common direction. Clicking, popping, or snapping noises may occur with disc reduction.
- In the closed mouth position, the TMJ disc is in an anterior position relative to the condyle within the glenoid fossa. During jaw opening the disc is "recaptured" by the condyle, and in the maximum opening position it is located with its intermediate band positioned between the condylar apex and the articular tubercle. The recapture of the disc during mouth opening produces a click sound, which is often audible also during jaw closing movement (i.e., reciprocal click). The click sound during jaw closing is due to the disc losing its correct relationship with the condyle, and is usually heard at a lower interincisal opening distance. A differential diagnosis should be considered with bone changes (e.g., osteophytes; deviations in form) producing a sound at the same interincisal

distance every time, due to the fixed obstacle.

(De Leeuw *et al.*, 2013; Schiffman *et al.*, 2014)

Diagnostic Criteria
DC/TMD criteria for **Disc displacement with reduction** (Schiffman *et al.*, 2014). Without imaging: sensitivity 0.34, specificity 0.92.

An intracapsular biomechanical disorder involving the condyle–disc complex. In the closed mouth position the disc is in an anterior position relative to the condylar head and the disc reduces upon opening of the mouth. Medial and lateral displacement of the disc may also be present. Clicking, popping, or snapping noises may occur with disc reduction. A history of prior locking in the closed position coupled with interference in mastication precludes this diagnosis.

History. Positive for at least one of the following:
1. In the last 30 days any TMJ noise(s) present with jaw movement or function.
   OR
2. Patient report of any noise present during the examination.

Examination. Positive for at least one of the following:
1. Clicking, popping, and/or snapping noise detected during both opening and closing, with palpation during at least one of three repetitions of jaw opening and closing.

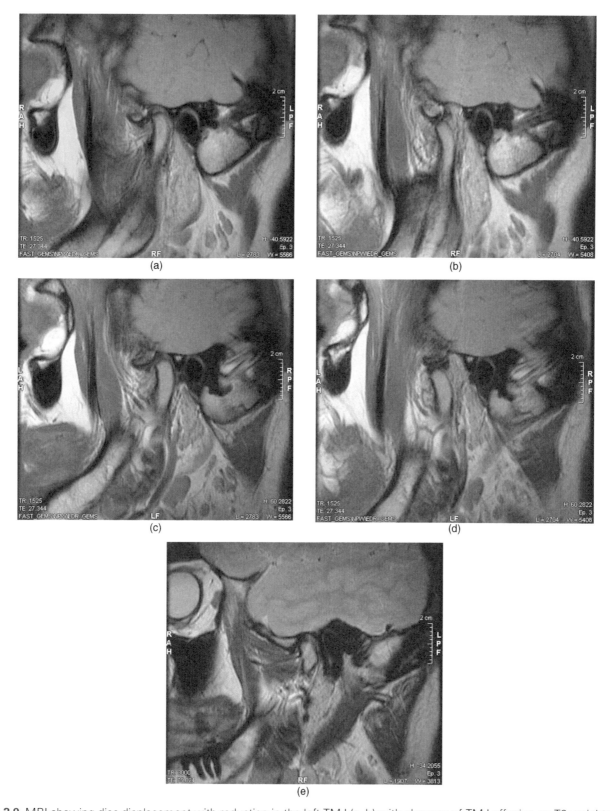

Figure 2.9 MRI showing disc displacement with reduction in the left TMJ (a, b) with absence of TMJ effusion on T2-weighted image (c) and normal disc positions in the right TMJ (d, e).

OR

2a. Clicking, popping, and/or snapping noise detected with palpation during at least one of three3 repetitions of opening or closing.
AND

2b. Clicking, popping, and/or snapping noise detected with palpation during at least one of three repetitions of right or left lateral movements, or protrusive movements.

Imaging. When this diagnosis needs to be confirmed, then TMJ MRI criteria are positive for both of the following:

1. In the maximum intercuspal position, the posterior band of the disc is located anterior to the 11:30 position and the intermediate zone of the disc is anterior to the condylar head.
AND

2. On full opening, the intermediate zone of the disc is located between the condylar head and the articular eminence.

Fundamental Points

- The diagnosis of disc displacement with reduction is mainly clinical, based upon history taking (i.e., patient's report of joint sounds), joint palpation (i.e., reciprocal joint sound at different interincisal distance during jaw opening and closing), and observation of jaw movements (i.e., deviation to the affected side). MRI may be used to confirm the clinical diagnosis and should then show an anteriorly displaced but with a reducing disc on mouth opening; see the "Diagnostic Criteria" box.
- Imaging should only be used when it has the possibility to change the diagnosis or the planned treatment. Panoramic radiographs add no useful information regarding TMJ disc disorders.
- MRI is the reference standard for assessment of soft tissues (i.e., TMJ disc position, joint effusion, etc.). The literature suggests that the agreement between MRI signs of disc displacement and the presence of audible click sounds is fairly weak (sensitivity of 0.33), and it is even weaker regarding the relationship between TMJ pain and MRI signs of effusion or structural changes.
- The treatment should be as conservative and reversible as possible. In the case of disc displacement with reduction in the absence of pain and jaw movement limitations, this means that counselling and reassurance is a recommended approach.

Self-study Questions

1. What is disc displacement with reduction?
2. How is a displacement with reduction diagnosed?
3. Should the displacement always be treated?
4. Is the severity of joint sound related to the disease severity?

References

De Leeuw R, Klasser GD (eds) (2013) *Orofacial pain: Guidelines for assessment, diagnosis, and management*, 5th edn Hanover Park, IL: Quintessence Publishing.
Schiffman E, Ohrbach R, Truelove E, et al. (2014) Diagnostic Criteria for Temporomandibular Disorders (DC/TMD) for clinical and research applications: recommendations of the International RDC/TMD Consortium Network and Orofacial Pain Special Interest Group. *J Oral Facial Pain Headache* **28**(1):6–27.

Answers to Self-study Questions

1. In the closed mouth position, the disc is in an anterior position relative to the condyle. During jaw opening the disc is recaptured by the condyle sliding on the articular tubercle, and in the open mouth position the disc is correctly located between the two bone surfaces. The disc recapture during jaw movement produces a click sound.

2. The diagnosis is based on history taking and clinical assessment, and may be confirmed by MRI.
DC/TMD criteria:
History. Positive for at least one of the following:
1. In the last 30 days any TMJ noise(s) present with jaw movement or function.
OR
2. Patient report of any noise present during the examination.

Examination. Positive for at least one of the following:

1. Clicking, popping, and/or snapping noise detected during both opening and closing, with palpation during at least one of three repetitions of jaw opening and closing.

OR

2a. Clicking, popping, and/or snapping noise detected

with palpation during at least one of three repetitions of opening or closing.

AND

2b. Clicking, popping, and/or snapping noise detected

with palpation during at least one of three repetitions of right or left lateral movements, or protrusive movements.

Imaging. When this diagnosis needs to be confirmed, then TMJ MRI criteria are positive for both of the following:

1. In the maximum intercuspal position, the posterior band of the disc is located anterior to the 11:30 position and the intermediate zone of the disc is anterior to the condylar head.

AND

2. On full opening, the intermediate zone of the disc is located between the condylar head and the articular eminence.

3. Asymptomatic disc displacement is not treated. Repositioning appliances or disc repositioning surgery have been shown to be ineffective to warrant permanent recapture.

4. There is no relationship between the strength of the clicking sound and severity of the condition. However, the sound may worry the patient and also influence their quality of life; for example, by preventing the patient from taking part in social events due to loud clickings that can be heard by other people. Attempts to reduce loud clickings and/or to decrease the frequency of the sound could be made with oral appliances, exercises, and joint viscosupplementation, but there is no literature to support this empirical evidence.

Case 2.4

Disc Displacement with Reduction with Intermittent Locking

Massimiliano Politi and Daniele Manfredini

A. Demographic Data and Reason for Contact

- Caucasian female, 24 years old (Figure 2.10).
- Referred to orofacial pain specialist due to transient jaw lock.

B. Symptom History

- Transient jaw lock, right side, that takes a few minutes to recover from each time.
- Pain intensity varies between 0 (at rest) and 6 (on locking, right TMJ) on a 0–10 NRS.
- Characteristic pain intensity 10 (NRS 0–100), current pain intensity 0 (NRS 0–10), pain-related disability 10 (NRS 0–100; GCPS) in the right TMJ.
- JFLS reveals limitation in mouth opening and chewing. Few and infrequent daytime parafunctions according OBCL.
- The patient began experiencing discomfort at around the age of 6–8 years.
- On a monthly interval, she could feel a sensation of grinding sand in her ears when she chew but cannot remember whether it was prompted by something particular or not. For several years she has experienced her jaw lock problem on a weekly basis.

C. Medical History

- No food intolerance or allergies.
- She broke her left tibia and damaged her knee ligaments in a bicycling accident 3 years ago. The medical report on the tibial fracture also diagnosed ligamentous laxity.

D. Psychosocial History

- Middle-class background; mother and father are both employers.
- Since she was young she has loved and engaged in horse riding.
- For the last 5 years she has worked as a shop assistant, spending many hours standing and not wearing appropriate shoes. She says that at the end

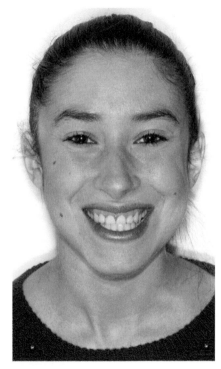

Figure 2.10 Frontal view of patient.

of the day she feels pain around the back of the neck and jaw soreness because she is always tense.

- The locking episodes were much more frequent 1–4 years ago and related to a period of working particularly hard and under constant pressure.
- Describes herself as a stable person normally but with limited stress management. Mild scores for depression (PHQ-9) and anxiety (GAD-7). Some physical symptoms (PHQ-15) but moderate level of stress (PSS-10). Good sleep quality (PSQL).
- GCPS grade I; that is, low intensity, low disability.
- No smoking, no alcohol consumption.

E. Previous Consultations and Treatments

- None in particular.

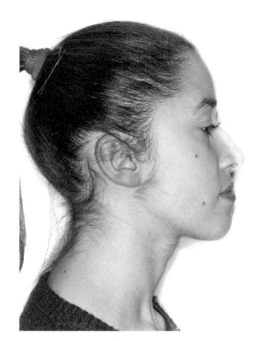

Figure 2.11 Lateral view of patient.

F. Extraoral Status

- Concave facial profile due to mandibular protrusion (Figure 2.11).
- Hypertrophy of masseter muscles by palpation.
- Maximum unassisted opening during an episode of locking is 15 mm (Figure 2.12a).
- Right TMJ clicking during jaw opening (late click) and closing movements (early click).
- Limitation on lateral mandibular movements (Figure 2.12b and c).

- No locking during examination.
- No TMJ pain during examination.

G. Intraoral Status

- Anterior crossbite (Figure 2.13a).
- Bilateral molar and canine Angle class III (Figure 2.13b).
- Negative overjet (Figure 2.13a).

H. Additional Examinations and Findings

- Radiographic examination requested by her previous dentists included panoramic radiograph and latero-lateral radiographs (Figure 2.14).
- MRI at open and closed mouth positions shows a reducing anteriorly displaced disc in the right TMJ (Figure 2.15a and b), but normal findings in the left TMJ (Figure 2.15c and d).

I. Diagnosis/Diagnoses

DC/TMD

- Bilateral disc displacement with reduction with intermittent locking.

J. Case Assessment

- Right TMJ disc displacement with intermittent locking in a patient with Angle class III.
- No TMJ pain on clicking during the examination, but the anamnestic information reveals occasions with TMJ pain on lockings. This is most likely a nociceptive-type pain due to mechanical intraarticular stimulus causing pain.
- No findings pointing towards concurrent arthritis.

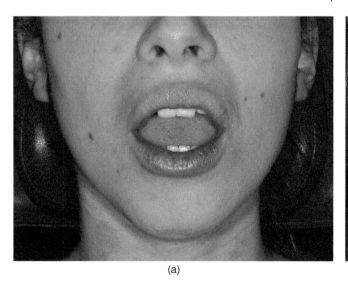
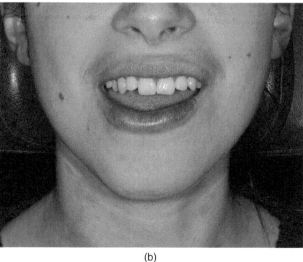

(a)   (b)

Figure 2.12 Mandibular movement capacity: maximum mouth opening capacity on locking 15 mm (a);, reduced laterotrusive capacity to the right (b) and left (c).

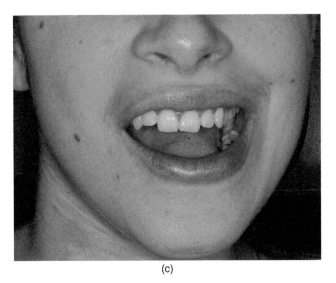

(c)

Figure 2.12 (*Continued*)

- There is an increased risk of development to disc displacement without reduction in cases with intermittent locking.

K. Evidence-based Treatment Plan including Aims

- Counselling, with the aim to reassure the patient.
- Jaw exercises, with the aim to avoid overloading the joint.

L. Prognosis and Discussion

- Prognosis for the disc displacement in itself is poor.
- There is an increased risk of development to disc displacement without reduction in cases with intermittent locking.
- The prognosis for increased function, less lockings, and less pain is good with the proposed treatment.

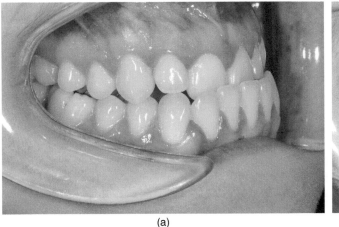

(a)

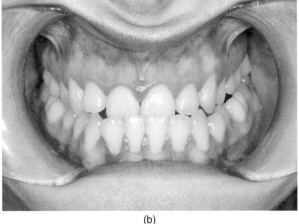

(b)

Figure 2.13 Angle class III and anterior crossbite. Lateral view (a) and frontal view (b).

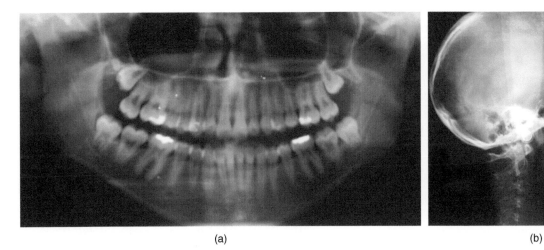

(a)

(b)

Figure 2.14 Panoramic (a) and lateral (b) radiographs of jaws.

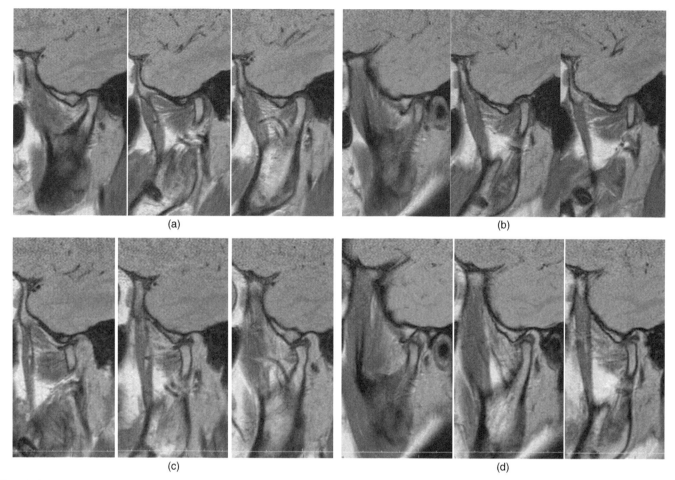

Figure 2.15 MRI TMJ findings. In the right TMJ the disc is located anteriorly to the condyle in the closed mouth position (a), but in a normal condition in the opened mouth position (b), indicating disc displacement with reduction. The left TMJ shows the disc in normal position in both the closed (c) and opened (d) mouth positions.

Background Information
- Intermittent locking is an intermediate stage between disc displacement with reduction (i.e., clicking joint) and disc displacement without reduction with limited opening (i.e., closed lock; Kalaykova *et al.*, 2011).
- Intermittent locking usually manifests with joint clicking because of an anterior disk displacement with reduction that sometimes is associated with limited mouth opening as a result of a transient lack of reduction. Intermittent locking accounted for 2.5–12% of all cases of TMD (Manfredini *et al.*, 2011; Takahara *et al.*, 2014).
- Data on risk factors are scarce. It is likely that parafunctions, especially in the form of jaw clenching, and anatomical factors may play a role in the onset of intermittent locking.

Parafunctional static loading may contribute to the temporary loss of reduction of an anteriorly displaced disc. Furthermore, there may be a relationship among the onset of intermittent locking, disc deformation, and degree of anterior displacement (Kalaykova *et al.*, 2011).

Diagnostic Criteria
DC/TMD citeria for **Disc displacement with reduction with intermittent locking** (Schiffman *et al.*, 2014). Without imaging: sensitivity 0.38, specificity 0.98.

An intracapsular biomechanical disorder involving the condyle–disc complex. In the closed mouth position the disc is in an anterior position relative to the condylar head, and the disc intermittently reduces with opening of the mouth. When the disc does not reduce with opening of the mouth, intermittent limited mandibular opening occurs. When limited opening occurs, a maneuver may be needed to unlock the TMJ. Medial and lateral displacement of the disc may also be present. Clicking, popping, or snapping noises may occur with disc reduction.

History. Positive for both of the following:

1a. In the last 30 days, any TMJ noise(s) present with jaw movement or function.

   OR

1b. Patient report of any noise present during the examination.

   AND

2. In the last 30 days, jaw locks with limited mouth opening, even for a moment, and then unlocks.

Examination. Positive for the following:

1. Disc displacement with reduction as defined in Case 2.3. Although not required, when this disorder is present clinically, examination is positive for inability to open to a normal amount, even momentarily, without the clinician or patient performing a specific manipulative maneuver.

Imaging. When this diagnosis needs to be confirmed:

1. The imaging criteria are the same as for disc displacement with reduction if intermittent locking is not present at the time of imaging. If locking occurs during imaging, then an imaging-based diagnosis of disc displacement without reduction will be rendered and clinical confirmation of reversion to intermittent locking is needed.

Fundamental Points

- Anamnestic information is fundamental: the diagnosis could not be made without the patient reporting an intermittent locking during the history taking, because it may happen that a patient does not experience jaw lock at the time they are examined.
- Intermittent locking may interfere with the activities of daily living.

Self-study Questions

1. How many episodes of jaw lock are needed to diagnose intermittent locking?

2. Why is it important to distinguish between disc displacement with reduction with or without intermittent lockings?

3. Why is MRI important for confirmation (if needed) of the diagnosis of disc displacement with reduction with intermittent locking?

References

Kalaykova S, Lobbezoo F, Naeije M (2011) Risk factors for anterior disc displacement with reduction and intermittent locking in adolescents. *J Orofac Pain* **25**:153–160.

Manfredini D, Guarda-Nardini L, Winocur E, *et al.* (2011) Research diagnostic criteria for temporomandibular disorders: a systematic review of Axis I epidemiologic findings. *Oral Surg Oral Med Oral Pathol Oral Radiol Endod* **112**(4):453–462.

Schiffman E, Ohrbach R, Truelove E, *et al.* (2014) Diagnostic Criteria for Temporomandibular Disorders (DC/TMD) for clinical and research applications: recommendations of the International RDC/TMD Consortium Network and Orofacial Pain Special Interest Group. *J Oral Facial Pain Headache* **28**(1):6–27.

Takahara N, Imai H, Nakagawa S, *et al.* (2014) Temporomandibular joint intermittent closed lock: clinic and magnetic resonance imaging findings. *Oral Surg Oral Med Oral Pathol Oral Radiol* **118**(4):418–423.

Answers to Self-study Questions

1. One.

2. Disc displacement with reduction with intermittent lockings has a much higher risk of developing into a disc displacement without reduction.

3. MRI has the ability to detect and show soft tissues like the disc.

Case 2.5

Disc Displacement without Reduction with Limited Opening

Stanimira I Kalaykova

A. Demographic Data and Reason for Contact
- Caucasian female, 22 years old, jaw feels stuck, cannot open mouth completely.

B. Symptom History
- Sudden onset of complaint 2 days ago.
- Limited mouth opening interferes with biting off large pieces of food and mouth hygiene, especially in the molar area; no other interferences with activities and participation.
- No pain, but an unpleasant pressing feeling in the right preauricular area.
- Prior to onset of current complaint, a history of:
  - Clicking TMJ sounds on the right side, according to patient since approximately 3 years.
  - In the last 6 months, a few occurrences of short-lasting, intermittent locking on the right side that the patient could solve by herself by moving the jaw first to the contralateral side and afterward opening the mouth. On movement, an audible click would occur after which the jaw would open completely.
- No other complaints from the masticatory system, except from the current complaint.
- The patient visits her dentist twice per year.
- Mouth hygiene consists of brushing twice per day and flossing.
- No history of trauma.
- The patient is aware of awake bruxism (jaw clenching).

C. Medical History
- Review of systems is negative.
- No allergies to medication; no seasonal allergies.
- No routine medications.
- No previous hospitalizations or surgeries; no emergency-room visits.

D. Psychosocial History
- Not married.
- The patient is a medical student.

- The patient shares a rental flat with two other students.
- Average socio-economic status.
- Active member of medical students' association.

E. Previous Consultations and Treatments
- No previous consultations and treatments regarding the current complaint.

F. Extraoral Status
- No asymmetries with the jaw in rest position.
- No swelling or redness.
- No signs of neurologic deficit or somatosensory abnormalities.
- Jaw movement capacity:
  - pain-free maximum mouth opening 24 mm;
  - active maximum mouth opening 25 mm with pressure feeling in the right preauricular area;
  - passive maximum mouth opening 26 mm with hard end-feel with pressure feeling in the right preauricular area;
  - protrusive movement 8 mm;
  - the jaw deviates toward the right side on mouth opening and protrusive movement;
  - laterotrusive movement toward the right side is 11 mm;
  - laterotrusive movement toward the left side is 6 mm.
- No audible or palpable TMJ sounds on movement.
- Manipulation by the clinician to allow reduction (unlock maneuver) is unsuccessful.
- Palpation of TMJ: pain free.
- Palpation of masticatory muscles: pain free.
- Neck: normal range of motion, pain free.

G. Intraoral Status
- Soft tissues:
  - linea alba present on inner aspect of cheeks right and left side;
  - gingiva and mucosa further in within normal limits.

- Dentition and hard tissues:
  - full dentition, except for all wisdom teeth (18, 28, 38, and 48);
  - no dental restorations present;
  - slight tooth wear in enamel within normal limits;
  - Angle class I occlusion;
  - overjet and overbite of 2 mm.

H. Additional Examinations and Findings

- None required.

I. Diagnosis/Diagnoses

DC/TMD

- Disc displacement without reduction with limited mouth opening in right TMJ.

J. Case Assessment

- Patient with restricted mouth opening capacity where the clinical examination points to a reduced translatory movement in the right TMJ.
- Anamnestic information reveals prior clickings in the right TMJ, intermittent lockings, and now no clickings but reduced mouth opening capacity; therefore, a very likely disc displacement without reduction.
- No other significant problems with the masticatory system.

K. Evidence-based Treatment Plan including Aims

- Treatment aims: restoration of oral function.
- Counselling, explanation about TMJ disc displacement.
- Mobilization aiming at gradual increase of condylar mobility and mouth opening.
- Physiotherapeutic exercise therapy ("Minagi" exercise therapy, or mouth opening exercise (passive stretch) and horizontal movement exercises (active movements)) (see Background Information box).

L. Prognosis and Discussion

- Good short-term prognosis since no TMJ pain is present on functional examination, no complicating factors in the patient's medical history, no complicating psychosocial factors, and the patient's young age.
- In the long term, with persistence of displaced disc position, intraarticular degenerative or adaptive changes might occur but with no significant risk of clinical signs and symptoms.

- A possible complication is development of arthralgia if too forceful mobilization is applied. The clinician should pay attention to pain response and the patient should carefully perform the mobilization exercises.

Background Information

Definition, prevalence, and pathophysiology

- DC/TMD defines disc displacement without reduction with limited mouth opening as "an intraarticular biomechanical disorder involving the condyle–disc complex." In the closed mouth position, the disc is located in an anterior (and/or medial or lateral) position relative to the condylar head, and the disc does not reduce with opening of the mouth. The disorder is associated with persistent limited mandibular opening that does not reduce with the clinician or patient performing a manipulative maneuver.
- Based on studies employing MRI, the prevalence of disc displacement without reduction is estimated to be 7–10%.
- In the pathophysiology of the loss of TMJ reduction capacity, a combination of biomechanical factors (e.g., parafunctional load of the TMJ and hypermobility), anatomical, and tissue-specific factors (e.g., disc deformation, joint lubrication) might be involved.
- Disc displacement with reduction with intermittent lockings has a high risk of developing into a disc displacement without reduction.

(Kalaykova et al., 2011; Naeije et al., 2013; Schiffman et al., 2014)

Physiotherapeutic exercise management

"Minagi" exercise therapy

- Place the thumb on the left maxillary canine and the forefinger on the right mandibular canine. Make maximal lateral gliding jaw movements to the left. Support the movements with the fingers. Make maximal jaw opening movements through the lateral border path on the left side.

Mouth opening exercise (passive stretch)

- Open the mouth as wide as you can. Place the thumbs of both hands on the maxillary anterior teeth and the forefingers on the mandibular anterior teeth. Stretch the fingers, thereby slightly increasing the mouth opening.

Afterwards, hold the mouth opening for 10 s. Repeat the exercises for 10 times. When stretching you may feel slight discomfort. In case you feel pain, please decrease the applied force.

Horizontal movement exercises (active movements)
- Bring the jaw as far as you can to the left; repeat 10 times. Bring the jaw as far as you can to the right; repeat 10 times. Bring the jaw as far as you can to the front; repeat 10 times.

(Minagi *et al.*, 1991; Yuasa and Kurita, 2001)

Diagnostic Criteria
DC/TMD criteria for **Disc displacement without reduction with limited opening** (Schiffman *et al.*, 2014). Without imaging: sensitivity 0.80, specificity 0.97.

An intracapsular biomechanical disorder involving the condyle–disc complex. In the closed mouth position the disc is in an anterior position relative to the condylar head, and the disc does not reduce with opening of the mouth. Medial and lateral displacement of the disc may also be present. This disorder is associated with persistent limited mandibular opening that does not resolve with the clinician or patient performing a specific manipulative maneuver. This is also referred to as "closed lock." Presence of TMJ noise (e.g., click with full opening) does not exclude this diagnosis.

History. Positive for both of the following:
1. Jaw locked or caught so that the mouth would not open all the way.
   AND
2. Limitation in jaw opening severe enough to limit jaw opening and interfere with ability to eat.

Examination. Positive for the following:
1. Maximum assisted opening (passive stretch) including vertical incisal overlap <40 mm. (Maximum assisted opening of <40 mm is determined clinically.)

Imaging. When this diagnosis needs to be confirmed, TMJ MRI criteria are positive for both of the following:
1. In the maximum intercuspal position, the posterior band of the disc is located anterior to the 11:30 position and the intermediate zone of the disc is anterior to the condylar head.
   AND
2. On full opening, the intermediate zone of the disc is located anterior to the condylar head.

Fundamental Points
- Clinical diagnostics based on oral history of jaw locking severe to interfere with eating and maximum assisted mouth opening <40 mm is highly specific for disc displacement without reduction with limited mouth opening.
- Imaging diagnostics is usually unnecessary. If confirmation is needed, MRI is the method of choice.
- Treatment aims consist of restoration of oral function by gradual increase of TMJ mobility and mouth opening. In case the condition is painful, pain reduction is an additional aim. See Case 2.1.
- Conservative approach consisting of counselling, mobilization jaw exercises, and in case of pain also medication is the first line of treatment. Minimally invasive surgical methods (e.g., intraarticular injections, arthrocentesis, or arthroscopy) can be considered as a second line of treatment in case of persistent signs and symptoms.
- The short-term prognosis is good. In the long term, with persistence of displaced disc position, intraarticular degenerative or adaptive changes might occur but with no significant risk of clinical signs and symptoms.

(De Leeuw *et al.*, 1995; Yuasa and Kurita, 2001; Sato *et al.*, 1997, 2001; Naeije *et al.*, 2013; Schiffman *et al.*, 2014)

Self-study Questions
1. Several alternative causes for limited mouth opening are considered in the differential diagnosis of the case presented. Why does disc displacement without reduction with limited mouth opening fit best the complaints of the patient described in the oral history?

2. According to the DC/TMD definition of disc displacement without reduction with limited mouth opening, manipulation to unlock the jaw performed

by the patient themselves, or by the clinician, is unsuccessful. How is this jaw manipulation performed?

3. Why is it recommended, in case of a painful disc displacement without reduction with limited mouth opening, to postpone mobilization exercises by a period of medication until pain has subsided?

4. What is the short-term natural course of disc displacement without reduction with limited mouth opening if left untreated?

References

De Leeuw R, Boering G, Stegenga B, de Bont LG (1995) Symptoms of temporomandibular joint osteoarthrosis and internal derangement 30 years after non-surgical treatment. *Cranio* **13**:81–88.

Kalaykova S, Lobbezoo F, Naeije M (2011) Effect of chewing upon disc reduction in the temporomandibular joint. *J Orofac Pain* **25**:49–55.

Minagi S, Nozaki S, Sato T, Tsuru H (1991) A manipulation technique for treatment of anterior disk displacement without reduction. *J Prosthet Dent* **65**:686–691.

Naeije M, Te Veldhuis AH, Te Veldhuis EC, *et al.* (2013) Disc displacement within the human temporomandibular joint: a systematic review of a 'noisy annoyance'. *J Oral Rehabil* **40**:139–158.

Sato S, Kawamura H, Nagasaka H, Motegi K (1997) The natural course of anterior disc displacement without reduction in the temporomandibular joint: follow-up at 6, 12, and 18 months. *J Oral Maxillofac Surg* **55**:234–238.

Sato S, Oguri S, Yamaguchi K, *et al.* (2001) Pumping injection of sodium hyaluronate for patients with non-reducing disc displacement of the temporomandibular joint: two year follow-up. *J Craniomaxillofac Surg* **29**:89–93.

Schiffman E, Ohrbach R, Truelove E, *et al.* (2014) Diagnostic Criteria for Temporomandibular Disorders (DC/TMD) for clinical and research applications: recommendations of the International RDC/TMD Consortium Network and Orofacial Pain Special Interest Group. *J Oral Facial Pain Headache* **28**:6–27.

Yuasa H, Kurita K (2001) Randomized clinical trial of primary treatment for temporomandibular joint disk displacement without reduction and without osseous changes: a combination of NSAIDs and mouth-opening exercise versus no treatment. *Oral Surg Oral Med Oral Pathol Oral Radiol Endod* **91**:671–675.

Answers to Self-study Questions

1. The patient describes a sudden onset of a mouth opening limitation. Moreover, the patient describes occurrence of clicking joint sounds that were intermittently replaced by silent (without clicking) short-lasting locking events. This anamnesis is typical for disc displacement without reduction and does not fit the majority of alternative differential diagnoses. The fact that the patient reports no pain complaints, no trauma in the history, and no (previous) comorbid medical conditions makes further some of the alternative differential diagnoses improbable.

2. The manipulation as an attempt to unlock a TMJ with an anterior disc displacement without reduction with limited mouth opening is performed with the patient sitting upright and leaning towards the headrest of the dental chair. The patient is instructed to relax the jaws as much as possible. The thumb of the clinician is placed intraorally, in the molar area on the affected side. The rest of the fingers form a grip to the jaw extraorally. Then the mandible on the affected sides is brought into caudal traction by pressing the thumb onto the molar area in a caudal direction, thereby increasing the space between the TMJ bony articulating surfaces. Then the jaw is pulled forward by keeping the condyle in a caudal position, thereby increasing the chance of surpassing the posterior band of the anteriorly displaced non-reducing disc.

   An alternative option is the "Minagi" exercise, noted in "M. Evidence-based Treatment Plan" and described in "Background Information."

3. The recommendation is given in order to reduce pain, which would otherwise decrease patient compliance throughout mobilization exercise therapy and therefore hamper recovery, and prevent possible (increase of) intraarticular inflammatory reaction.

4. If left untreated, the signs and symptoms tend to diminish over time despite the permanently displaced position of the articular disc. Mouth opening limitation, deviation toward the affected side, and possible secondary pain decreases in time in most patients.

Case 2.6

Disc Displacement without Reduction without Limited Opening

Stanimira I Kalaykova

A. Demographic Data and Reason for Contact

- Caucasian female, 27 years old, seeks for "My jaw locked some time ago and now I can't open my mouth as much as I used to do."

B. Symptom History

- Sudden onset of pain and difficulties opening the mouth 2 months ago during mealtime.
- Acute, painful limited mouth opening at onset of complaints where the limited mouth opening initially interfered with eating.
- Pain decreased and disappeared the first 3 weeks; today, no pain.
- Mouth opening limitation decreased somewhat with time.
- Prior to onset of current complaint, a history of:
  - Clicking TMJ sounds on the left side since approximately 5 years.
  - In the last 12 months, several occasions of short-lasting, intermittent locking on the left side that would disappear by itself. On movement, an audible click would occur after which the jaw would open completely.
- The patient visits her dentist twice per year.
- No history of trauma.
- The patient is aware of sleep bruxism.

C. Medical History

- Review of systems is negative.
- No allergies to medication; mild seasonal allergies.
- No routine medications.
- No previous hospitalizations or surgeries; no emergency-room visits.

D. Psychosocial History

- Not married.
- The patient does secretarial work.
- The patient lives in a rental flat.
- Average socio-economic status.

E. Previous Consultations and Treatments

- None.

F. Extraoral Status

- No asymmetries with the jaw in rest position.
- No signs of neurologic deficit or somatosensory abnormalities.
- Jaw movement capacity:
  - mouth opening – pain-free maximum mouth opening 30 mm, active maximum mouth 41 mm, passive maximum mouth opening 43 mm but no pain on mandibular movement;
  - protrusive and both laterotrusive movements 10 mm.
- No audible or palpable TMJ sounds on movement.
- No TMJ palpation pain.
- Nonfamiliar palpation pain of masticatory muscles.
- Neck: normal range of motion, pain-free movements and palpation.

G. Intraoral Status

- Soft tissues:
  - linea alba present on inner aspect of cheeks right and left side.
- Dentition and hard tissues:
  - full dentition, except for lower wisdom teeth (38 and 48);
  - no dental restorations present;
  - occlusal and incisal tooth-wear grade 2 present in the front teeth;
  - Angle class I occlusion;
  - overjet and overbite of 2 mm.

H. Additional Examinations and Findings

- MRI confirmed disc displacement without reduction (Figure 2.16).

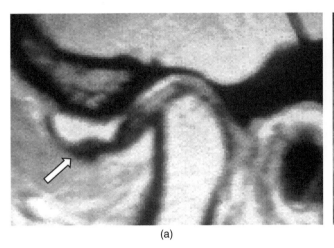
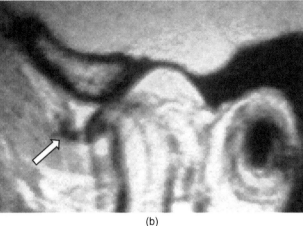

(a)   (b)

Figure 2.16 MRI scan showing disc displacement without reduction in the left TMJ. The disc (arrow) is located anteriorly to the condyle head, both in the closed (a) and open (b) mouth positions.

I. Diagnosis/Diagnoses
DC/TMD

- Disc displacement without reduction without limited mouth opening in left TMJ.

J. Case Assessment

- Patient has no pain, no occlusal changes, and acceptable mandibular movement capacity. The movement capacity may, however, be less than it was before the permanent disc displacement occurred but must be considered as acceptable.
- The patient may be worried about what has happened and what to expect in the future.

K. Evidence-based Treatment Plan including Aims

- Counselling and patient information.
- No other treatment needed.

L. Prognosis and Discussion

- Good short- and long-term prognosis due to no complicating factors in the patient's medical history or psychosocial history, and the patient is young.

Background Information

- DC/TMD defines disc displacement without reduction without limited mouth opening as "an intraarticular biomechanical disorder involving the condyle–disc complex. In the closed mouth position the disc is located in an anterior (and/or medial or lateral) position relative to the condylar head, and the disc does not reduce with opening of the mouth. This disorder is not associated with current limited mouth opening."
- Based on studies employing MRI, the prevalence of disc displacement without reduction is estimated to be 7–10%.
- Treatment seeking is usually associated with arthralgia, if present, secondary to disc displacement without reduction without limited mouth opening.

(Sandler *et al.*, 1998; Naeije *et al.*, 2013; Schiffman *et al.*, 2014)

Diagnostic Criteria

DC/TMD criteria for **Disc displacement without reduction without limited opening** (Schiffman *et al.*, 2014). Without imaging: sensitivity 0.54, specificity 0.79.

An intracapsular biomechanical disorder involving the condyle–disc complex. In the closed mouth position the disc is in an anterior position relative to the condylar head, and the disc does not reduce with opening of the mouth. Medial and lateral displacement of the disc may also be present. This disorder is associated with persistent limited mandibular opening that does not resolve with the clinician or patient performing a specific manipulative maneuver. This is also referred to as "closed lock." Presence of TMJ noise (e.g., click with full opening) does not exclude this diagnosis.

History. Positive for both of the following:

1. Jaw locked or caught so that the mouth would not open all the way.
AND
2. Limitation in jaw opening severe enough to limit jaw opening and interfere with ability to eat.

Examination. Positive for the following:

1. Maximum assisted opening (passive stretch) including vertical incisal overlap ≥40 mm. (Maximum assisted opening of ≥40 mm is determined clinically.)

Imaging. When this diagnosis needs to be confirmed, TMJ MRI criteria are positive for both of the following:

1. In the maximum intercuspal position, the posterior band of the disc is located anterior to the 11:30 position and the intermediate zone of the disc is anterior to the condylar head.
AND
2. On full opening, the intermediate zone of the disc is located anterior to the condylar head.

Fundamental Points

Diagnosis, treatment, and prognosis

- Clinical diagnostics based on oral history of jaw locking severe to interfere with eating and maximum assisted mouth opening ≥40 mm has low sensitivity (0.54) and specificity (0.79) for recognition of disc displacement without reduction with limited mouth opening.
- If needed, imaging diagnostics are required to confirm the clinical diagnosis. MRI is the method of choice to depict the location of the articular disc.
- The short-term prognosis is good. In the long term, with persistence of the displaced disc position, intraarticular degenerative or adaptive changes will most likely occur but with no significant risk of clinical signs and symptoms.

(De Leeuw *et al.*, 1995; Naeije *et al.*, 2013; Vos *et al.*, 2013; Schiffman *et al.*, 2014)

Self-study Questions

1. Which information from the oral history in the case presented is suggestive of disc displacement without reduction without limited mouth opening?

2. Which is the method of choice for TMJ imaging to confirm disc displacement without reduction without limited mouth opening needs to be applied?

3. Based on which criteria is the MRI diagnosis of disc displacement without reduction set?

References

De Leeuw R, Boering G, Stegenga B, de Bont LG (1995) Symptoms of temporomandibular joint osteoarthrosis and internal derangement 30 years after non-surgical treatment. *Cranio* **13**:81–88.

Naeije M, Te Veldhuis AH, Te Veldhuis EC, *et al.* (2013) Disc displacement within the human temporomandibular joint: a systematic review of a 'noisy annoyance'. *J Oral Rehabil* **40**:139–158.

Sandler NA, Buckley MJ, Cillo JE, Braun TW (1998) Correlation of inflammatory cytokines with arthroscopic findings in patients with temporomandibular joint internal derangements. *J Oral Maxillofac Surg* **56**:534–543.

Schiffman E, Ohrbach R, Truelove E, *et al.* (2014) Diagnostic Criteria for Temporomandibular Disorders (DC/TMD) for clinical and research applications: recommendations of the International RDC/TMD Consortium Network and Orofacial Pain Special Interest Group. *J Oral Facial Pain Headache* **28**:6–27.

Vos LM, Huddleston Slater JJ, Stegenga B (2013) Lavage therapy versus nonsurgical therapy for the treatment of arthralgia of the temporomandibular joint: a systematic review of randomized controlled trials. *J Orofac Pain* **27**:171–179.

Answers Self-study to Questions

1. The patient's complaints have started with a jaw lock with a sudden onset accompanied by pain and cessation of joint clicking sounds. In time, a gradual increase of mouth opening has occurred.

2. The method of choice is MRI as it is able to depict the articular TMJ disc.

3. Disc displacement without reduction is diagnosed based on MRI when both of the following criteria are satisfied: (1) in the maximum intercuspal position, the posterior disc band of the disc is located anterior to the 11:30 position and the intermediate zone of the disc is anterior to the condylar head, and (2) on full mouth opening, the intermediate zone of the disc is located anterior to the condylar head.

C: Hypomobility

Case 2.7

Fibrous Ankylosis

Tore Bjørnland

A. Demographic Data and Reason for Contact

- Male, 52 years old.
- Referred from general practitioner to oral and maxillofacial surgeon because of inability to perform dental and periodontal treatment.

B. Symptom History

- Pain on function in both TMJs for 15 years.
- Decreasing mandibular range of motion.
- Unable to chew regular food.
- Unable to have regular dental work done.

C. Psychosocial History

- Married, four children.
- Works in oil-related business as a chef.
- Smokes 20 cigarettes a day.
- On sick leave because of knee pain.
- No depression or anxiety.

D. Medical History

- Ankylosing spondylitis diagnosed at age of 33.
- Affects peripheral joints, especially knees, hands, and TMJs.
- Total hip prosthesis at age of 47.
- Medication: diclofenac 75 mg two times daily.
- Periodontal disease.
- Some fillings and prosthetic restorations.
- Unable to have dental treatment done the last 4 years.

E. Previous Consultations and Treatments

- No previous consultations for TMJ problems.

F. Extraoral Status

- Slight mandibular asymmetry: mandible 4 mm to the right.
- No lateral excursions or protrusion.

G. Intraoral Status

- Periodontal disease with involvement of all teeth.
- Loss of molars in upper jaw.
- Bleeding on probing.
- Dental calculus.
- Dental plaque.
- Frontal open bite 4 mm, occlusion only on premolars (Figure 2.17).
- Pain from TMJ on opening.

H. Additional Examinations and Findings

- Radiological examination of neck with flexion and extension revealed no erosions and subluxations, but a possible fibro-osseous ankylosis between C3 and C4.
- Examination of general health, including blood samples, revealed an elevated C-reactive protein (CRP) of 33 g/L and erythrocyte sedimentation rate (ESR) of 25 mm/h. Other blood tests were within normal limits.
- Panoramic radiograph, TMJ MRI and computed tomography (CT) showed limited translatory movements bilaterally (Figure 2.18).
- CT with angiography showed, in addition to erosions and ankylosis, no embedded arteries.
- Resorption of the cranial base on left TMJ.
- Caries.
- Periodontal disease.

I. Diagnosis/Diagnoses

Expanded DC/TMD

- Bilateral TMJ fibrous ankylosis.

DC/TMD

- Bilateral TMJ arthralgia.

Other

- Systemic ankylosing spondylitis.

J. Case Assessment

- Nutritional challenges. The patient could not attend regular meals with friends (e.g. at restaurants). He was unable to eat regular food without use of a food

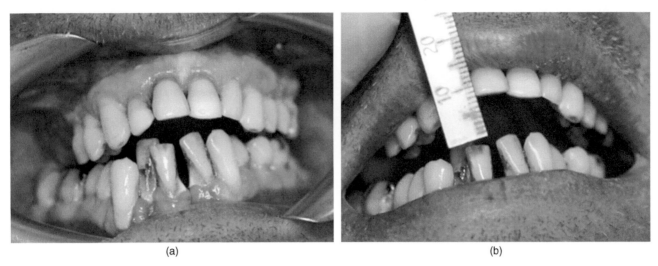

Figure 2.17 (a) Intraoral picture of 52-year-old man with ankylosing spondylitis with occlusion on only both sides premolars. Anterior open bite 4 mm. (b) Maximal range of motion increases the inter-incisal distance to 8 mm.

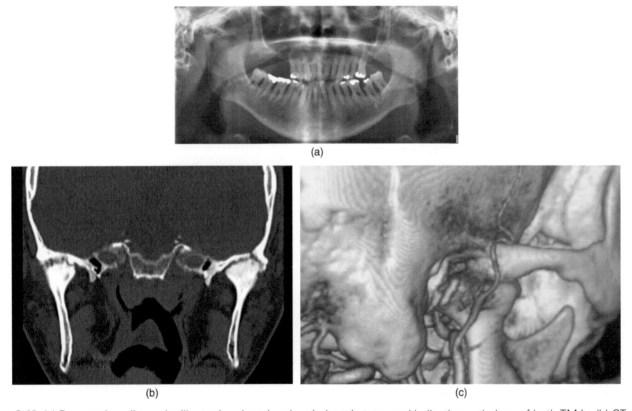

Figure 2.18 (a) Panoramic radiography illustrating dental and periodontal status and indicating pathology of both TMJs. (b) CT showing fibro-osseous changes in both TMJs. Left side with perforation to the cranial fossa. (c) CT with intravenous angiography of right-side TMJ with the maxillary and superficial temporal arteries in close relation to the TMJ. The arteries are not embedded by bone, and there is no stenosis in the arteries. Resorption of the superior and posterior part of the condyle is also observed.

processer. In particular, as a chef in the petroleum production sector in the North Sea he could no longer maintain his professional career.

- Involvement of neck. This is of great importance if it is necessary to undergo general anaesthesia and intubation.
- Possible bilateral facial nerve paraesthesia after TMJ procedures may be a complication and, furthermore, cause eye problems, especially if it occurs bilaterally.
- After years with minimal use of masticatory muscles, they may be atrophied and the muscles will need comprehensive physical exercise to regain mobility and strength.
- Fibro-osseous or bony ankylosis with involvement of the cranial fossa may be a serious complication and may give intracranial infections.

K. Evidence-based Treatment Plan including Aims

Treatment goals

- Periodontal treatment.
- Dental treatment, inclusive of oral implants and prosthodontic restorations.
- Dental hygiene instructions.
- Physical therapy.
- To achieve the possibility to open jaw.

Management

- Bilateral ankylosis resection with interpositional dermis–fat graft. Procedure on left side as first operation and the right side operated 3 months later. Fat collected from the belly. Osteotomies were performed. No leakage of cerebrospinal fluid. After resection of the ankylotic condyles the maximum assisted opening was increased to 40 mm (Figures 2.19 and 2.20).

L. Prognosis and Discussion

- No facial nerve paraesthesia was observed after the operations. The occlusion was stable with no vertical anterior open bite and 4 mm horizontal open bite. Physical therapy was instituted once a week, together with general physical therapy of the other joints involved. Dental and periodontal treatments were started. The plan to do implant surgery and prosthodontic treatment was not done since the patient was very satisfied with the situation.
- Re-ankylosis is possible in cases with both unilateral and bilateral fibrous or bony ankylosis. Treatment decision is difficult. Should one use ankylosis resection with ramus–condyle unit reconstruction with a prosthetic total joint or interpositional arthroplasty?
- Treatment of TMJ ankylosis with total joint prosthesis may be more predictable with regard to achieving a good occlusion compared with interpositional arthroplasty. On the other hand, total joint replacement often gives less lateral and protrusive mandibular motion.
- The reason for operation of the two sides with a 3 month interval was first the possibility of involvement of the cranial fossa on the left side, evaluation of the occlusion after resection of one side and evaluation of possible facial paraesthesia. If some complications had appeared on the one side, there was the option to cancel the operation on the other side.

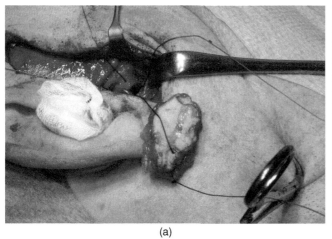
(a)

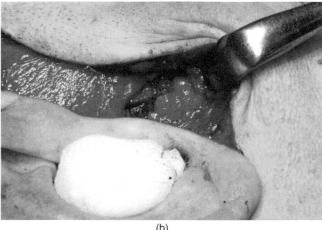
(b)

Figure 2.19 (a) Right-side ankylosis resection with placement of dermis–fat graft secured with sutures to the zygomatic arch. (b) After right TMJ ankylosis resection and placement of dermis–fat graft in the TMJ space.

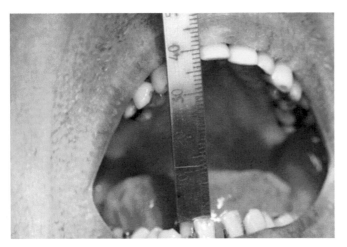

Figure 2.20 Maximal range of motion 40 mm at 6 months after bilateral TMJ ankylosis resection and placement of dermis–fat graft.

- If re-ankylosis appears, one has to consider reoperation where the use of total joint replacement may be necessary.
- Facial nerve paraesthesia – if bilateral this may be a serious complication due to dryness of the eyes, with possible blindness as a result.
- Perforation to the cranial fossa may be a serious complication in cases where the arthritic process has resorbed the articular fossa.
- Alternative treatment plans could be either alloplastic total joint prosthesis or resection of ankylotic condyle with bone transplantation from rib, hip or fibula.

Background Information
- Fibrous ankylosis of the TMJ is a rare condition that may affect one or both TMJs (Loveless *et al.*, 2010).
- The aetiology may be trauma, iatrogenic causes due to previous surgical interventions or to inflammatory diseases such as immunological diseases (e.g. rheumatoid arthritis, ankylosing spondylitis, juvenile idiopathic arthritis) (Loveless *et al.*, 2010).
- The ankylosis will in most cases appear gradually with decreased mandibular motion as one of the clinical signs. Pain may or may not be a present.
- Erosion, destruction, bone remodelling and bone formation may be seen in the development of the fibrous ankylosis.
- Radiographically, an orthopantomogram may give the first indication of pathology of the TMJs.

- CT or CBCT is the best radiographic examination for TMJ ankylosis. MRI may give additional information about active inflammation. CT with angiography is recommended to evaluate possible vessels inside the ankylosed part of the TMJ.
- Erosion of the fossa may be a part of the process, and the cranial fossa may be involved in the resorption and bone remodelling.
- Even if there is ankylosis, the patient may have some degree of mandibular movement because of the elasticity of the mandible.

Diagnostic Criteria
Expanded DC/TMD criteria for **TMJ fibrous ankylosis** (Peck *et al.*, 2014). Sensitivity and specificity have not been established.

In fibrous ankylosis there are no gross bony changes, and the predominant radiographic finding is absence of ipsilateral condylar translation on opening. Note that fibrous ankylosis may be considered a more severe form of TMJ adhesions/adherence.

History. Positive for the following:
1. History of progressive loss of jaw mobility.

Examination. Positive for all of the following:
1. Severely limited range of motion on opening. AND
2. Uncorrected jaw deviation to the affected side on opening. AND
3. Marked limited laterotrusion to the contralateral side.

Imaging. CT/CBCT is positive for both of the following:
1. Imaging findings of decreased ipsilateral condylar translation on opening. AND
2. Imaging findings of a disc space between ipsilateral condyle and eminence.

Criteria for DC/TMD **Arthralgia** (Schiffman *et al.*, 2014), see Case 2.1.

Classification of diagnostic criteria for ankylosing spondylitis does not include TMJ symptoms, but includes both radiological and clinical criteria of especially sacroiliitis grading and clinical criteria of low back pain and limitation of lumbar spine (Raychaudhuri and Deodhar, 2014).

Fundamental Points

- When the patient has a general diagnosis of ankylosing spondylitis, TMJ ankylosis should most probably be part of the general diagnosis. There might, however, be other reasons for TMJ ankylosis: trauma, infection or iatrogenic reasons.
- Surgical excision of the ankylosed part is necessary to achieve normal range of motion (Dimitroulis, 2004, 2013; Loveless *et al.*, 2010; Mercuri, 2012; Aagaard and Thygesen, 2014; Lotesto *et al.*, 2016).
- Before surgery one has to evaluate neck stiffness or resorptions with radiographic examinations of the neck with extension and flexion.
- Intubation as part of the general anaesthesia may be difficult; therefore, tracheotomy may be planned before surgery.
- Interpositional grafts are necessary to avoid re-ankylosis (Dimitroulis, 2004).
- Total joint replacement has to be considered (Loveless *et al.*, 2010; Mercuri, 2012; Aagaard and Thygesen, 2014; Lotesto *et al.*, 2016).
- Postoperative physiotherapy and mandibular exercises are important in order to avoid re-ankylosis.

Self-study Questions

1. Describe the aetiology of fibrous ankylosis.
2. Give examples of the clinical signs of fibrous ankylosis.
3. What kind of imaging is necessary in establishing the diagnosis and what additional imaging is necessary before treatment?
4. What kind of treatment is necessary for fibrous ankylosis?

Referencess

Aagaard E, Thygesen T (2014) A prospective, single-centre study on patient outcomes following temporomandibular joint replacement using a custom-made Biomet TMJ-prosthesis. *Int J Oral Maxillofac Surg* **43**:1229–1235.

Dimitroulis G (2004) The interpositional dermis–fat graft in the management of temporomandibular joint ankylosis. *Int J Oral Maxillofac Surg* **33**:675–760.

Dimitroulis G (2013) A new surgical classification for temporomandibular disorders. *Int J Oral Maxillofac Surg* **42**:218–222.

Lotesto A, Miloro M, Mercuri LG, Sukotjo C (2016) Are oral and maxillofacial surgery residents trained adequately in alloplastic TMJ total joint replacement? *J Oral Maxillofac Surg* **74**(4):712–718.

Loveless T, Bjornland T, Dodson TB, Keith DA (2010) Efficacy of temporomandibular joint ankylosis surgical treatment. *J Oral Maxillofac Surg* **68**:1276–1282.

Mercuri LG (2012) Alloplastic temporomandibular joint replacement: rationale for the use of custom devices. *Int J Oral Maxillofac Surg* **41**:1033–1040.

Peck CC, Goulet JP, Lobbezoo F, *et al.*(2014) Expanding the taxonomy of the diagnostic criteria for temporomandibular disorders. *J Oral Rehabil* **41**(1):2–23.

Raychaudhuri SP, Deodhar A (2014) The classification and diagnostic criteria of ankylosing spondylitis. *J Autoimmun* **48–49**:128–133.

Schiffman E, Ohrbach R, Truelove E, *et al.* (2014) Diagnostic Criteria for Temporomandibular Disorders (DC/TMD) for clinical and research applications: recommendations of the International RDC/TMD Consortium Network and Orofacial Pain Special Interest Group. *J Oral Facial Pain Headache* **28**(1):6–27.

Answers to Self-study Questions

1. The aetiology may be trauma, iatrogenic causes such as previous surgical interventions or inflammatory diseases such as immunological diseases (e.g. rheumatoid arthritis, ankylosing spondylitis, juvenile idiopathic arthritis).

2. Reduced range of motion and lateral excursion to the contralateral side. Pain may be or not be part of the clinical signs. Open bite may occur if there is much resorption of the condyle. Growth disturbances may occur if the ankylosis takes place in a growing child.

3. CT or CBCT is the best radiographic examination for TMJ ankylosis. MRI may give additional information about active inflammation. CT with angiography is recommended to evaluate possible vessels inside the ankylosed part of the TMJ. Before surgery one has to evaluate neck stiffness or resorptions with radiographic examinations of the neck with extension and flexion.

4. Surgical excision of the ankylosed part is necessary to achieve normal range of motion. Interpositional grafts are necessary to avoid re-ankylosis. Total joint replacement has to be considered. Postoperative physiotherapy and mandibular exercises are important in order to avoid re-ankylosis.

Case 2.8

Bony Ankylosis

Tore Bjørnland

A. Demographic Data and Reason for Contact

- Vietnamese female, 18 years old, lives in Vietnam.
- Contact made from general medical practitioner to a Norwegian charity organization for the possibility of oral and maxillofacial surgery in Norway.
- Can come to Norway for a limited time to do necessary treatment.

B. Symptom History

- Cannot open mouth for as long as she can remember; cannot brush teeth.
- Toothache.
- Not satisfied with chin.
- Sleep apnoea.
- Nutritional challenges.

C. Medical History

- Fell down from table and hit the chin at 1 year of age; no treatment.
- No allergies.
- No routine medications.
- No previous hospitalizations or surgeries.
- Difficulties in eating and gaining weight.
- Not possible to have dental treatment performed.
- Often pain from decayed teeth.
- Not able to move the jaw (assisted or unassisted) as long as she can remember.
- No known organic disease.

D. Psychosocial History

- Patient lives with mother, father and two brothers.
- Not satisfied with teeth.
- Not satisfied with facial aesthetics.
- No depression or anxiety.

E. Previous Consultations and Treatment

- She has had some extractions.
- Some fillings in incisors.
- Teeth erupted until met by teeth in opposite jaw.
- Probably no treatment for TMJ ankylosis so far.

F. Extraoral Status

- Severe mandibular micrognathia (Figure 2.21).
- Asymmetry; mandible more pronounced to the left.
- No mandibular movement (assisted or unassisted).

G. Intraoral Status

- Upper and lower teeth in contact; not possible to move mandible.
- Several remaining roots.
- Loss of upper front teeth.

H. Additional Examinations and Findings

- Panoramic radiograph, lateral cephalogram, CT (Figures 2.22 and 2.23).
- Appointment with anaesthesiologist in order to evaluate nasal intubation or tracheotomy before surgery.

I. Diagnosis/Diagnoses
Expanded DC/TMD

- Left TMJ osseous ankylosis.

Other

- Sequela after mandibular fracture.
- Sleep apnoea.
- Mandibular micrognathia.
- Periodontitis.
- Caries.

J. Case Assessment

- Nutritional challenges. The patient has never had regular meals, only soft liquids. Necessary to give nutritional information and teaching.
- Since the patient should return home shortly after the end of the surgical treatment, there was limited time for dental rehabilitation.
- Only the most necessary treatment will be possible to perform before the patient has to return home.

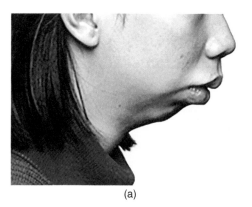
(a)

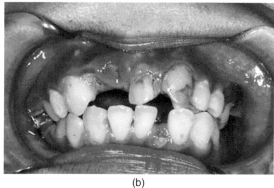
(b)

Figure 2.21 (a) Profile of 18-year-old female with bony ankylosis of left TMJ. (b) No mandibular movements. Teeth had erupted until they met the antagonizing teeth. Manifest caries and endodontic problems.

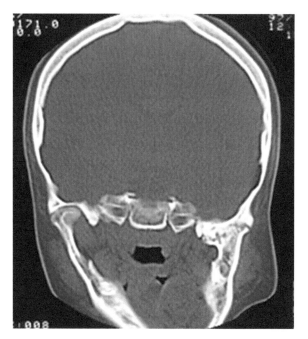

Figure 2.22 CT with ankylosis of left TMJ, which also shows deviation of the mandible to affected side and asymmetry.

- In TMJ ankylosis the maxillary artery and other vessels in the TMJ area may be embedded in the ankylosed TMJs. During surgery, excessive bleeding from the ankylosed bone may occur. It is therefore important to evaluate the maxillary artery by CT with angiography.
- Facial paraesthesia is a complication that may occur after all TMJ surgery but is more frequent in ankylosis cases.
- Re-ankylosis may occur. There may, therefore, be a need for another surgical intervention.
- In the treatment planning we have to consider ankylosis resection, interpositional arthroplasty with temporalis myofascial flap or dermis–fat

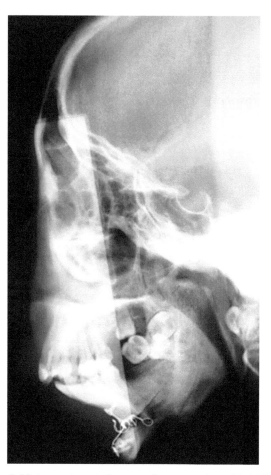

Figure 2.23 Lateral cephalogram after resection of left TMJ ankylotic part, genioplasty and removal of eight roots.

transplantation or reconstruction with a prosthetic total joint in the treatment of this patient.

K. Evidence-based Treatment Plan including Aims

Treatment goals

- Healthy dentition.

- Adequate dental hygiene.
- Normal mandibular movement capacity.
- Normal facial appearance and profile.

Management

- Simultaneous condylectomy with temporalis myofascial flap.
- Removal of infected roots.
- Genioplasty.
- Dental restorations.
- Physical therapy of masticatory muscles.

L. Prognosis and Discussion

- In this case, orthodontic treatment after the condylectomy and removal of dental roots should be considered. Endodontic treatment should also be considered.
- After dental treatment and alignment of teeth, bimaxillary surgery could then have been performed to enhance the facial profile and correct the asymmetry.
- In the present case, only limited time was available for treatment since the patient had to go back to the family for different reasons. The postoperative result, however, was adequate in relation to the patient's expectations and the preoperative starting point (Figure 2.24).
- Surgical treatment of TMJ bony ankylosis is challenging, and so far the surgical treatments are based on case studies and are not evidence based. Surgical treatment of ankylosed TMJs should preferably be centralized to a few institutions.
- There is a possibility of re-ankylosis. Therefore, care has to be taken to cautiously remove a sufficient volume of the ankylosed condyle. The range of motion has to be checked during surgery to evaluate how much the maximal range of motion can be after surgery. In this case, the masticatory muscles had not been used for chewing and there was a severe atrophy of the muscles. Training and physical therapy are therefore a crucial part of the postoperative treatment.
- The postoperative range of motion was 25 mm at 1 week, and it had increased to 37 mm at 3 months. The profile was acceptable and the patient was happy with the result. No complications such as facial nerve paraesthesia were seen.

Background Information

- Bony ankylosis of the TMJ is a very rare condition that most often affects one TMJ (Loveless *et al.*, 2010).
- The aetiology may be untreated condylar fractures, other trauma, iatrogenic causes such as previous surgical interventions or inflammatory diseases such as immunological diseases (e.g. rheumatoid arthritis, ankylosing spondylitis, juvenile idiopathic arthritis) (Loveless *et al.*, 2010).
- The ankylosis will in most cases appear gradually with decreased range of motion as one of the clinical signs. Pain may or may not be present.
- Radiographically, a panoramic radiograph may give the first indication of pathology of the TMJs.
- CT or CBCT is the best radiographic examination to detect TMJ bony ankylosis. MRI may give additional information about any active inflammation. CT with angiography is recommended to evaluate possible vessels inside the ankylosed part of the TMJ.

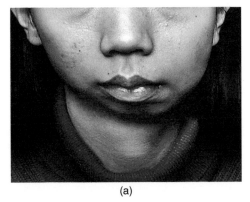
(a)

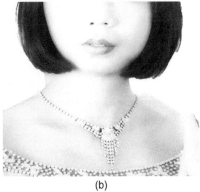
(b)

Figure 2.24 (a) Preoperative facial view. (b) Picture sent to surgeon 1 year after surgery from her residential home.

- CT signs of erosion, destruction, bone remodelling and bone formation may be seen in the development of the bony ankylosis.
- Even if there is bony ankylosis, the patients may have some degree of range of motion because of the elasticity of the mandible.
- If bony ankylosis appears in a growing child, severe maxilla–mandibular growth disturbances may appear.

Diagnostic Criteria

Expanded DC/TMD criteria for **Osseous ankylosis** (Peck et al., 2014). Sensitivity and specificity have not been established.

Bony ankylosis results from the union of the bones of the TMJ by proliferation of bone cells; this may cause complete immobility of that joint. It is characterized by radiographic evidence of bone proliferation with marked deflection to the affected side and marked limited laterotrusion to the contralateral side.

History. Positive for the following:
1. History of progressive loss of jaw mobility.

Examination. Positive for the following:
1. Absence of or severely limited jaw mobility with all movements.

Imaging. CT/CBCT is positive for the following:
1. Imaging-based evidence of bone proliferation with obliteration of part or all of the joint space.

Fundamental Points

- Severly reduced mouth opening capacity and lateral excursion to the contralateral side are important clinical signs of ankylosis.
- Erosion of the fossa may be a part of the process and the cranial fossa may be involved in the resorption and bone remodelling (Loveless et al., 2010).
- In bony ankylosis of the TMJ, surgical excision of the ankylosed part is necessary to achieve normal range of motion (Dimitroulis, 2004; Loveless et al., 2010, Mercuri, 2012; Aagaard and Thygesen, 2014).
- Before surgery one has to evaluate neck stiffness or resorptions with radiographic

examinations of the neck with extension and flexion.
- Intubation as part of the general anaesthesia may be difficult and, therefore, tracheotomy should be considered before surgery.
- Interpositional grafts are necessary to avoid re-ankylosis (Dimitroulis, 2004).
- Total joint replacement has to be considered as an alternative treatment (Loveless et al., 2010; Mercuri, 2012; Aagaard and Thygesen, 2014; Lotesto et al., 2016).
- Postoperative physiotherapy and mandibular exercises are important in order to avoid re-ankylosis (Loveless et al., 2010).
- Dental rehabilitation may be necessary in cases of long-standing ankylosis.
- Reconstructive jaw surgery or orthognathic surgery may be indicated to achieve normal jaw relations and aesthetics.

Self-study Questions

1. Describe the aetiology of bony ankylosis.
2. Give examples of the clinical signs of bony ankylosis.
3. What kind of imaging is necessary in establishing the diagnosis and what additional imaging in necessary before treatment?
4. What kind of treatment is necessary in the treatment of bony ankylosis?

References

Aagaard E, Thygesen T (2014) A prospective, single-centre study on patient outcomes following temporomandibular joint replacement using a custom-made Biomet TMJ-prosthesis. *Int J Oral Maxillofac Surg* **43**:1229–1235.

Dimitroulis G (2004) The interpositional dermis–fat graft in the management of temporomandibular joint ankylosis. *Int J Oral Maxillofac Surg* **33**:675–760.

Lotesto, A, Miloro M, Mercuri LG, Sukotjo C (2016) Are oral and maxillofacial surgery residents trained adequately in alloplastic TMJ total joint replacement? *J Oral Maxillofac Surg* **74**(4):712–718.

Loveless T, Bjornland T, Dodson TB, Keith DA (2010) Efficacy of temporomandibular joint ankylosis surgical treatment. *J Oral Maxillofac Surg* **68**:1276–1282.

Mercuri LG (2012) Alloplastic temporomandibular joint replacement: rationale for the use of custom devices. *Int J Oral Maxillofac Surg* **41**:1033–1040.

Peck CC, Goulet JP, Lobbezoo F, et al. (2014) Expanding the taxonomy of the diagnostic criteria for temporomandibular disorders. *J Oral Rehabil* **41**(1):2–23.

Answers to Self-study Questions

1. The aetiology may be untreated condylar fractures trauma, iatrogenic causes such as previous surgical interventions or inflammatory diseases such as immunological diseases (e.g. rheumatoid arthritis, ankylosing spondylitis, juvenile idiopathic arthritis).

2. Highly reduced range of motion and lateral excursion to the contralateral side. Pain may be or not be part of the clinical signs. Open bite may occur if there is much resorption of the condyle. Growth disturbances may occur if the ankylosis takes place in a growing child. It might be difficult to differentiate between fibrous and bony ankylosis

3. CT or CBCT is the best radiographic examination for TMJ ankylosis. MRI may give additional information about active inflammation. CT with angiography is recommended to evaluate possible vessels inside the ankylosed part of the TMJ. Before surgery one has to evaluate neck stiffness or resorptions with radiographic examinations of the neck with extension and flexion.

4. Surgical excision of the ankylosed part is necessary to achieve normal range of motion. Interpositional grafts are necessary to avoid re-ankylosis. Total joint replacement has to be considered. Postoperative physiotherapy and mandibular exercises are important in order to avoid re-ankylosis.

Case 2.9

Hypomobility: Coroniod Process Hyperplasia

Tore Bjørnland and Fredrik Hallmer

A. Demographic Data and Reason for Contact

- Male student, 29 years old.
- Referred from general dental practitioner because of decreased mandibular motion and difficulties of receiving dental care.

B. Symptom History

- Decreasing mandibular range of motion the last 8–10 years.
- Difficulty in having regular dental work done.

C. Psychosocial History

- Student, living by himself.
- Describes himself as a calm person with good stress management. Normal scores for depression (PHQ-9), no anxiety (GAD-7). No physical symptoms (PHQ-15) and moderate level of stress (PSS-10). Good sleep quality (PSQI).

D. Medical History

- Migraine.
- No allergies.
- No routine medications.
- No previous hospitalizations or surgeries.

E. Previous Consultations and Treatments

- No previous consultations for TMJ problems.
- Referred to oral and maxillofacial surgeon for examination and possible treatment.
- Has had some dental fillings.
- Difficulty in having dental treatment done the last year.

F. Extraoral Status
Face
- Facial asymmetry with left-side deviation of the chin.

Temporomandibular joint
- No joint sounds.
- No pain on palpation.

Masticatory muscles
- No pain on jaw opening or palpation.

Jaw movement capacity

- Limited mandibular motion; unassisted opening 20 mm.
- Limited lateral excursion, 5 mm to each side.
- Limited protrusion, 2 mm.
- No TMJ pain on mandibular movement.
- Deviation to the right on mouth opening.

G. Intraoral Status
Soft tissues
- Normal findings oral mucosa, no bleeding on probing.

Hard tissues
- Complete dentition with few restorations. No caries.

Occlusion
- Bilateral contacts premolars and molars in intercuspal position. Canine and anterior guidance.

H. Additional Examination and Findings
- Panoramic radiography and CT show elongated right coronoid process (Figure 2.25).

I. Diagnosis/Diagnoses
Expanded DC/TMD
- Coronoid hyperplasia.

J. Case Assessment
- There were nutritional challenges because of problems with opening mouth and chewing. The patient had chosen to eat food of low nutritional value during the period of restricted jaw opening.
- After a long time with restricted mandibular opening the masticatory muscles may have atrophied. Therefore, comprehensive physical therapy may be needed, both by physical therapist and self-assisted training.

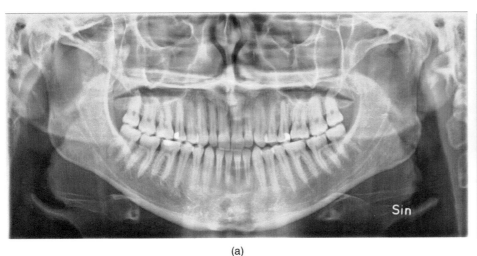
(a)

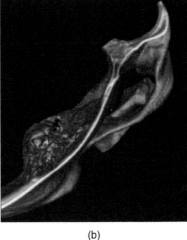
(b)

Figure 2.25 (a) Panoramic radiography illustrates dental and periodontal status and indicates pathology of right coronoid process. (b) CT showing hyperplasia of the right coronoid process interfering with the zygomatic arch.

- Coronoid hyperplasia may reappear after surgical excision.

K. Evidence-based Treatment Plan including Aims

Treatment goals

- To achieve the possibility to open jaw normally without pain.
- Dental hygiene instructions.
- Physical therapy.

Management

- Coronoidotomy of the right coronoid processes.
- An intraoral approach was performed where the right coronoid process was exposed. A coronoidotomy where the hyperplastic coronoid was sectioned and a 5 mm segment was resected.
- Jaw exercises.

L. Prognosis and Discussion

- Surgery is the standard treatment option with the goal to eliminate mechanical obstruction of the coronoid process interfering with the zygomatic arch at mouth opening. An intraoral approach was chosen to minimize scares and risk of facial nerve damage. Either coronoidectomy or coronoidotomy are performed. If coronoidectomy is performed the coronoid process is resected, whereas in a coronoidotomy the process is sectioned and left. Less postoperative morbidity has been reported in cases with a coronoidotomy; on the other hand, there is a higher recurrence rate due to risk of reattachment of the coronoid process.

- No facial nerve paresthesia was observed after the operation. The occlusion was stable with no vertical anterior or horizontal open bite. Postoperative physiotherapy was instituted the first weeks with stretching exercises for the preservation of the increased mouth opening. At 6 months postoperatively the patient had increased maximal mouth opening (38 mm).
- Reattachment of the coronoid process and regeneration of the coronoid process after coronoidectomy or coronoidotomy might occur. In this case, radiological findings 3 years after surgery showed regrowth and a new hyperplasia of the coronoid process (Figure 2.26).

Background Information

- Coronoid hyperplasia is a rare condition that may affect one or both coronoids.
- The etiology is unknown, but muscular hyperactivity or trauma may be reasons for the hyperplasia. In cases with condylar destruction one may observe coronoid elongation or hyperplasia.
- The etiology of mandibular hypomobility can be classified into:
  - intracapsular – this group may have internal derangement, degenerative arthritis, intracapsular fracture, infection;
  - extracapsular, like coronoid hyperplasia – other causes include, muscle contracture, radiation, fibrosis, scarring from trauma or prior surgery;
  - neurologic (e.g., traumatic brain injury, tetany);

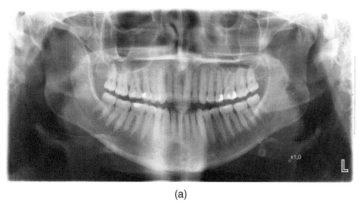

(a)

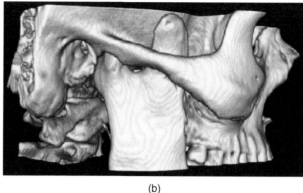

(b)

Figure 2.26 (a) Panoramic radiography 3 years after coronoidotomy shows regeneration of the right coronoid process. (b) CT showing regeneration of the coronoid process 3 years after coronoidotomy and a new hyperplasia of the right coronoid process.

- psychogenic, hysterical trismus or conversion reaction.
- Decreased mouth opening capacity as one of the clinical signs may appear gradually. Pain may or may not be present.

Diagnostic Criteria

Expanded DC/TMD criteria for **Coronoid hyperplasia** (Peck *et al.*, 2014). Sensitivity and specificity have not been established.

Progressive enlargement of the coronoid process that impedes mandibular opening when it is obstructed by the zygomatic process of the maxilla.

History. Positive for the following:
1. Complaint of limitation of jaw opening.

Examination. Positive for the following:
1. Reduction of active and passive maximum jaw opening.

Imaging. CT/CBCT is positive for the following:
1. An elongated coronoid process which approximates the posterior aspect of the zygomatic process of the maxilla on opening.

Fundamental Points

- Radiographically, a panoramic radiograph may give the first indication of pathology of the TMJs.
- CT or CBCT is the best radiographic examination to diagnose coronoid hyperplasia.

- Muscular hyperactivity has to be evaluated.
- Rare diseases, such as fibrodysplasia ossificans progressiva, have to be excluded.
- Surgical excision of the hyperplastic part is necessary to achieve normal mandibular movement capacity.
- Intubation as part of the general anesthesia may be difficult and, therefore, tracheotomy may be planned before surgery.
- Postoperative physiotherapy and mandibular exercises are important in order to avoid re-ankylosis.

(McLoughlin *et al.*, 1995; Piedra, 1995; Kubota *et al.*, 1999; Mulder *et al.*, 2012)

Self-study Questions

1. Describe the differential diagnosis to coronoid hyperplasia.
2. What may be the etiology of coronoid hyperplasia?
3. What kind of imaging is necessary in establishing the diagnosis?
4. What kind of treatment is necessary in the treatment of coronoid hyperplasia?

References

Kubota Y, Takenoshita Y, Takamori K, *et al.* (1999) Levandoski panographic analysis in the diagnosis of hyperplasia of the coronoid process. *Br J Oral Maxillofac Surg* **37**:409–411.

McLoughlin PM, Hopper C, Bowley NB (1995) Hyperplasia of the mandibular coronoid process: an analysis of 31 cases and a review of the literature. *J Oral Maxillofac Surg* **53**:250–255.

Mulder CH, Kalaykova SI, Gortzak RA (2012) Coronoid process hyperplasia: a systemic review of the literature from 1995. *Int J Oral Maxillofac Surg* **41**:1483–1489.

Peck CC, Goulet JP, Lobbezoo F, *et al.* (2014) Expanding the taxonomy of the diagnostic criteria for temporomandibular disorders. *J Oral Rehabil* **41**(1):2–23.

Piedra I (1995) The Levandoski panoramic analysis in the diagnosis of facial and dental asymmetries. *J Clin Pediatr Dent* **20**:15–21.

Answers to Self-study Questions

1. The differential diagnosis may be hypomobility of muscular origin, different TMJ disturbances such as disc displacement, arthritis, osteoarthritis.

2. The etiology is unknown, but muscular hyperactivity or trauma may be reasons for the hyperplasia. In cases with condylar destruction one may observe coronoid elongation or hyperplasia. Rare diseases, such as fibrodysplasia ossificans progressiva, may also give coronoid hyperplasia and reduced range of motion.

3. A panoramic radiograph should be the first X-ray to be taken. CT or CBCT is the next radiographic examination to be considered.

4. Surgical excision of the hyperplastic coronoid process is necessary to achieve normal opening capacity. Postoperative physiotherapy and mandibular exercises are important in order to avoid re-ankylosis.

D: Degenerative Joint Diseases

Case 2.10

Degenerative Joint Disease

Per Alstergren

A. Demographic Data and Reason for Contact

- Male, 44 years of age (Figure 2.27).
- Born in Bosnia, immigrated to Sweden 24 years ago.
- Referred to orofacial pain specialist from general practitioner due to TMJ pain and sounds.

B. Symptom History

- Today, pain from right TMJ at rest, movement, and chewing.
- Chewing and mouth opening worsens the pain. Rest, diclofenac and ibuprofen may decrease the pain.
- Pain intensity varies between 1 (at rest) and 5 (on chewing hard food) on a 0–10 NRS.
- Characteristic pain intensity 10 (NRS 0–100), current pain intensity 1 (NRS 0–10), pain-related disability 23 (NRS 0–100; GCPS).
- JFLS reveals limitation in mouth opening and chewing. No apparent daytime parafunctions according OBCL.
- No headache. No neck pain.
- Grating sounds from the right TMJ.
- Debut with grating sounds in the right TMJ 7 years ago. Since 2 years ago, intermittent pain as described earlier from the right TMJ and increasing grating sounds.
- Trauma to the left side of the face at a soccer game 12 years ago. Initially pain in the right TMJ and mouth opening difficulties that subsided during 2 weeks.
- Six months ago the patient noticed occlusal changes with a gradual loss of occlusal contacts, especially in the front. Today, no contacts in the front.

C. Medical History

- Hypothyreosis.
- Diffuse and undiagnosed knee joint pains.
- Medication: diclofenac a few times a week against the knee and TMJ pain.

D. Psychosocial History

- Married, three children (21, 15, and 12 years of age).

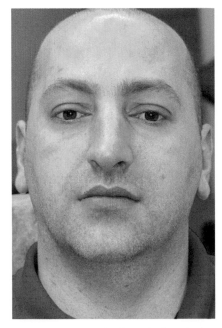

Figure 2.27 Male, 44 years old. Born in Bosnia, immigrated to Sweden 24 years ago. Referred to orofacial pain specialist from general practitioner due to TMJ pain and sounds.

- Works as a chef in a high school; enjoys his work but finds it very stressful. Few sick-leave days in general.
- In his spare time: house renovation, gym, family, and friends.
- Describes himself as person that easily gets stressed and with inadequate stress management. Mild scores for depression (PHQ-9) and anxiety (GAD-7). Some physical symptoms (PHQ-15; 7 p) but moderate level of stress (PSS-10). Normal catastrophizing (Patient Catastrophizing Scale (PCS)). Good sleep quality (PSQI).
- GCPS grade I; that is, low pain intensity and low disability.
- No smoking, moderate alcohol consumption.

E. Previous Consultations and Treatments

- Several visits to this general dental practitioner. Tried splint but with limited success.

F. Extraoral Status

Asymmetries

- No apparent swelling or other facial asymmetries. No redness. No increased skin temperature over either TMJ.

Somatosensory abnormalities

- Normal findings bilaterally for the trigeminal nerve regarding touch, cold. and pinprick.

Temporomandibular joint

- Familiar palpation pain on the right side. Normal translatory movement on both sides. Familiar pain from the right TMJ on mouth opening; laterotrusion to both sides and on protrusion.
- Palpable crepitus from the right TMJ.

Masticatory muscles

- Familiar palpation pain in right masseter and temporalis muscle. No referred pain.

Jaw movement capacity

- Maximum mouth opening without pain is 29 mm, maximum unassisted opening is 45 mm with familiar pain in right TMJ, and maximum assisted mouth opening is 50 mm with familiar pain in the right TMJ. Right laterotrusion 14 mm (no familiar pain), left laterotrusion 10 mm with familiar pain in the right TMJ and masseter muscle, and protrusion 9 mm with familiar pain in the right TMJ.

Neck examination

- Normal range of motion; no familiar neck pain on movement or palpation.

G. Intraoral Status

Soft tissues

- Normal findings.

Hard tissues and dentition

- Complete dentition (except for 46) with some fillings.

Occlusion

- Dentition: 17–27, 37–45, 47. Hard occlusion shows contacts on the following teeth in the upper jaw: 17, 24–27 (Figure 2.28).

H. Additional Examinations and Findings

- CBCT of the right TMJ shows condyle and temporal eminence flattening, v-shaped temporal eminence, condylar bone loss, and condylar osteophytes (Figure 2.29). Normal findings on the left side.

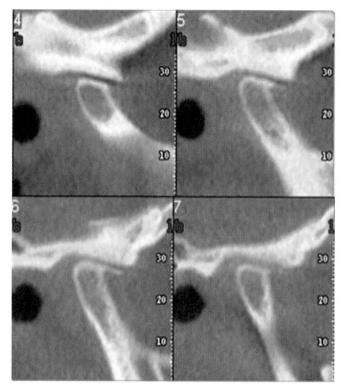

Figure 2.28 Dentition: 17–27, 37–45, 47. Hard occlusion shows contacts on the following teeth in the upper jaw: 17, 24–27.

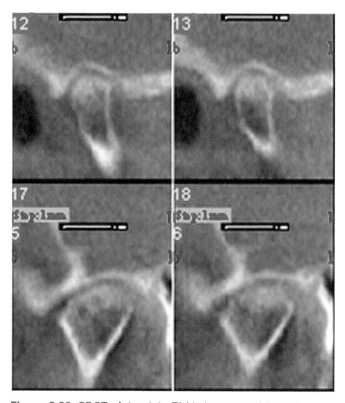

Figure 2.29 CBCT of the right TMJ shows condyle and temporal eminence flattening, v-shaped temporal eminence, condylar bone loss, and condylar osteophyte. Normal findings on the left side.

I. Diagnosis/Diagnoses
DC/TMD

- Right TMJ degenerative joint disease.
- Arthralgia in the right TMJ.
- Myalgia of the masticatory muscles.

Expanded DC/TMD

- Arthritis, right TMJ.

J. Case Assessment

- Degenerative joint disease in the right TMJ with a probable secondary arthritis due to the finding of arthralgia, including TMJ pain on mandibular movements (see Case 2.2).
- Radiographic examination shows typical signs of degenerative joint disease in the right TMJ: condyle and temporal eminence flattening, v-shaped temporal eminence, condylar bone loss, and condylar osteophytes, supporting the diagnosis of degenerative joint disease.
- Minor masticatory muscle myalgia that was not part of the main complaint. However, it may point to a muscle tension situation that in turn may have contributed to the degenerative joint disease by excessive TMJ loading.
- Bone tissue changes in combination with the ongoing inflammatory activity in the right TMJ are a likely cause of the changes in occlusion.

K. Evidence-based Treatment Plan including Aims

- After information and counselling, the first priority is to stop the inflammatory activity in the right TMJ. The aim would be to eliminate the pain and the ongoing cartilage and bone tissue destruction in the joint. See Case 2.2 for detail. In overview, anti-inflammatory treatment (intraarticular corticosteroids or NSAIDs) supplemented with a treatment modality that has the possibility to reduce the risk of a relapse of the arthritis. For example, jaw exercise.
- When the inflammatory activity is substantially reduced and under control, the occlusal changes should be addressed. The aim for this part should be adequate chewing ability and stable, comfortable occlusion. Treatment options range from no treatment and natural normalization of the occlusion, via occlusal adjustment, prosthodontic therapy, orthodontic therapy, surgery, or combinations of these. The goal here must be increased or normalized chewing capacity. Also, the treatment should be minimal since there is an increased risk of future arthritic episodes that may have the possibility to further change the occlusion.

L. Prognosis and Discussion

- The prognosis is very much dependent on how well it will be possible to stop the inflammatory activity. The supposedly long duration of arthritis, including pain and later occlusal changes due to the bone tissue destruction, is a negative prognostic factor. The short-term prognosis for treatment of arthritis must be considered as good, especially if intraarticular corticosteroids are used. However, the long-term prognosis is unclear and depends on how well the inflammation will be controlled, also over time.

Background Information

- Degenerative joint disease is primarily a noninflammatory progressive and degenerative cartilage disease resulting in degradation of load-bearing cartilage tissue and remodeling of underlying bone tissue. However, the etiology of the majority of TMJ degenerative joint disease is complex and multifactorial or unknown.
- The terms degenerative joint disease, osteoarthritis, osteoarthrosis, and arthrosis are often used interchangeably. In DC/TMD, these terms have all been replaced with the umbrella term "degenerative joint disease." Future research will hopefully clarify this matter.
- Degenerative joint disease is frequently associated with arthritis. This association is bidirectional; that is, degenerative joint disease can cause arthritis and arthritis can cause degenerative joint changes.
- Degenerative joint disease can initiate and maintain a secondary arthritis due to an intraarticular discharge of short cartilage collagen fragments from the damaged cartilage surface. These fragments may be discharged as part of the degenerative process or by joint movement and loading, especially if the cartilage surface is damaged. Short collagen fragments cause inflammation by an unspecific immune system reaction. Indeed, one commonly used animal model of rheumatoid arthritis uses intraarticular injections of short collagen fragments to cause chronic arthritis.
- Degenerative joint disease is the most common joint disease with a prevalence in the TMJ of 8–16% in the general population. The

prevalence increases with age but is also related to genetic factors, disc displacement, loss of molar support, trauma, and loading, where loading can both prevent and contribute to degenerative joint disease.

- Given the limited understanding of its pathogenesis and the low healing potential of avascular cartilage, no effective therapy is available for restoring the structures of TMJ with progressive osteoarthritis.

(De Souza *et al.*, 2012; Wang *et al.*, 2015; Ahmad and Schiffman, 2016)

Diagnostic Criteria

Expanded DC/TMD criteria for **Degenerative joint disease** (Peck *et al.*, 2014). Without imaging: sensitivity 0.55, specificity 0.61.

A degenerative disorder involving the joint characterized by deterioration of articular tissue with concomitant osseous changes in the condyle and/or articular eminence. Degenerative joint disease can be subclassified: degenerative joint disease without arthralgia is osteoarthrosis, and degenerative joint disease with arthralgia is osteoarthritis. Flattening and/or cortical sclerosis are considered indeterminate findings for degenerative joint disease and may represent normal variation, aging, remodeling or a precursor to frank degenerative joint disease. Degenerative joint disease can result in malocclusions, including an anterior open bite, especially when present bilaterally, or contralateral posterior open bite when present unilaterally.

1. Osteoarthrosis

History. Positive for at least one of the following:
1. In the last 30 days any TMJ noise(s) present with jaw movement or function.
   OR
2. Patient report of any noise present during the examination.
   Examination. Positive for the following:
1. Crepitus detected with palpation during maximum unassisted opening, maximum assisted opening, lateral or protrusive movements.
   Imaging. When this diagnosis needs to be confirmed, TMJ CT/CBCT criteria are positive for at least one of the following:
1. Subchondral cyst(s).
   OR
2. Erosion(s).
   OR
3. Generalized sclerosis.
   OR
4. Osteophyte(s).
   Rheumatologic consultation when needed:
1. Negative for rheumatologic disease.

2. Osteoarthritis

History. Positive for both of the following:
1a. In the last 30 days any TMJ noise(s) present with jaw movement or function.
   OR
1b. Patient report of any noise present during the examination.
   AND
2. Arthralgia.
   Examination. Positive for both of the following:
1. Crepitus detected with palpation during maximum unassisted opening, maximum assisted opening, right or left lateral movements, or protrusive movements.
   AND
2. Arthralgia.
   Imaging. TMJ CT/CBCT criteria are positive for at least one of the following:
1. Subchondral cyst(s).
   OR
2. Erosion(s).
   OR
3. Generalized sclerosis.
   OR
4. Osteophyte(s).
   Rheumatologic consultation when needed:
1. Negative for rheumatologic disease.
   Criteria for DC/TMD **Myalgia**, see Case 3.3; and for **Arthralgia**, see Case 2.1 (Schiffman *et al.*, 2014). Expanded DC/TMD criteria for **Arthritis**, see Case 2.2 (Peck *et al.*, 2014).

Fundamental Points

- The relation between degenerative changes as detected by CT or MRI and clinical symptoms is very weak.
- Loading of the joint is one, but far from the only, factor for development and maintenance of degenerative joint disease. Regarding the knee joint, long-distance runners have less degenerative changes, probably due to the repetitive character of movements and loading. On the other hand, football players have more degenerative changes despite running quite long distances, probably due to the more intense, unpredictable and uneven loading of the joint surfaces. If this applies to the TMJ as well is unknown.
- Treatment should be primarily symptomatic. This may comprise counselling, anti-inflammatory treatment, jaw exercises, splint, and so on.
- Severe degenerative joint disease may cause occlusal changes, usually anterior open bite or harder contacts on the affected side.
- Some patients have coarse crepitus that causes limitations of daily activities and quality of life. Intraarticular injections with hyaluronic acid have been shown to be safe and provide symptom relief regarding the knee joint. Hyaluronic acid improves the hydrodynamics of the damaged cartilage and it has anti-inflammatory effects. There are a few studies on the use of hyaluronic acid in TMJ but with divergent results, although there seems to be some benefit.

(Manfredini *et al.*, 2010)

Self-study Questions

1. How are degenerative joint disease and arthritis related?
2. Describe treatment options for degenerative joint disease.
3. How common is TMJ degenerative joint disease?
4. When should you consider occlusal therapy in a patient with TMJ degenerative joint disease and occlusal changes?

References

Ahmad M, Schiffman EL (2016) Temporomandibular joint disorders and orofacial pain. *Dent Clin North Am* **60**(1):105–124.

De Souza RF, Lovato da Silva CH, Nasser M, *et al.* (2012) Interventions for the management of temporomandibular joint osteoarthritis. *Cochrane Database Syst Rev* (**4**):CD007261.

Manfredini D, Piccotti F, Guarda-Nardini L (2010) Hyaluronic acid in the treatment of TMJ disorders: a systematic review of the literature. *Cranio* **28**(3):166–176.

Peck CC, Goulet JP, Lobbezoo F, *et al.* (2014) Expanding the taxonomy of the diagnostic criteria for temporomandibular disorders. *J Oral Rehabil* **41**(1):2–23.

Schiffman E, Ohrbach R, Truelove E, *et al.* (2014) Diagnostic Criteria for Temporomandibular Disorders (DC/TMD) for clinical and research applications: recommendations of the International RDC/TMD Consortium Network and Orofacial Pain Special Interest Group. *J Oral Facial Pain Headache* **28**(1):6–27.

Wang XD, Zhang JN, Gan YH, Zhou YH (2015) Current understanding of pathogenesis and treatment of TMJ osteoarthritis. *J Dent Res* **94**(5):666–673.

Answers to Self-study Questions

1. Degenerative joint disease is frequently associated with arthritis. This association is bidirectional; that is, degenerative joint disease can cause arthritis and arthritis can cause degenerative joint changes.

2. Anti-inflammatory treatment (if there is an associated arthritis, may need NSAIDs, intraarticular corticosteroids, hyaluronic acid, etc.), jaw exercises, behavioral therapy, splint. The prognosis for treating the degenerative joint diseases in itself is poor but good regarding reducing symptoms.

3. Degenerative joint disease is the most common joint disease with a prevalence in the TMJ of 8–16% in the general populatione. The prevalence increases with age but is also related to genetic factors, disc displacement, loss of molar support, trauma, and loading, where loading can both prevent and contribute to degenerative joint disease.

4. If (i) there is no inflammatory activity in either TMJs, (ii) there are no ongoing changes in the occlusion, (iii) the patient experiences an uncomfortable occlusion or chewing difficulties, and (iv) there are objective occlusal changes that can explain chewing difficulties or uncomfortable occlusion.

E: Systemic Arthritides

Case 2.11

Rheumatoid Arthritis with Temporomandibular Joint Involvement

Per Alstergren

A. Demographic Data and Reason for Contact
- Female, 39 years of age.
- Born in Sweden to Swedish parents.
- Referred to orofacial pain specialist from rheumatologist due to TMJ pain and a question of whether the TMJ is affected by her rheumatoid arthritis.

B. Symptom History
- Today, bilateral TMJ and jaw pain at rest, movement, and chewing. Left side worst. Difficulties opening mouth wide due to pain.
- Chewing and mouth opening worsens the pain. Rest and ibuprofen may decrease the pain. Usually morning stiffness and associated TMJ pain in the jaws that clears during the morning. Otherwise no apparent fluctuation of pain intensity during the day or night.
- Pain intensity varies between 2 at rest and 6 on mouth opening (NRS 0–10).
- Characteristic pain intensity 35 (NRS 0–100), current pain intensity 3 (0–10 NRS), pain-related disability 15 (NRS 0–100; GCPS).
- JFLS reveals limitation in mouth opening and chewing. Few and infrequent daytime parafunctions according to OBCL.
- Patient reports that she cannot enjoy eating food anymore, mainly due to the TMJ pain. She is very disturbed by this fact.
- No headache.
- Grating sounds from both TMJs.
- Debut (TMJ pain) 1 year ago during a general relapse of the rheumatoid arthritis that probably was triggered by a temporary stop in medication (due to an infection). Since then the TMJ pain is as described earlier despite the rheumatoid arthritis going into remission 2 months later when the patient started her current medication.
- Since 6 months a gradual loss of occlusal contacts in the front. Today, no contacts in the front,

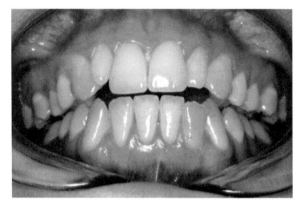

Figure 2.30 Anterior open bite developed during the last 6 months due to bilateral TMJ cartilage and bone tissue destruction by rheumatoid arthritis.

but no chewing difficulties (except for the pain) (Figure 2.30).
- No facial trauma.

C. Medical History
- Rheumatoid factor (RF)-positive and anti-citrullinated antibodies (ACPA)-positive rheumatoid arthritis diagnosed 3 years ago, but symptoms from the fingers since 6 years ago. Joint areas most affected: fingers, feet, and wrists.
- Systemic inflammatory activity: in general low the last 2 years after beginning current medication regime. Before that, high systemic inflammatory activity as assessed by inflammatory markers in blood (ESR, CRP, RF, and ACPA).
- The systemic inflammatory activity increased dramatically during 2 months a year ago, with increased pain in most joints, when the patient had to stop medication due to a severe bronchitis. The patient restarted medication after that and the systemic inflammatory activity returned to low.
- Previous smoker, stopped 4 years ago.
- Medication: methotrexate, Humira® and Folacin®.

D. Psychosocial History

- Married, two children (8 and 12 years of age).
- Works 80% as a secretary. Few sick-leave days in general. Enjoys work and home life very much. Spends as much time as possible together with the family. Likes travel, cycling, and walks.
- Describes herself as a stable person. Normal scores for depression (PHQ-9) and anxiety (GAD-7). Some physical symptoms (PHQ-15), but low level of stress (PSS-10). Good sleep quality (PSQI).
- GCPS grade I; that is, low pain intensity, low disability.
- No smoking, almost no alcohol consumption.

E. Previous Consultations and Treatments

- Her rheumatologist has treated her the last 3 years, since diagnosis, regarding her rheumatoid arthritis in general. Treatment has included pharmacology, physiotherapy, and counselling. No specific treatment of the TMJ.
- Regular annual visits to her dentist, but no specific assessment or treatment of the TMJ.

F. Extraoral Status

Asymmetries

- No apparent swelling or other facial asymmetries. No redness.

Somatosensory abnormalities

- Normal findings regarding touch, cold, and pinprick, except for extraoral cold hypersensitivity in the left maxillary branch of the trigeminal nerve.

Temporomandibular joint

- Bilateral and TMJ familiar pain on mouth opening, laterotrusion to the left, and on protrusion.
- Bilateral familiar palpation pain.
- Bilateral reduced translatory movement.
- Palpable crepitus from both TMJs.

Masticatory muscles

- Bilateral and familiar palpation pain masseter and temporal muscles. No referred pain.
- No masticatory muscle pain on mandibular movement.

Jaw movement capacity

- Maximum mouth opening without pain is 15 mm, maximum unassisted opening is 28 mm, and maximum assisted mouth opening is 45 mm.
- Right laterotrusion 10 mm, left laterotrusion 9 mm, and protrusion 8 mm.

Neck examination

- Normal range of motion, familiar neck pain on movement or palpation but no spreading of the pain toward the orofacial region.

G. Intraoral Status

Soft tissues

- Normal.

Hard tissues and dentition

- Complete dentition with few and minor fillings (Figure 2.30).

Occlusion

- Dentition: 17–27, 37–47. Hard occlusion shows contacts on the following teeth in the upper jaw: 17, 16, 26, 27 (Figure 2.30).

H. Additional Examinations and Findings

- The occlusal changes motivate a radiographic examination. The purpose would be to identify structural changes due to an inflammatory processes in both TMJs that may explain the anterior open bite and signs of ongoing inflammatory activity.
- The radiographic examination was performed by a radiologist using a bilateral CBCT of both TMJs. This examination showed substantial structural changes in both TMJs with signs of condylar erosions and loss of compact bone on both condyles, bilateral condyle bone loss, condylar flattening, and sclerosis, as well as bilateral osteophytes (Figure 2.31).

I. Diagnosis/Diagnoses

Expanded DC/TMD

- Systemic arthritides.
- Bilateral TMJ arthritis.

DC/TMD

- Myalgia of the masticatory muscles.

J. Case Assessment

- Most probably a bilateral TMJ involvement of rheumatoid arthritis causing TMJ arthritis with pain and tissue destruction. In turn, this has limited the patient's possibility to enjoy food and reduced her chewing capacity.
- Bilateral TMJ crepitus as well as bilateral radiographic signs of structural changes in accordance with TMJ rheumatoid arthritis and with signs of probable ongoing inflammatory activity (erosions, loss of compact bone).

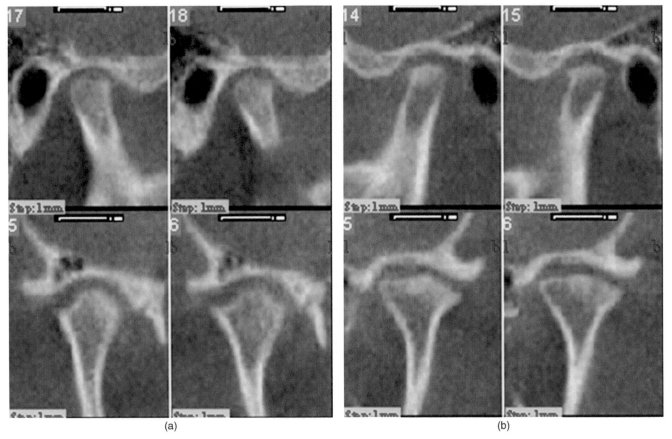

Figure 2.31 Bilateral CBCT of the TMJs showed substantial structural changes in right (a) and left (b) TMJs with signs of condylar erosions and loss of compact bone on both condyles, bilateral condyle bone loss, condylar flattening, and sclerosis, as well as bilateral osteophytes.

- There are no indications of other factors that may have caused the bilateral TMJ arthritis.
- Very low psychosocial factors.
- The patient also had myalgia in the masticatory muscles. Myalgia is a common finding in rheumatoid arthritis, especially close to the joints. This seems to be the case also for the TMJ and masticatory muscles. There are no other indications of a muscle tension problem.

K. Evidence-based Treatment Plan including Aims

- The main problem is the bilateral TMJ arthritis due to rheumatoid arthritis. The long-term prognosis for the TMJ is highly dependent on the systemic treatment and the systemic inflammatory activity. It is, however, not uncommon with one or a few joints with active inflammation despite an appropriate systemic medication and in general low systemic inflammatory activity. Our findings and assessment must therefore be communicated with the rheumatologist.

- The initial treatment should be anti-inflammatory with the goal to stop the inflammatory activity in both TMJs. For this, intraarticular corticosteroids are highly indicated. As always, pharmacological anti-inflammatory treatment has to be combined with a treatment modality that has the possibility to reduce the risk of a relapse of the arthritis (e.g., jaw exercise, splint).
- Initial treatment: anti-inflammatory treatment of both TMJs. Treatment options range from intraarticular corticosteroids, NSAIDs per os, de-loading of the joint (splint), and jaw exercise (Kopp and Wennerberg, 1981; Fredriksson *et al.*, 2006).
- When the inflammatory activity is substantially reduced and under control, the occlusal changes should be addressed. The aim for this part should be adequate chewing ability and stable, comfortable occlusion, but only if the patient still experience such problems. Sometimes, the occlusion can normalize by itself in about 2 months if the inflammatory activity in the TMJ can be inhibited properly.

L. Prognosis and Discussion

- The prognosis is very much dependent on how well it will be possible to stop the inflammatory activity and her systemic inflammatory activity.
- The patient is RF-positive and ACPA-positive, which are two strong negative prognostic factors. However, the short-term prognosis for treatment of arthritis must be considered as good.
- The long-term prognosis is unclear and depends to a great extent on how well the systemic inflammatory activity can be controlled by her systemic treatment.

Background Information

- Rheumatoid arthritis is a chronic, autoimmune, autoinflammatory, progressive disorder that can affect and damage joints, but also other tissues. In some people, the condition also can damage a wide variety of body systems, including the skin, eyes, lungs, heart, and blood vessels.
- The worldwide prevalence of rheumatoid arthritis is 0.8–1.2%, with a higher prevalence in the Western Hemisphere. The TMJ is involved in 30–50% of patients with rheumatoid arthritis.
- An autoimmune and autoinflammatory disorder, rheumatoid arthritis occurs when the immune system mistakenly attacks the body's own tissues. In turn, this causes a strong immune system reaction, including inflammation, in the synovial membranes in the joints.
- This reaction usually causes an intraarticular inflammatory milieu that can eventually result in pain (especially during joint movement and loading), cartilage and bone tissue destruction, and joint deformity.
- The inflammation associated with rheumatoid arthritis is what can damage other parts of the body as well.
- While new types of medications have improved treatment options dramatically, severe rheumatoid arthritis can still cause physical disabilities.
- TMJ involvement of rheumatoid arthritis can have a substantial impact on daily activities and quality of life.

(Tegelberg and Kopp, 1987; Hochberg et al., 2010; Doria et al., 2012; Ahmed et al., 2013)

Diagnostic Criteria

Expanded DC/TMD criteria for **Systemic arthritides** (Peck et al., 2014). Sensitivity and specificity have not been established.

Joint inflammation resulting in pain or structural changes caused by a generalized systemic inflammatory disease, including rheumatoid arthritis, juvenile idiopathic arthritis, spondyloarthropathies (ankylosing spondylitis, psoriatic arthritis, infectious arthritis, Reiter's syndrome), and crystal-induced disease (gout, chondrocalcinosis). Other rheumatologically related diseases that may affect the TMJ include autoimmune disorders and other mixed connective tissue diseases (scleroderma, Sjögren's syndrome, lupus erythematosus). This group of arthritides therefore includes multiple diagnostic categories that are best diagnosed and managed by rheumatologists regarding the general/systemic therapy. Clinical signs and symptoms of ongoing chronic (TMJ) inflammation are variable among patients and often over time for a single patient. They can vary from no sign/symptom to only pain to only swelling/exudate to only tissue degradation to only growth disturbance. Resorption of condylar structures may be associated with malocclusion, such as a progressive anterior open bite. Note that imaging in early stages of the disease may not demonstrate any osseous findings.

History. Positive for both of the following:

1. Rheumatologic diagnosis of a systemic inflammatory joint disease.
   AND
2. a. In the past month, any TMJ pain present.
      OR
   b. TMJ pain which worsens with episodes/exacerbations of the systemic inflammatory joint disease.

Examination. Positive for both of the following:

1. Rheumatologic diagnosis of a systemic joint disease.
   AND
2. a. Arthritis signs and symptoms.
      OR
   b. Crepitus detected with palpation during maximum unassisted opening, maximum assisted opening, right or left lateral movements, or protrusive movements

Imaging. If osseous changes are present, TMJ CT/CBCT or MRI is positive for at least one of the following:

1. Subchondral cyst(s).
   OR
2. Erosion(s).
   OR
3. Generalized sclerosis.
   OR
4. Osteophyte(s).

DC/TMD criteria for **Myalgia** (Schiffman *et al.*, 2014), see Case 3.3. Expanded DC/TMD criteria for TMJ **Arthritis** (Peck *et al.*, 2014), see Case 2.2.

Fundamental Points

- Inflammation of the articular tissues in the TMJ may result in pain as well as cartilage and bone tissue destruction (Alstergren *et al.*, 2008).
- The inflammatory process is rapid and highly unspecific, but when chronic the signs and symptoms of arthritis can lie on a continuum from no signs/symptom to a combination of pain, swelling/exudate, tissue degradation, and/or growth disturbance. The presentation at any time point may include none or one or more of these signs and symptoms (Peck *et al.*, 2014). This means that some patients have pain but no tissue destruction, whereas others may show severe tissue destruction but no pain. This makes the diagnostic process more difficult.
- In systemic arthritides, TMJ pain on jaw movements has been found to be strongly related to an inflammatory intraarticular milieu (Alstergren and Kopp, 1997; Alstergren *et al.*, 2008). TMJ pain on jaw movement may thus in the future be proven as a useful clinical symptom or sign when attempting to diagnose TMJ arthritis.
- Regarding treatment and prognosis, the most important factor for long-term prognosis is how well the systemic inflammatory activity can be controlled, usually by adequate systemic pharmacological treatment. This usually requires systemic pharmacological treatment by the rheumatologist. However, in cases of progressing inflammatory activity in the TMJ despite low systemic inflammatory activity and

no other symptomatic joints, efficient local treatment of the TMJ to minimize the local inflammatory activity is very important.

- Biologics (e.g. the tumor necrosis factor (TNF) inhibitors Humira and Enbrel®, as well as other newer biologics) have revolutionized and substantially improved treatment outcome in rheumatology. This treatment also has effect on the TMJ (Kopp *et al.*, 2005).
- Intraarticular corticosteroid treatment has been found to be efficient and safe as adjunct treatment of rheumatoid arthritis leading to significant pain relief and functional improvement for months up to 1 year (Cheng and Abdi, 2007; Cheng *et al.*, 2012). If intraarticular treatment with corticosteroids is provided, it should always be combined with another treatment modality; for example, jaw exercise or de-loading of the joint.
- In general, jaw exercise and de-loading are the most important nonpharmacological treatments to consider. In addition, jaw exercise, de-loading of the TMJ by behavioral therapy and splint and, in some patients, occlusal therapy may be indicated.
- Occlusal adjustment (grinding, prosthodontic therapy, orthodontic therapy, and/or surgery) may be considered in severe cases. In those cases, the only goal should be to increase the chewing ability. However, this should only be considered when the inflammatory activity in the TMJ is under control.

Self-study Questions

1. How common is TMJ involvement in rheumatoid arthritis?
2. Rheumatoid arthritis is an autoimmune disease. What does that mean?
3. Give three examples of treatments for the TMJ in rheumatoid arthritis.
4. What is the most important factor for the long-term outcome regarding TMJ rheumatoid arthritis?

References

Ahmed N, Mustafa HM, Catrina AI, Alstergren P (2013) Impact of temporomandibular joint pain in rheumatoid arthritis. *Mediators Inflamm* **2013**:597419.

Alstergren P, Kopp S (1997) Pain and synovial fluid concentration of serotonin in arthritic temporomandibular joints. *Pain* **72**(1–2):137–143.

Alstergren P, Fredriksson L, Kopp S (2008) Temporomandibular joint pressure pain threshold is systemically modulated in rheumatoid arthritis. *J Orofac Pain* **22**(3):231–238.

Cheng J, Abdi S (2007) Complications of joint, tendon, and muscle injections. *Tech Reg Anesth Pain Manag* **11**(3):141–147.

Cheng OT, Souzdalnitski D, Vrooman B, Cheng J (2012) Evidence-based knee injections for the management of arthritis. *Pain Med* **13**(6):740–753.

Doria A, Zen M, Bettio S, *et al.* (2012) Autoinflammation and autoimmunity: bridging the divide. *Autoimmun Rev* **12**(1):22–30.

Fredriksson L, Alstergren P, Kopp S (2006) Tumor necrosis factor-alpha in temporomandibular joint synovial fluid predicts treatment effects on pain by intra-articular glucocorticoid treatment. *Mediators Inflamm* **2006**(6):59425.

Hochberg MC, Silman AJ, Smolen JS, *et al.* (eds) (2010) *Rheumatology*. St Louis, MO: Elsevier.

Kopp S, Wenneberg B (1981) Effects of occlusal treatment and intraarticular injections on temporomandibular joint pain and dysfunction. *Acta Odontol Scand* **39**(2):87–96.

Kopp S, Alstergren P, Ernestam S, *et al.* (2005) Reduction of temporomandibular joint pain after treatment with a combination of methotrexate and infliximab is associated with changes in synovial fluid and plasma cytokines in rheumatoid arthritis. *Cells Tissues Organs* **180**(1):22–30.

Peck CC, Goulet JP, Lobbezoo F, *et al.* (2014) Expanding the taxonomy of the diagnostic criteria for temporomandibular disorders. *J Oral Rehabil* **41**(1):2–23.

Schiffman E, Ohrbach R, Truelove E, *et al.* 2014. Diagnostic Criteria for Temporomandibular Disorders (DC/TMD) for clinical and research applications: recommendations of the International RDC/TMD Consortium Network and Orofacial Pain Special Interest Group. *J Oral Facial Pain Headache* **28**(1):6–27.

Tegelberg A, Kopp S (1987) Clinical findings in the stomatognathic system for individuals with rheumatoid arthritis and osteoarthrosis. *Acta Odontol Scand* **45**(2):65–75.

Answers to Self-study Questions

1. The worldwide prevalence of rheumatoid arthritis is 0.8–1.2% with a higher prevalence in the Western Hemisphere. The TMJ is involved in 30–50% of patients with rheumatoid arthritis.

2. Autoimmune means that your own immune system does not recognize your other cells as your own; that is, your self-tolerance is impaired. Instead, the immune system thinks you have foreign antigens and tries to eliminate those by initiating a strong immune system reaction, including inflammation.

3. Intraarticular corticosteroid, jaw exercise, and splint.

4. Regarding treatment and prognosis, the most important factor for long-term prognosis is how well the systemic inflammatory activity can be controlled, usually by adequate systemic pharmacological treatment. This usually requires systemic pharmacological treatment by the rheumatologist. However, in cases of progressing inflammatory activity in the TMJ despite low systemic inflammatory activity and no other symptomatic joints, efficient local treatment of the TMJ to minimize the local inflammatory activity is very important.

Case 2.12

Juvenile Idiopathic Arthritis

Randy Cron and Britt Hedenberg-Magnusson

A. Demographic Data and Reason for Contact

- Caucasian female, 14 years old.
- Jaw pain.
- Referred to orofacial pain specialist from dentistry.
- X-ray revealed condylar head flattening.

B. Symptom History

- One year of left jaw pain and stiffness with decreased mouth opening.
- Earache.
- Bilateral hip pain.
- Morning stiffness and gelling.

C. Medical History

- History of oral ulcers and wheezing with seasonal allergies.
- Past medical history includes surgical removal of left shoulder cyst at age 5 years.
- Family history notable for maternal grandmother with rheumatoid arthritis.

D. Psychosocial History

- Lives with mother (paralegal) and stepfather (works for pool company).
- Enjoys history in school.
- Hobbies include reading, volleyball, music, running, and texting.
- No history of psychiatric disorders or psychological distress.

E. Previous Consultations and Treatments

- Dentist evaluated TMJ pain by clinical examination and panoramic imaging.
- Oral surgeon also evaluated her TMJ pain.
- No prior treatments.

F. Extraoral Status

- Normal general physical exam.

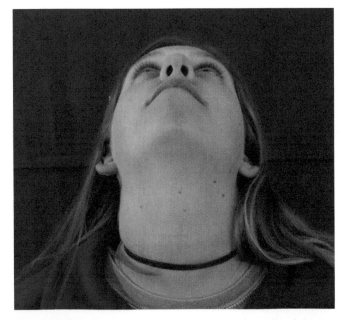

Figure 2.32 Left side of mandible is shorter than the right.

- Musculoskeletal exam reveals slight (0.5 cm) leg length discrepancy and generalized hypermobility at first exam.
- Later exam dates revealed arthritis in several joints, including knee, hip, and sacroiliac.
- Left side of mandible shorter than right (Figure 2.32).

G. Intraoral Status

- Maximal incisal opening at first visit was 42 mm (Figure 2.33).
- Slight deviation of jaw to right with mouth opening (Figure 2.34).
- Increased condylar movement of the left TMJ.
- Post-normal tooth relation on the left side.
- Stable occlusion.

H. Diagnosis/Diagnoses

Expanded DC/TMD

- Systemic arthritides.

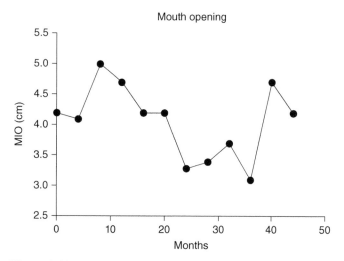

Figure 2.33 Maximal incisal opening over time.

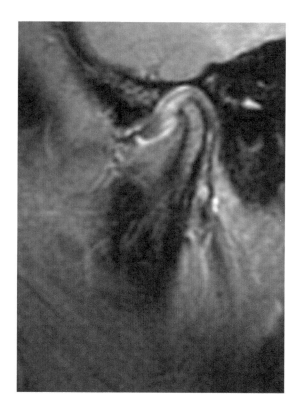

Figure 2.35 TMJ MRI at onset revealing acute and chronic left TMJ arthritis.

- Idiopathic chondrolysis is in differential diagnosis, which may ultimately be JIA.
- TMD with orofacial pain as a cause of parafunctional activity is in differential diagnosis and could be a reason to insert behavioral and relieving treatment as a complement.
- TMJ arthritis in children also occurs in other rheumatic disorders (e.g., sarcoidosis, Sjögren's, mixed connective tissue disease, dermatomyositis), but for this patient there were no signs/symptoms to suggest these diseases as the cause of her TMJ arthritis (Stoll and Cron, 2015).

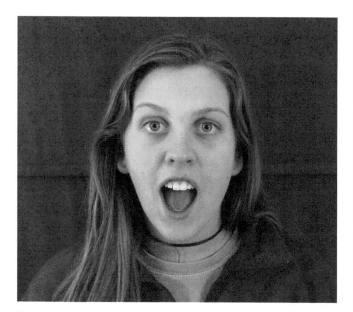

Figure 2.34 Deviation with mouth opening.

DC/TMD
- Arthralgia left TMJ.

Other
- Juvenile idiopathic arthritis (JIA).

I. Additional Examinations and Findings
- TMJ MRI with contrast revealed: normal right TMJ; left TMJ with anterior flattening of condyle, small erosions, pannus anteriorly, and mild periarticular contrast enhancement (Figure 2.35).

J. Case Assessment
- Likely JIA as cause of TMJ pain, based on imaging and history of other joint pain.

K. Evidence-based Treatment Plan including Aims
- Stop progression of ongoing TMJ inflammation.
- Minimize TMJ pain associated with TMJ arthritis.
- Maintain mouth opening and function.
- Systemic anti-arthritis therapy, including biologic agents (e.g., TNF inhibitors) (Stoll et al., 2015).
- Intraarticular long-acting corticosteroids (Ringold and Cron, 2009).
- Oral functional appliances may help to reduce pain, improve jaw movement, and maintain normal mandible and mid-face growth in children with JIA

when used routinely over several years (Portelli *et al.*, 2014; Stoll and Cron, 2015).

L. Prognosis and Discussion

- Guarded prognosis in terms of TMJ arthritis in JIA as it remains a difficult-to-treat joint (Stoll and Cron, 2015).
- TMJ arthritis can progress (as noted on MRI) despite aggressive systemic therapy for JIA (Stoll *et al.*, 2015).
- TMJ arthritis may or may not respond to systemic therapy or to intraarticular immunosuppression (corticosteroids or TNF inhibitors) (Stoll *et al.*, 2015).
- Undertreated or unresponsive progressive TMJ arthritis in growing children can lead to micrognathia, mid-face growth disturbances, facial asymmetry, poor mouth opening, and TMJ pain at rest, or with activity (e.g., eating, speaking; Arabshahi and Cron, 2006).
- Over the following 2 years, she received intraarticular corticosteroids to her left TMJ on two occasions.
- In addition, her TMJ arthritis and JIA (other joints) were managed with systemic TNF inhibitors, eventually switch to co-stimulatory blockade (CTLA-4-Ig).
- Two years later, TMJ MRI showed normal right TMJ, left TMJ condyle flattening with erosions over the majority of the articular surface, bone marrow edema, 4 mm effusion, diffuse synovial thickening, increased pannus, and disc displacement anteriorly and medially (Figure 2.36).

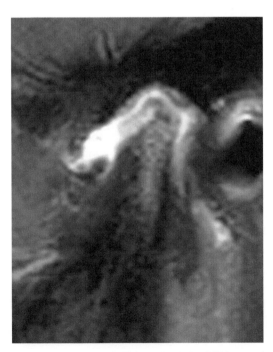

Figure 2.36 Worsening left TMJ arthritis by MRI over time.

- Her TMJ symptoms are markedly improved after therapy.

Background Information

- As many as 80% of children with JIA have TMJ arthritis, including at disease onset (75%) (Ringold and Cron, 2009).
- TMJ arthritis at onset has often been considered asymptomatic, but TMJ pain or facial pain, as well as decreased TMJ mobility, seem to be important risk factors (Ringold and Cron, 2009; Leksell *et al.*, 2012).
- Deviation to the involved, or more involved, side with mouth opening is a strong predictor of TMJ arthritis. The patient reported herein unusually demonstrated deviation toward the unaffected TMJ with mouth opening despite having a shorter mandible on the affected side (Stoll and Cron, 2015).
- The most sensitive diagnostic tool for detecting TMJ arthritis in children with JIA is MRI with contrast. Ultrasound and clinical exam are neither sensitive nor specific for detection of early TMJ arthritis in children with JIA with current methods (Ringold and Cron, 2009).
- Chronic bony changes (e.g., condylar head flattening and erosions) on MRI are highly specific for TMJ arthritis in the setting of children with JIA, but mild synovial enhancement with contrast may be a normal finding. Pannus seen on MRI, however, is always abnormal (Stoll and Cron, 2015).

Diagnostic Criteria

Expanded DC/TMD criteria for **Systemic arthritides** (Peck *et al.*, 2014). Sensitivity and specificity have not been established.

Joint inflammation resulting in pain or structural changes caused by a generalized systemic inflammatory disease, including rheumatoid arthritis, JIA, spondyloarthropathies (ankylosing spondylitis, psoriatic arthritis, infectious arthritis, Reiter's syndrome), and crystal-induced disease (gout, chondrocalcinosis). This group of arthritides therefore includes multiple diagnostic categories that are best diagnosed and managed by rheumatologists regarding the general/systemic therapy.

Clinical signs and symptoms of ongoing chronic (TMJ) inflammation are variable among patients and often over time for a single patient. They can vary from no sign/symptom to only pain to only swelling/exudate to only tissue degradation to only growth disturbance. Resorption of condylar structures may be associated with malocclusion such as a progressive anterior open bite. A diagnostic instrument should aim to identify patients with chronic inflammation early and accurately, should not exclude patients with chronic arthritis of long duration, and should not only diagnose rheumatoid arthritis but the whole range of chronic inflammatory states. Note that imaging in early stages of the disease may not demonstrate any osseous findings.

History. Positive for both of the following:
1. Rheumatologic diagnosis of a systemic inflammatory joint disease.
   AND
2. a. In the past month, any TMJ arthralgia.
      OR
   b. TMJ pain which worsens with episodes/exacerbations of the systemic inflammatory joint disease.

Examination. Positive for both of the following:
1. Rheumatologic diagnosis of a systemic joint disease.
   AND
2. a. Arthritis signs and symptoms (see Case 2.2).
      OR
   b. Crepitus detected with palpation during maximum unassisted opening, maximum assisted opening, right or left lateral movements, or protrusive movements.

Imaging. If osseous changes are present, TMJ CT/CBCT or MRI is positive for at least one of the following:
1. Subchondral cyst(s).
   OR
2. Erosion(s).
   OR
3. Generalized sclerosis.
   OR
4. Osteophyte(s).
   DC/TMD criteria for **TMJ arthralgia** (Schiffman *et al.*, 2014), see Case 2.1.

Fundamental Points

- TMJ arthritis in JIA remains one of the most difficult joints to treat.
- TMJ arthritis affects the quality of life, including jaw pain, chewing difficulties, and micrognathia (due to mandibular growth disturbance).
- There is a wide range of normal maximal incisal opening measurements in children (from 30 to 70 mm).
- Maximal incisal opening over time can be used to monitor response to therapy in individual JIA patients with TMJ arthritis (Figure 2.33).
- Pain levels at rest, movement, and loading over time can be used to monitor TMJ arthritis activity.
- There is some evidence that ongoing inflammation and/or repeated intraarticular corticosteroid treatments may contribute to hypertrophic bone formation and/or decreased mandible growth (Leksell *et al.*, 2012, 2015; Stoll and Cron, 2015; Stoll *et al.*, 2015).
- There are no formal diagnostic criteria for TMJ arthritis in children with JIA, but TMJ MRI with contrast is currently the most sensitive and specific tool diagnostically.
- Chronic TMJ arthritis MRI findings include condylar head flattening, bony erosions, pannus formation, and disc abnormalities.
- Acutely active TMJ arthritis MRI findings include excess joint fluid/effusion, synovial enhancement, and bone marrow edema (Stoll and Cron, 2015).
- Clinical examination findings consistent with TMJ arthritis include pain at rest and pain upon jaw movement and loading, palpatory pain, limited mouth opening, lateral deviation with mouth opening, facial asymmetry, micrognathia, and open frontal bite (Pedersen *et al.*, 2008, Leksell *et al.*, 2012; Stoll and Cron, 2015).

Self-study Questions

1. What is the best way to diagnose early TMJ arthritis in children with JIA?

2. What are some of the acute and chronic findings of TMJ arthritis in children with JIA as noted on MRI with contrast and in clinic?

3. What effect can active TMJ arthritis have on growth of children with JIA?

4. What are potential treatment options for TMJ arthritis in children with JIA?

References

Arabshahi B, Cron RQ (2006) Temporomandibular joint arthritis in juvenile idiopathic arthritis: the forgotten joint. *Curr Opin Rheumatol* **18**(5):490–495.

Leksell E, Ernberg M, Magnusson B, *et al.* (2012) Orofacial pain and dysfunction in children with juvenile idiopathic arthritis: a case–control study. *Scand J Rheumatol* **41**(5):375–378.

Leksell E, Hallberg U, Magnusson B, *et al.* (2015) Perceived oral health and care of children with juvenile idiopathic arthritis: a qualitative study. *J Oral Facial Pain Headache* **29**(3):223–230.

Peck CC, Goulet JP, Lobbezoo F, *et al.* (2014) Expanding the taxonomy of the diagnostic criteria for temporomandibular disorders. *J Oral Rehabil* **41**(1):2–23.

Pedersen TK, Küseler A, Gelineck J, Herlin T (2008) A prospective study of magnetic resonance and radiographic imaging in relation to symptoms and clinical findings of the temporomandibular joint in children with juvenile idiopathic arthritis. *J Rheumatol* **35**(8):1668–1675.

Portelli M, Matarese G, Militi A, *et al.* (2014) Temporomandibular joint involvement in a cohort of patients with juvenile idiopathic arthritis and evaluation of the effect induced by functional orthodontic appliance: clinical and radiographic investigate. *Eur J Paediatr Dent* **15**(1):63–66.

Ringold S, Cron RQ (2009) The temporomandibular joint in juvenile idiopathic arthritis: frequently used and frequently arthritic. *Pediatr Rheumatol Online J* **7**:11.

Schiffman E, Ohrbach R, Truelove E, *et al.* (2014) Diagnostic Criteria for Temporomandibular Disorders (DC/TMD) for clinical and research applications: recommendations of the International RDC/TMD Consortium Network and Orofacial Pain Special Interest Group. *J Oral Facial Pain Headache* **28**(1):6–27.

Stoll ML, Cron RQ (2015) Temporomandibular joint arthritis in juvenile idiopathic arthritis: the last frontier. *Int J Clin Rheumatol* **10**(4):273–286.

Stoll ML, Cron RQ, Saurenmann RK (2015) Systemic and intra-articular anti-inflammatory therapy of temporomandibular joint arthritis in children with juvenile idiopathic arthritis. *Semin Orthod* **21**(2):125–133.

Answers to Self-study Questions

1. TMJ MRI with contrast is the most sensitive and specific modality for detecting TMJ arthritis in children with JIA (present in up to 80% at diagnosis of JIA). TMJ arthritis is often asymptomatic early during disease. Ultrasound and clinical exam are neither specific nor sensitive for diagnosing TMJ arthritis in children with JIA.

2. TMJ MRI with contrast can reveal acutely active signs of arthritis, including bone marrow edema, synovial enhancement, and effusions. More chronic signs of TMJ arthritis as noted on MRI include pannus, condylar head flattening and erosions, and disc abnormalities. Clinical signs include restricted and painful mandibular movement deviating to the affected side, tenderness to palpation over the affected TMJ, and occlusal changes.

3. TMJ arthritis in children with JIA can lead to micrognathia, asymmetric facies, abnormalities in mid-face growth, poor mouth opening, and pain/dysfunction with mouth opening/chewing/talking.

4. Aggressive systemic therapy likely benefits TMJ arthritis (less overall severe micrognathia noted anecdotally since the introduction of biologic therapies for JIA), but TMJ arthritis continues in many children despite systemic therapy. Other treatment options include intraarticular corticosteroids, and in highly refractory cases intraarticular anti-TNF treatment. Functional oral appliances will not treat TMJ inflammation, but they assist in pain relief, functional training, and maintaining normal mandible and mid-face growth.

F: Other Temporomandibular Joint Disorders

Case 2.13

Neoplasms of the Temporomandibular Joint: Benign Osteochondroma of the Coronoid Process

Eiro Kubota

A. Demographic Data and Reason for Contact

- Japanese male, 38 years old, with limited mouth opening.

B. Symptom History

- Limitation of mouth opening occurred 10 years ago, and it has gradually advanced.
- The cause of limitation of the mouth opening was unknown.
- Pain localized to the left preauricular region when opening the mouth.
- No tenderness on masticatory muscles and TMJ proper.
- Maximum mouth opening became 12 mm recently.
- Visited dental clinic 10 years ago with chief complaint of limited mouth opening.

C. Medical History

- Review of system is negative.
- No allergies to medication.
- No routine medications.
- No previous hospitalizations or surgeries.

D. Psychosocial History

- Married, no children, satisfied with home situation.
- High socio-economic status.
- He felt a little stress, but has no depression according to PHQ-9 and no anxiety according to GAD-7.
- Nonsmoking, moderate alcohol consumption.

E. Previous Consultations and Treatments

- The patient noticed difficulty of mouth opening and consulted dentist.
- No dental problems that cause the limitation of mouth opening were pointed out.
- Referred to hospital for further examination to rule out any disorders by a CT scan.

F. Extraoral Status

Weight and height

- Within normal limits.

Facial asymmetry

- Within normal limits.

Swelling or redness

- No swelling of the preauricular region.

Neurologic findings

- Within normal limits.

Motor function abnormalities

- Movement of the extremities are within normal limits.

Temporomandibular Joint

- Pain on the left TMJ when opening the mouth.

Masticatory muscles

- No pain on palpation.

Jaw movement capacity

- Maximum mouth opening 12 mm.

Neck

- Within normal limits.

G. Intraoral Status

Soft tissues

- Within normal limits.

Hard tissues

- No caries, but several restorations on several teeth.

Occlusion

- Within normal limits.

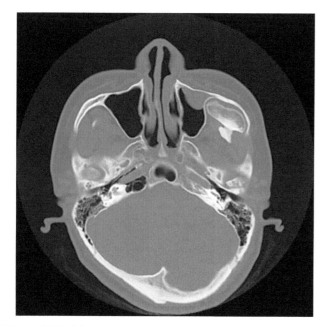

Figure 2.37 A large osteochondroma arising from the coronoid process occupied the infratemporal fossa. The tumor interferes with the zygoma and lateral wall of the maxilla.

H. Additional Examinations and Findings

- CT, MRI, and tumor scintigram should be required (Figure 2.37).
- Consult anesthesiologist for the need of tracheotomy when intubating.

I. Diagnosis/Diagnoses
Expanded DC/TMD

- Benign neoplasm in the TMJ.
- TMJ osseous ankylosis.

J. Case Assessment

- Medically the patient was healthy. The pain in the preauricular region is not stress related.
- There were no signs of dental infections and no suspicion of soft tissue tumors or inflammation.
- To rule out other disorders that cause limitation of mouth opening, CT examination was done.
- Tumor of the coronoid process (osteochondroma) was diagnosed after resection of the lesion.

K. Evidence-based Treatment Plan including Aims

- Resection of the tumor.

L. Prognosis and Discussion

- The primary dentist treated the patient with physical therapy and NSAIDs, but the limitation of mouth opening was not due to TMD.

- CT or MRI images would be of great help for differential diagnosis of these kinds of disorders.
- Because of this being a benign tumor, prognosis is good after resection.

Background Information

- Osteochondroma, sometimes called osteocartilagenous exostosis, is the most common benign tumor of bone. It represents 35% of all benign bone tumors.
- The clinical signs and symptoms do not distinguish this tumor from other slow-growing tumors or tumor-like masses of the condyle. In particular, it is difficult to distinguish from condylar hyperplasia.
- Histopathologically, the tumor contains trabecular bone with a rim of cartilage. The chondrocytes can form rows that are perpendicular to the surface of the lesion, and they may overlie a zone of endochondral ossification.
- Radiographically, the tumor usually shows a globular pattern with distorted condylar morphology, whereas in condylar hyperplasia the condylar head is simply symmetrically enlarged and the condylar neck is usually lengthened.
- If osteochondroma occurs on a condyle, a slowly developing asymmetry is associated with ipsilateral deviation of the chin and unilateral posterior open bite.

(Unni and Carrie, 2010)

Diagnostic Criteria

Expanded DC/TMD criteria for **Neoplasm in jaw, benign** (Peck *et al.*, 2014). Sensitivity and specificity have not been established.

- Neoplasms of the joint result from tissue proliferation with histologic characteristics, and may be benign (e.g., chondroma or osteochondroma) or malignant (e.g., primary or metastatic). They are uncommon but well documented. They may present with swelling, pain during function, limited mouth opening, crepitus, occlusal changes, and/or sensory-motor changes. Facial asymmetry with a midline shift may occur as the lesion expands. Diagnostic imaging, typically using CT/CBCT and/or MRI, and biopsy are essential when a neoplasm is suspected.

Histopathological criteria for osteochondroma
- Periosteum appears as pink fibrous capsule. Cartilage resembles disorganized growth plate with ossification toward base. Medullary cavity merges with that of underlying bone (http://pathologyoutlines.com/).

  Expanded DC/TMD criteria For **TMJ osseous ankylosis** (Peck *et al.*, 2014), see Case 2.8

3

Fundamental Points
- A slowly developing limitation of mouth opening is a clinical sign of the osteochondroma of the coronoid process. A slowly developing asymmetry associated with ipsilateral deviation of the chin and unilateral posterior open bite are the most common clinical signs of this tumor.
- Osteochondroma contains trabecular bone with a rim of cartilage. The chondrocytes can form rows that are perpendicular to the surface of the lesion, and they may overlie a zone of endochondral ossification (Figure 2.38).
- Complete excision of the lesion is necessary. Condylectomy or coronoidectomy was the most frequently performed procedure.

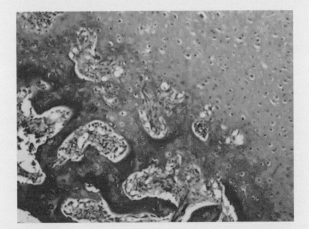

Figure 2.38 Histopathological findings of the osteochondroma. The tumor contains trabecular bone with a rim of cartilage. The chondrocytes can form rows that are perpendicular to the surface of the lesion, and they may overlie a zone of endochondral ossification.

- In case of condylar osteochondroma, minor occlusal abnormalities may require correction by orthodontics, while major ones require reconstruction with costochondral graft, ramus osteotomy, or a joint prosthesis.

(Karras *et al.*, 1996; Aydin, 2001; Wolford *et al.*, 2002)

Self-study Questions
1. Which imaging analyses are necessary for the diagnosis of this disease?
2. Which blood analyses are required to differentially diagnose the neoplasm out of the other joint diseases of the TMJ?
3. Which symptoms are characteristic of this tumor?
4. Which treatment options are available to this patient?

References

Aydin MA (2001) Osteochondroma of the mandibular condyle: report of 2 cases treated with conservative surgery. *J Oral Maxillofac Surg* **59**:1082–1089.

Karras SC, Wolford LM, Cottrell DA (1996) Concurrent osteochondroma of the mandibular condyle and ipsilateral cranial base resulting in temporomandibular joint ankylosis: report of case and review of the literature. *J Oral Maxillofac Surg* **54**:640–646.

Peck CC, Goulet JP, Lobbezoo F, *et al.* (2014) Expanding the taxonomy of the diagnostic criteria for temporomandibular disorders. *J Oral Rehabil* **41**(1):2–23.

Unni KK, Carrie (eds) (2010) *Dahlin's bone tumors. General aspects and data on 11,087 cases*, 6th edn. Philadelphia, PA: Lippincott-Raven.

Wolford LM, Mehra P, Franco P (2002) Use of conservative condylectomy for treatment of osteochondroma of the mandibular condyle. *J Oral Maxillofac Surg* **60**: 262–268.

Answers to Self-study Questions
1. When TMJ neoplasm is first considered, plane X-ray, CT, MRI, ^{99m}Tc-scintigram, ^{67}Ga-scintigram, and also fluorodeoxyglucose positron emission tomography (FDG-PET) (in case of malignancy) analyses are mandatory for the diagnosis. In slow-growing benign osteochondroma the ^{67}Ga-scintigram is usually negative, but positive for ^{99m}Tc-scintigram.
2. To differentially diagnose other diseases that develop ankylosis, such as rheumatoid arthritis, psoriatic arthritis, or ankylosing spondylitis, RF and ACPA levels in addition to blood cell count and CRP should

be examined. These values are all within normal limits in case of the tumor.

3. If the tumor occurrs on the coronoid process, the tumor interferes with the zygoma and lateral wall of the maxilla when opening the mouth, and the patient gradually develops limited mouth opening. If the osteochondroma occurrs unilaterally on the condyle, the patient shows slowly developing asymmetry associated with ipsilateral deviation of the chin and unilateral posterior open bite.

4. Coronoidectomy is a first choice in the case of the osteochondroma on the coronoid process, but if the tumor occurs on the condyle, condylectomy is the most frequently performed procedure. In case of condylar osteochondroma, minor occlusal abnormalities may require correction by orthodontics, while major ones require reconstruction with costochondral graft, ramus osteotomy, or a joint prosthesis.

Case 2.14

Neoplasms of the Temporomandibular Joint: Malign Chondrosarcoma of the Condyle

Eiro Kubota

A. Demographic Data and Reason for Contact

- Japanese male, 37 years old, referred from general practitioner due to swelling of the right cheek and preauricular region and unusual appearance in panoramic radiograph in the right TMJ region.

B. Symptom History

- Increasing swelling of the right cheek and preauricular region since 2 months.
- No pain.

C. Medical History

- Review of system is negative.
- No allergies to medication.
- No routine medications.
- No previous hospitalizations or surgeries.

D. Psychosocial History

- Married.
- Above-average socio-economic status.

E. Previous Consultations and Treatments

- Visited dental clinic 1 month ago and consulted regarding the swelling of the preauricular region.
- Unusual appearance in panoramic radiograph in the right TMJ region (Figure 2.39).

F. Extraoral Status

Weight and height

- Within normal limits.

Facial asymmetry

- Asymmetry with diffuse preauricular swelling on the right side.

Neurologic findings

- Sensory paresthesia for touch and cold in the right mental region.

Motor function abnormalities

- Movement of the extremities is within normal limits.

Temporomandibular joint

- Palpation reveals elastic hard mass, 30 mm in diameter, in the right TMJ region.
- Palpation pain.

Masticatory muscles

- No palpation pain.

Jaw movement capacity

- Maximum unassisted mouth opening 32 mm.
- No mandibular movement pain.

Neck

- Within normal limits; no movement or palpation pain.

G. Intraoral Status

Soft tissues

- Within normal limits.

Hard tissues

- No caries, but restorations on several teeth.

Occlusion

- Within normal limits.

H. Additional Examinations and Findings

- CT (Figure 2.40a) and MRI scans (Figure 2.40b–d) show typical appearance of chondrosarcoma.

I. Diagnosis/Diagnoses

Expanded DC/TMD

- Malignant neoplasm in the TMJ.

Other

- Chondrosarcoma of the condyle.

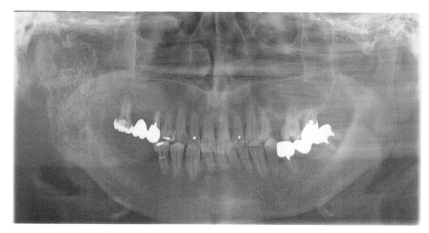

Figure 2.39 Panoramic radiograph showing abnormal patters over the right TMJ, zygomatic arch, and mandibular ramus.

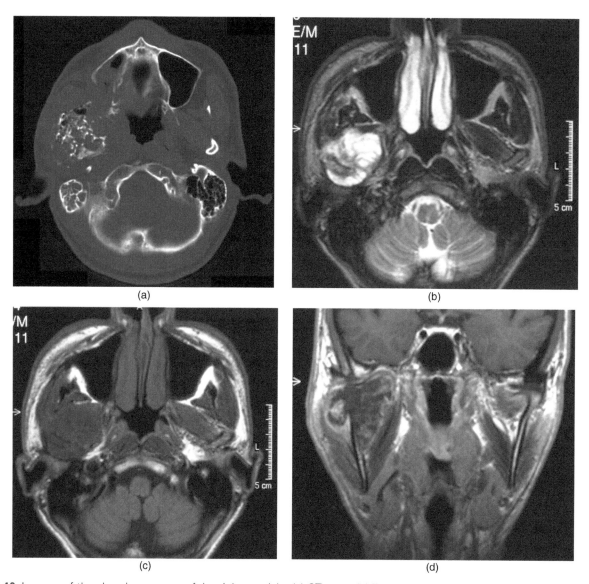

(a)

(b)

(c)

(d)

Figure 2.40 Images of the chondrosarcoma of the right condyle: (a) CT scan, (b) T2-weighted axial MRI image, (c) T1-weighted axial, and (d) coronal MRI images.

J. Evidence-based Treatment Plan, including Aims

Aim

- Immediate removal of malign tissue.

Treatment

- Resection of the tumor.

K. Prognosis and Discussion

- Prognosis is poor regarding survival, especially in a high-grade lesion like this.
- Individualized treatment based on the principles of resection achieving clear margins and consideration of adjuvant radiotherapy or chemotherapy may improve the prognosis.

Background Information

- Chondrosarcoma of the head and neck is rare, although it constitutes 40% of the reported TMJ sarcomas. In terms of the bony skeleton, head and neck lesions account for only 1%.
- The production of malignant cartilage along with cellular pleomorphism are the hallmarks of the chondrosarcoma. No osteoid formation is observed.
- Histopathologically, cellularity is increased with a myxomatous matrix, and the cartilage cells tend to be large, and may contain multiple nuclei or a large nucleus (Figure 2.41).

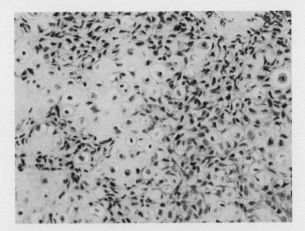

Figure 2.41 Histopathological finding of the chondrosarcoma. Cellularity is increased with a myxomatous matrix and the cartilage cells tend to be large. The cells may contain multiple nuclei or a large nucleus.

- Chondrosarcoma develops from mesenchymal stem cells, which show partial chondroblastic differentiation. Typically, it is a slow-growing tumor and the majority is low grade.
- High-grade tumors may metastasize to regional lymph nodes. Low-grade tumors have an excellent prognosis, but recurrences are often observed.
(Plesh *et al.*, 2005)

Diagnostic Criteria

Expanded DC/TMD criteria for **Neoplasm in jaw**, malignant (Peck *et al.*, 2014). Sensitivity and specificity have not been established.

- Neoplasms of the joint result from tissue proliferation with histologic characteristics, and may be benign (e.g., chondroma or osteochondroma) or malignant (e.g., primary or metastatic). They are uncommon but well documented. They may present with swelling, pain during function, limited mouth opening, crepitus, occlusal changes, and/or sensory-motor changes. Facial asymmetry with a midline shift may occur as the lesion expands. Diagnostic imaging, typically using CT/CBCT and/or MRI, and biopsy are essential when a neoplasm is suspected.

Histopathological diagnostic criteria for chondrosarcoma

- A lobular growth pattern with hypercellularity. Cells are usually pleomorphic and may be binucleated.

Fundamental Points

- Swelling is a consistent finding, and pain or discomfort are also noted. Limited mouth opening and diminished hearing have also been described.
- Failure of local control of the tumor is the cause of death for most patients, and lung is the most common site of distant metastasis.
- Surgery is the first choice of treatment, but if the tumor has spread beyond the condyle, parotidectomy, removal of zygomatic arch and temporal bone, as well as skull base resection may be required.

- Chondrosarcoma is not sensitive to radiation, but it has recently been advocated as an appropriate adjuvant therapy for patients who have unresectable tumors, high-grade lesions, or positive margins.

(Arlen *et al.*, 1970; Richter *et al.*, 1974; Harwood *et al.*, 1980)

Self-study Questions

1. Which imaging analyses are necessary for the diagnosis of the disease?

2. Which blood analyses are required to differentially diagnose the neoplasm out of the other inflammatory diseases of the TMJ?

3. Which symptoms are characteristic of this malignant tumor?

4. Which treatment options are available to this patient?

References

Arlen M, Tollefsen HR, Huvos AG, Marcove RC (1970) Chondrosarcoma of the head and neck. *Am J Surg* **120**:456–460.

Harwood AR, Drajbach JL, Fornasier VL (1980) Radiotherapy of chondrosarcoma of bone. *Cancer* **45**:2769–2777.

Peck CC, Goulet JP, Lobbezoo F, *et al.* (2014) Expanding the taxonomy of the diagnostic criteria for temporomandibular disorders. *J Oral Rehabil* **41**(1):2–23.

Plesh O, Sinishi SE, Crawford PB, Gansky SA (2005) Diagnosis based on the Research Diagnostic Criteria for Temporomandibular Disorders in a biracial population of young women. *J Orofac Pain* **19**:65–75.

Richter KJ, Freeman NS, Quick DA (1974) Chondrosarcoma of the temporomandibular joint: report of case. *J Oral Surg* **32**:777–781.

Answers to Self-study Questions

1. When TMJ neoplasm is first considered, CT, MRI, ^{99m}Tc-scintigram, ^{67}Ga-scintigram, and also FDG-PET (in case of malignancy) analyses are mandatory for the diagnosis. In slow-growing tumor, ^{67}Ga-scintigram is usually negative, but positive for ^{99m}Tc-scintigram. If it were a malignant tumor, FDG-PET analysis is informative.

2. When the lesion is associated with inflammation, white blood cell counts and CRP level would be increased. In the case of gout or rheumatoid arthritis, blood uric acid level or RF as well as ACPA levels would be increased. In the case of tumor, these values are all within normal limits.

3. Sensory abnormality on the right mental region is a sign of tumor involvement of the inferior alveolar nerve, and may indicate malignant tumor.

4. Surgery is the first choice, but if the tumor has spread beyond the condyle, parotidectomy, removal of zygomatic arch and temporal bone, as well as skull base resection may be required.

Case 2.15

Synovial Chondromatosis

Lars Eriksson and Peter Abrahamsson

A. Demographic Data and Reason for Contact
- A 48-year-old Caucasian woman.
- Presence of pain and swelling over the right TMJ.

B. Symptom History
- For more than a year diffuse pain on the right side of the face, especially in front of the right ear.
- The pain is aggravated when chewing tough food, and the patient has experienced reduced motion capacity of the lower jaw.
- During the last few months a minor swelling in front of the right ear has occurred, as well as frequent popping and clicking in the right TMJ.

C. Medical History
- Negative, except for moderate hypertension.
- Regularly takes medicine to normalize the blood pressure.
- No previous hospitalizations.
- Increased need for analgesics in the course of time.

D. Psychosocial History
- Married for 20 years with two teenagers living at home.
- Working as a social welfare officer in a stressful position.
- Normal scores for depression (PHQ-9) and anxiety (GAD-7). No physical symptoms (PHQ-15) and moderate level of stress (PSS-10).
- GCPS grade I; that is, low intensity, low disability.
- Nonsmoking, moderate alcohol consumption.
- No history of psychological distress and has moderate sleep quality.

E. Previous Consultations and Treatments
- ENT consultation has shown normal status.
- The patient's dentist has recommended avoidance of tough food and the patient was given a bite splint 6 months ago to use at night without any obvious effect on the symptoms.

F. Extraoral Status
Face
- No asymmetries noted, except minor swelling over the right TMJ.
- No abnormal neurologic findings noticeable.

Temporomandibular joint
- Minor swelling; moderate palpation pain over the right joint without any signs of infection.
- During maximal mouth opening movements a "bumpy" motion is palpated over the right joint, and slight crepitation and occasionally clicking are heard

Masticatory muscles
- Familiar pain on palpation of masseter and temporalis muscles on the right side.
- No referred pain.

Jaw movement capacity
- Maximal mouth opening 38 mm with a slight deviation to the right, laterotrusion to the right 7 mm and to the left 4 mm, and protrusion 5 mm with slight deviation to the right.

Neck
- Normal range of motion, but the right sternocleidomastoideus muscle is sore at palpation.

G. Intraoral Status
Soft tissues
- Within normal limits.

Hard tissues
- Full dentition except for missing lower first molar left side. Moderate abrasion of all cuspids.

Occlusion
- Normal bite with a stable occlusion.

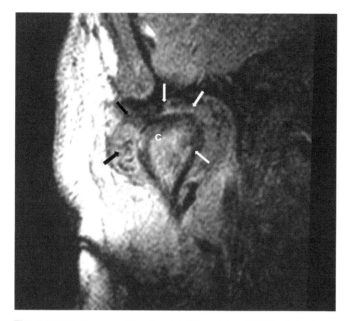

Figure 2.42 Preoperative frontal T1-weighted MRI of right TMJ showing distension of the joint capsule and multiple loose bodies in an intraarticular soft tissue mass (arrows) surrounding the condyle (C).

H.   Additional Examination and Findings

- Because of the swelling over the right TMJ, MRI seems most appropriate as this technique has shown to give more information than CT of soft tissue involvement (disc included), loose calcified or not calcified bodies, and intraarticular fluid.
- The MRI examination revealed distension of the lateral joint capsule, fluid in the joint and several loose bodies of varying size, and calcification in the upper joint compartment suggestive of synovial chondromatosis (Figure 2.42).
- Except for MRI, arthroscopy can be a diagnostic alternative or an additional examination to MRI with these types of pathological changes.

I.   Diagnosis/Diagnoses
Expanded DC/TMD

- Synovial chondromatosis, right TMJ.

DC/TMD

- Degenerative joint disease, right TMJ.
- Masticatory muscle myalgia.

J.   Case Assessment

- The minor swelling that was moderately sore to palpation over the right TMJ without any signs of

infection, the "bumpy" motion palpated over the joint, and crepitation and occasional clicking in the right TMJ indicated intraarticular changes.
- The somewhat reduced maximal mouth opening and the difference in laterotrusive movements with reduced lateral movement to the left supported the suspicion of a right intraarticular obstacle.
- Medically the patient was healthy except for a moderate hypertension, which could not explain the patient's actual symptoms.
- Tentative diagnoses could be myalgia because of the painful masticatory muscles on the right side, combined with degenerative condylar changes on the right side indicated by the crepitation in that joint. The slight swelling might further indicate edema in the joint capsule and/or an arthritis with excess of fluid in the joint. In addition, the occasional clicking in the right joint might indicate intraarticular loose bodies. As synovial chondromatosis has been reported to be the most common pseudotumor in the TMJ, with the symptoms exhibited in this patient an extended examination with MRI seemed to be indicated to reveal any intraarticular soft tissue changes.

K.   Evidence-based Treatment Plan including Aims

- The aim is to remove the chondroid changes.
- The treatment options for synovial chondromatosis are open or arthroscopic surgery. The aim is to reduce/eliminate pain and normalize reduced mouth opening if present. Open surgery is most frequently used and usually involves exposure of the joint via a preauricular approach. Free fragments should be removed, paying attention to the anterior and medial recess where a number of fragments may hide (Figure 2.43). Synovial areas with evident chronic inflammation may be resected and if the disc is severely deformed or perforated it can be excised

L.   Prognosis and Discussion

- The prognosis of open surgical removal via a preauricular incision seems to be good, and relapse is very seldom reported. Surgical removal of the pathological changes with arthroscopic technique, which is less invasive, may be used as an alternative to open surgery but a disadvantage with this method is that it is difficult to retrieve major intraarticular loose bodies or a destroyed disc (Lim *et al.*, 2011; Figure 2.44).

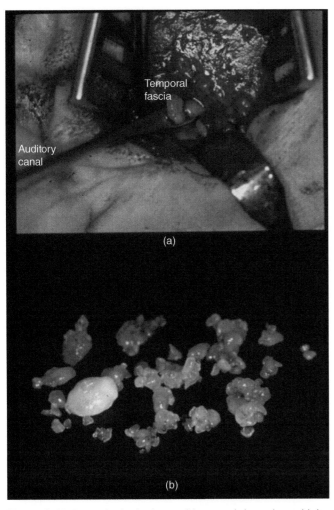

Figure 2.43 Preauricular incison with turned-down lateral joint capsule. Loose bodies (arrow) visible after opening of the upper joint compartment (A). Extirpated loose bodies of varying size and shape all found in the upper joint compartment (B).

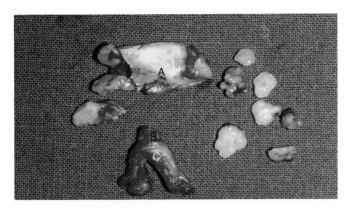

Figure 2.44 A and B indicate two halves of an extirpated surgically divided deformed disc with a major perforation (C) surrounded by loose cartilage bodies.

Background Information

- Synovial chondromatosis is a rare condition that usually affects a single joint; for example, the knee, hip, or elbow, but the TMJ may also be affected. Most cases of synovial chondromatosis occur in middle-aged people, and concerning the TMJ it has been reported to be more common in women than in men (Holmlund *et al.*, 2003). In a review of 285 pseudotumors and tumors of the TMJ published in 181 articles of 15 journals included in *Journal Citation Reports* the distribution of pseudotumors was clearly the most numerous, representing over two-thirds of the lesions. Synovial chondromatosis accounted for 61.8% of the pseudotumors (Poveda-Roda *et al.*, 2013)
- Two forms of the disease have been recognized: primary and secondary. In the primary form, which is uncommon, the etiology is not known; however, a response to repetitive, low-grade trauma has been proposed. The secondary synovial chondromatosis is more common and arises as a result of an inflammatory or noninflammatory arthropathy (Coleman *et al.*, 2013).
- Synovial chondromatosis is a non-neoplastic disease characterized by metaplasia of the connective tissue leading to chondrogenesis in the synovial membrane (Matsumura *et al.*, 2012). Part of the chondrified tissue enters the

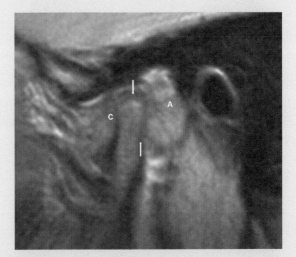

Figure 2.45 Preoperative lateral T1-weighted MRI of a TMJ showing a major intraarticular soft tissue mass (arrows) posterior to the condyle (C) and anterior to the auditory canal (A).

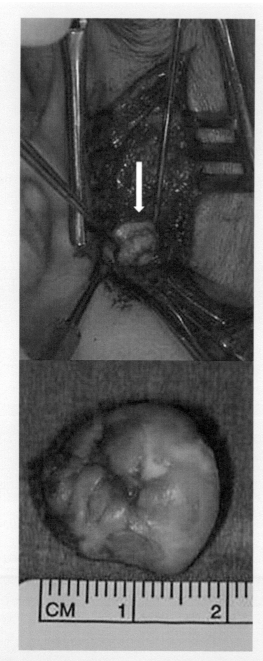

Figure 2.46 Extirpation via a preauricular approach of an intraarticular loose body (arrow) shown in Figure 2.45.

joint cavity and undergoes chronic calcification, leading to formation of a joint loose body of cartilage tissue (Yokota *et al.*, 2008). Milgram (1977) divided the process into three stages. In stage 1 there is active intrasynovial disease only, with no loose bodies; in stage 2, transitional lesions with both active intrasynovial proliferation and free loose bodies occur; and in stage 3, multiple free osteochondral bodies with

no demonstrable intrasynovial disease can be observed. (Milgram, 1977). Even a major single loose body can be formed (Figures 2.45, 2.46, and 2.47).

- Concerning the risk of malignancy of synovial chondromatosis, there are somewhat divergent opinions. According to Pau *et al.* (2013) the disease is considered to be metaplastic and shows no malignant tendencies, but can become locally aggressive, erode the cranial base, and even spread intracranially, whereas according to Coleman *et al.* (2013), malignancy, even if very rare, can arise in synovial chondromatosis or de novo within the synovial membrane.

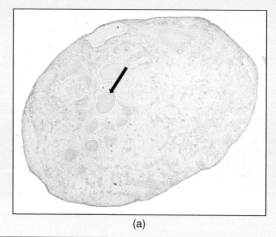

(a)

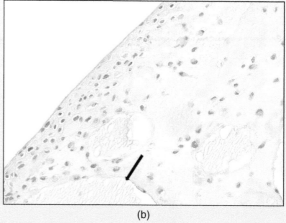

(b)

Figure 2.47 (A) Section of a roundish nodule with variable cellularity and pools of fluid (arrow). (B) Section from the periphery of the nodule in (A) showing a hypercellular area with fairly small chondrocytes and pools of fluid (arrow). H&E stain.

Diagnostic Criteria

Expanded DC/TMD criteria for **Synovial chondromatosis** (Peck *et al.*, 2014). Sensitivity and specificity have not been established.

Cartilaginous metaplasia of the mesenchymal remnants of the synovial tissue of the joint. Its main characteristic is the formation of cartilaginous nodules that may be pedunculated and/or detached from the synovial membrane, becoming loose bodies within the joint space. Calcification of the cartilage can occur (i.e., osteochondromatosis). The disease may be associated with malocclusion, such as a progressive ipsilateral posterior open bite. Imaging is needed to establish the diagnosis.

History. Positive for at least one of the following:
1. Report of preauricular swelling.
   OR
2. Arthralgia.
   OR
3. Progressive limitation of mouth opening.
   OR
4. In the past month, any joint noise(s) present.

Examination. Positive for at least one of the following:
1. Preauricular swelling.
   OR
2. Arthralgia.
   OR
3. Maximum assisted opening (passive stretch) <40mm, including vertical incisal overlap,
   OR
4. Crepitus.

Imaging. TMJ MRI or CT/CBCT is positive for at least one of the following:
1. MRI – multiple chondroid nodules, joint effusion, and amorphous iso-intensity signal tissues within the joint space and capsule.
   OR
2. CT/CBCT – loose calcified bodies in the soft tissues of the TMJ.

Laboratory testing. Histological examination confirms cartilaginous metaplasia.

DC/TMD criteria for **Degenerative joint disease**, see Case 2.10; for **Myalgia**, see Case 3.3; and for **Arthralgia**, see Case 2.1 (Schiffman *et al.*, 2014).

Fundamental Points

Issues important for diagnosis, treatment plan, and management of the case

- A careful history, including general health, medication, and pain and functional disturbances in the jaws and neck.
- Extraoral clinical examination with palpation of jaw and neck muscles and the TMJs with registration of soreness.
- Registration of joint sounds, clicking, and crepitation if any.
- Assessment by palpation of irregularities in condylar movements during opening, lateral, and closing movements.
- Measurement of maximal opening, protrusion, and laterotrusion.
- Preliminary diagnoses supplemented with at first hand MRI examination for extended information of the actual swelling over the joint.
- Depending on the MRI findings, radiographic examination of the actual joint might be indicated for detailed studies of the hard tissue components,
- Information that a surgical procedure is necessary to get rid of the intraarticular pathological changes,

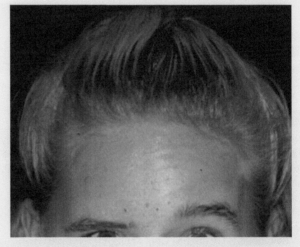

Figure 2.48 Postoperative weakness of the frontal branch of the right facial nerve leading to problems to raise the eyebrow and frown on the surgical side.

- Preoperative information, including a presentation of the surgical method to be used and pros and cons with the method and the evaluated time for postoperative hospitalization.
- Information that the disc if severely deformed or perforated will be removed.
- Information on the risk, even if minimal, for facial nerve weakness of above all the frontal nerve branch leading to problems to raise the eyebrow and frown on the surgical side (Figure 2.48). Information of the risk of developing joint crepitation, if the disc is removed.
- The need for postoperative training of jaw movements, especially translatory movements, and if necessary by the aid of a physiotherapist, as well as the expected time for sick leave.

Self-study Questions

1. Describe the etiology of synovial chondromatosis.

2. Give examples of three clinical signs or symptoms that can occur with TMJ synovial chondromatosis. Give a suggestion of a differential diagnosis with similar signs or symptoms.

3. Describe how loose cartilage bodies occur at synovial chondromatosis.

4. Is synovial chondromatosis a benign or a malignant condition?

5. Give an example of two possible surgical methods for treatment of synovial chondromatosis.

6. Give an example of a postoperative nerve complication that might occur after a preauricular incision to the TMJ.

References

Coleman H, Chandraratnam E, Morgan G, *et al.* (2013) Synovial chondrosarcoma arising in synovial chondromatosis of the temporomandibular joint. *Head Neck Pathol* **7**(3):304–309.

Holmlund AB, Eriksson L, Reinholt FP (2003) Synovial chondromatosis of the temporomandibular joint. Clinical, surgical and histological aspects. *Int J Oral Maxillofac Surg* **32**(2):143–147.

Lim SW, Jeon SJ, Choi,SS, Choi KH (2011) Synovial chondromatosis in the temporomandibular joint: a case with typical imaging features and pathological findings. *Br J Radiol* **84**(1007):e213–e216.

Matsumura Y, Nomura J, Nakanishi K, *et al.* (2012) Synovial chondromatosis of the temporomandibular joint with calcium pyrophosphate dihydrate crystal deposition disease (pseudogout). *Dentomaxillofac Radiol* **41**(8):703–707.

Milgram JM (1977) Synovial osteochondromatosis: a histopathological study of thirty cases. *J Bone Joint Surg Am* **59**(6):792–801.

Pau M, Bicsák A, Reinbacher KE, *et al.* (2014) Surgical treatment of synovial chondromatosis of the temporomandibular joint with erosion of the skull base: a case report and review of the literature. *Int J Oral Maxillofac Surg* **43**(5):600–605.

Peck CC, Goulet JP, Lobbezoo F, *et al.* (2014) Expanding the taxonomy of the diagnostic criteria for temporomandibular disorders. *J Oral Rehabil* **41**(1):2–23.

Poveda-Roda R, Bagán JV, Sanchis JM, Margaix M (2013) Pseudotumors and tumors of the temporomandibular joint. A review. *Med Oral Patol Oral Cir Bucal* **18**(3):e392–e402.

Schiffman E, Ohrbach R, Truelove E, *et al.* (2014) Diagnostic Criteria for Temporomandibular Disorders (DC/TMD) for clinical and research applications: recommendations of the International RDC/TMD Consortium Network and Orofacial Pain Special Interest Group. *J Oral Facial Pain Headache* **28**(1):6–27.

Yokota N, Inenaga C, Tokuyama T, *et al.* (2008) Synovial chondromatosis of the temporomandibular joint with intracranial extension – case report. *Neurol Med Chir (Tokyo)* **48**(6):266–270.

Answers to Self-study Questions

1. Two forms of the disease have been recognized: primary and secondary. In the primary form, which is uncommon, the etiology is not known; however, a response to repetitive, low-grade trauma has been proposed. The secondary synovial chondromatosis form is more common and arises as a result of an inflammatory or noninflammatory arthropathy.

2. The most common clinical signs and symptoms that might occur are unilateral pain, limitation of mouth opening, clicking and/or crepitation in the joint, and swelling over the joint. The symptoms are not specific for the diagnosis and can be found in, for example, patients with TMJ osteoarthritis or TMJ disc displacement.

3. Cartilage tissue is generated in the synovia, and part of the chondrified tissue enters the joint cavity and undergoes chronic calcification, leading to formation of a joint loose body of cartilage tissue. The process involves three stages. In the first stage, chondrogenesis occurs in the synovial membrane. In the second stage, chondrogenetic tissue begins to enter or be released into the joint cavity with formation of edematous synovial connective tissue and a loose body. In the third stage, chondrogenesis in the synovial membrane disappears and only a loose body can be observed. In most cases several

loose cartilage bodies occur, but even a single major loose body can be formed.

4. A benign condition, even if a recurrence may occur. Malignant transformation has been described but the risk seems to be very low.

5. Open surgery via a preauricular approach, which is the most common method. Arthroscopic surgery might be an alternative, but removal of major intraarticular loose bodies can technically be problematic with this method.

6. Palsy of the frontal branch of the facial nerve might occur, even if the risk for permanent palsy is minimal, leading to problems to raise the eyebrow and frown on the surgical side.

Case 2.16

Mandibular Condylar Fracture

Peter Abrahamsson and Lars Eriksson

A. Demographic Data and Reason for Contact
- A 71-year-old Caucasian woman presenting after an accidental fall with pain and minor swelling over the left cheek, a nonfitting bite, and laceration of the lower lip.

B. Symptom History
- The patient tripped while walking and hit the right side of the chin when falling on the pavement the day before the examination.
- There was no loss of consciousness.
- The patient had no problems from the TMJs or masticatory muscles before the accident, but is now complaining of limited mouth opening, a nonfitting bite, and a feeling of a preauricular swelling on the left side, and even pain in the jaws, temple, and in front of the ear on the left side, especially with jaw movements.

C. Medical History
- Is under examination by her general practitioner because of suspected hypertension and osteoporosis.
- No medication.
- No previous hospitalizations.

D. Psychosocial History
- Socially active retired teacher living with her husband in a bungalow.
- Normal scores for depression (PHQ-9) and anxiety (GAD-7). A few physical symptoms (PHQ-15) and normal level of stress (PSS-10).
- Nonsmoking, moderate alcohol consumption.
- No history of psychological distress and has moderate sleep quality.

E. Previous Consultations and Treatments
- Examination at the Accident and Emergency Department excluded head injuries and fractures other than a suspected jaw fracture. A laceration of the lower lip was sutured and the patient was referred to the Department of Oral and Maxillofacial Surgery.

F. Extraoral Status
- The mandible deviates to the left. Shorter ramus height on the left side compared with the right side.
- Swelling and redness of the lower lip and chin.
- Nothing abnormal in neurologic findings.
- Minor swelling and palpation pain of the left TMJ and condylar neck. Condylar translatory motion not possible to palpate on the left side during mouth opening.
- Bilateral and familiar palpation pain in temporalis and masseter muscles.
- Maximal unassisted mouth opening 29 mm with deviation to the left, laterotrusion to the right 1 mm and to the left 8 mm, and protrusion 5 mm with deviation to the left. Familiar pain in the left TMJ on all jaw movements.
- Neck has normal range of motion; no pain.

G. Intraoral Status
Soft tissues
- Minor hematoma on the inner side of the lower lip.

Hard tissues and dentition
- Complete dentition. Enamel fracture of the upper right lateral incisor, and fractured buccal cusps on the second premolar and first molar in the left upper jaw.

Occlusion
- Anterior and lateral (right side) open bite with contacts only in the left molar region.

Saliva
- Nothing remarkable.

H. Additional Examination and Findings
- CT scan is an appropriate technique for both detailed information of mandibular fractures and for illustration of any displaced segments. A left subcondylar fracture with a lateral displacement was found (Figure 2.49).

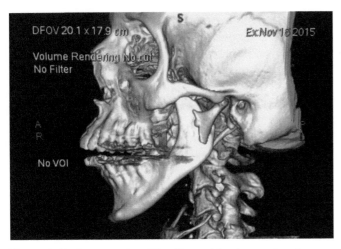

Figure 2.49 Preoperative CT-radiographic picture showing a left subcondylar fracture with a lateral displacement of the condylar fragment (C).

I. Diagnosis/Diagnoses

Expanded DC/TMD

- Left condylar fracture. Other mandibular fractures may not be excluded at this point.

DC/TMD

- Masticatory muscle myalgia.
- Left TMJ arthralgia.

Other

- Fractured teeth.

J. Case Assessment

- The combination of an acute trauma, changed occlusion, and painful and reduced mandibular motion capacity with difference in maximal laterotrusive movements between the right and left side prompted a suspicion of a condylar fracture.
- The suspicion was strengthened by the lack of palpable condylar movements on the left side, difference in ramus height between the right and left side, and palpation pain of the left TMJ region.
- A clinical differential diagnosis based on pain, altered occlusion, and impaired laterotrusion after a trauma is an acute traumatic arthritis of the TMJ. When this happens there is usually a swelling in the TMJ on the affected side and changes of the occlusion with primary contacts on the contralateral side, as an edema in the traumatized joint will press the condylar head in a caudal direction. At laterotrusion there is usually a normal range of motion to the affected side and an impaired range of motion to the opposite side. These facts make this differential diagnosis less likely.

- The combination of a trauma, reduced motion capacity, and deviation of the lower jaw and changed occlusion makes an additional radiographic examination indicated in order to check for fractures.

K. Evidence-based Treatment Plan including Aims

- The aim for treatment of condylar fractures is to normalize the occlusion during healing. This can be done by the aid of either closed treatment or open surgery. If a condyle is minimally displaced or not displaced, closed treatment is the method of choice.
- During closed treatment, minor occlusal changes may be initially observed for some days. Usually, the occlusion will be normalized spontaneously. However, if not, it may have to be guided with nonrigid or rigid fixation attached to alternatively arch bars, brackets, or intermaxillary fixation screws (Figure 2.50).
- Major displacement of a fractured condyle resulting in a more disturbed occlusion is nowadays frequently reduced and fixated by open surgery, allowing anatomic repositioning and immediate postoperative function of the jaw. Usually, an extraoral approach is then used. When the fracture is exposed it can be reduced and fixated with titanium plates and screws (Figures 2.51 and 2.52). If so, the occlusion is usually temporarily fixated during the surgical procedure.

L. Prognosis and Discussion

- The prognosis of closed treatment of condylar fractures as well as for open surgery is, in general, good. In some cases it is not feasible to expect an anatomic reduction of the condylar fracture, but minimal to moderate displacement of the condylar segment generally results in adequate postoperative function and occlusion. A prerequisite for that is that a

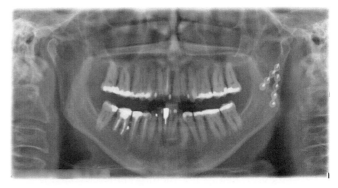

Figure 2.50 Postoperative panoramic radiograph showing repositioned condylar fracture on the left side fixated with two titanium plates and screws.

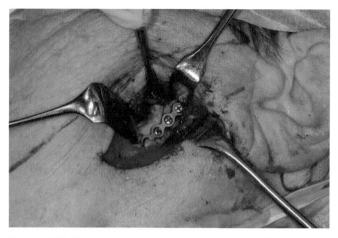

Figure 2.51 Fracture site exposed via a submandibular incision. The subcondylar fracture reduced to correct position (arrow) and fixated with titanium plates and screws.

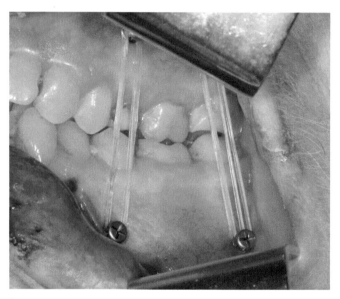

Figure 2.52 Intermaxillary fixation with elastics attached to screws in the alveolar process for guidance of a bite with a fractured condyle to correct occlusion.

proper occlusal relationship is established during the period of healing of the fracture.

- Generally, intermaxillary fixation is used in adults for a maximum of 2–3 weeks. In children, intermaxillary fixation is unusual but can in specific cases be used for 10–14 days, followed by a period of aggressive functional rehabilitation (Tucker, 1998). In particular, at intracapsular fractures early mobilization is essential to avoid intraarticular adhesions.
- Patients with displaced fractured condyles should, according to a systematic review and meta-analysis by Al-Moraissi and Ellis (2015), be treated with open

reduction with internal fixation as this handling provides a superior clinical outcome compared with closed treatment. A disadvantage with open reduction is the risk of damage to the facial nerve, resulting in paralysis and the risk of formation of scars and infection. In children, open surgery is usually not indicated for treatment of condylar fractures as their capacity to remodel a displaced condyle to normal configuration is excellent.

Background Information

- The incidence of condylar fractures has been estimated to be about 1/1000 persons. In a retrospective analysis of more than 4000 mandibular fractures the majority of patients were men (83%) with a mean age of 38 years, and condyle or subcondylar fractures occurred in 18% of the mandibular fractures. Most injuries occurred in the summer months (Morris *et al.*, 2015). In a study of mandibular fractures treated at a Swedish university hospital from 1999 to 2008, 70% of the patients were men and 50% were aged 16–30 years (Ramadhan *et al.*, 2014).
- According to Ramadhan *et al.* (2014), the most common reasons for mandibular fractures were interpersonal violence (24%), falls (23%), and traffic accidents (19%), while Morris *et al.* (2015) reported that low-velocity blunt injuries caused 62% and high-velocity blunt injuries 31% of the mandibular fractures in their study.
- Condylar fractures are divided into three sites: the condylar head (intracapsular), the condylar neck (extracapsular), and the subcondylar region (Zachariades *et al.*, 2006). Unilateral condylar fractures represented two-thirds of the condylar fractures, and 19% of the condyles were nondisplaced, 12% deviated, and 69% displaced.
- Significant differences in treatment outcome have been reported by Al-Moraissi and Ellis (2015) between open reduction and closed treatment with rigid internal fixation regarding maximal interincisal opening, laterotrusive movements, protrusive movement, malocclusion, pain, and chin deviation on mouth opening. Even though the incidence of facial injury is high, it is difficult to collect data, particularly when long-term evaluation is required, as rates of compliance and attendance

at follow-up tend to be low (O'Connor *et al.*, 2015). The number of large-scale studies is therefore small. A concerted effort to collaborate nationally and across different specialties to undertake larger studies will help to improve the outcome. Quality of life based on patient satisfaction after open versus closed treatment for mandibular condyle fractures should also be better evaluated (Kommers *et al.*, 2013).

- Ankylosis of the TMJ is a feared complication. Often it is due to hemarthrosis, occurring at condylar head fractures within the joint capsule, that is responsible for the ankylosis (Hackenberg *et al.*, 2014). At these types of fractures early mobilization of the jaw is essential. At subcondylar fractures, fractures situated below the attachment of the joint capsule, closed treatment with intermaxillary fixation can be used with a minor risk of ankylosis.

Diagnostic Criteria

Expanded DC/TMD criteria for **Fracture** (Peck *et al.*, 2014). Sensitivity and specificity have not been established.

A nondisplaced or displaced break in bone involving the joint (i.e., temporal bone and/or mandible). The fracture may include the cartilage. The most common is the subcondylar fracture. The condition may result in a malocclusion (e.g., contralateral posterior open bite) and impaired function (e.g., uncorrected ipsilateral deviation with opening; restricted contralateral jaw movement), and typically results from a traumatic injury.

History. Positive for both of the following:
1. Trauma to the orofacial region.
   AND
2. Preauricular swelling.
   OR
3. Arthralgia.
   OR
4. Limited mouth opening.

Examination. Positive for at least one of the following, consistent with the history findings:
1. Preauricular swelling.
   OR
2. Arthralgia.
   OR

3. Maximum assisted opening (passive stretch) <40 mm including vertical incisal overlap.
   Imaging. CT/CBCT is positive for the following:
1. Evidence of fracture.
   DC/TMD criteria for **Myalgia**, see Case 3.3, and for **Arthralgia**, see Case 2.1 (Schiffman *et al.*, 2014).

Fundamental Points

Issues important for diagnosis, treatment plan, and management of the case

- Patient information of clinical findings and treatment plan, including advantages and disadvantages with the method to be used, is very important.
- Information on the risk, even if minimal, for facial nerve weakness at open surgery with extraoral entry.
- The need for postoperative training of jaw movements, if necessary by the aid of a physiotherapist, as well as the expected time for sick leave must be explained.

Self-study Questions

1. Describe three symptoms indicating that a condylar fracture can be suspected.
2. What is the advantage with CT scan at condylar fractures?
3. What is the aim for the treatment of condylar fractures?
4. Give three methods used for treatment of condylar fractures?
5. Motivate the different treatment techniques.
6. Is open surgery indicated for treatment of condylar fractures in children? Motivate.

References

Al-Moraissi EA, Ellis E, III, (2015) Surgical treatment of adult mandibular condylar fractures provides better outcomes than closed treatment: a systematic review and meta-analysis. *J Oral Maxillofac Surg* **73**(3):482–493.

Hackenberg B, Lee C, Caterson EJ (2014) Management of subcondylar mandible fractures in the adult patient. *J Craniofac Surg* **25**(1):166–171.

Kommers SC, van den Bergh B, Forouzanfar T (2013) Quality of life after open versus closed treatment for mandibular condyle fractures: a review of literature. *J Craniomaxillofac Surg* **41**(8):221–225.

Morris C, Bebeau NP, Brockhoff H, *et al.* (2015) Mandibular fractures: an analysis of the epidemiology and patterns of injury in 4,143 fractures. *J Oral Maxillofac Surg* **73**(5):951.e1–951.e12.

O'Connor RC, Shakib K, Brennan PA (2015) Recent advances in the management of oral and maxillofacial trauma. *Br J Oral Maxillofac Surg* **53**(10):913–921.

Peck CC, Goulet JP, Lobbezoo F, *et al.* (2014) Expanding the taxonomy of the diagnostic criteria for temporomandibular disorders. *J Oral Rehabil* **41**(1):2–23.

Ramadhan A, Gavelin P, Hirsch JM. Sand LP (2014) A retrospective study of patients with mandibular fractures treated at a Swedish university hospital 1999–2008. *Ann Maxillofac Surg* **4**(2):178–181.

Schiffman E, Ohrbach R, Truelove E, *et al.* (2014) Diagnostic Criteria for Temporomandibular Disorders (DC/TMD) for clinical and research applications: recommendations of the International RDC/TMD Consortium Network and Orofacial Pain Special Interest Group. *J Oral Facial Pain Headache* **28**(1):6–27.

Tucker MR (1998) Management of facial fractures. In: Peterson LJ, Ellis E, III, Hupp JR, Tucker MR (eds), *Contemporary oral and maxillofacial surgery*, 3rd edn. St Louis, MO: Mosby; pp 587–611.

Zachariades N, Mezitis M, Mourouzis C, *et al.* (2006) Fractures of the mandibular condyle: a review of 466 cases. Literature review, reflections on treatment and proposals, *J Craniomaxillofac Surg* **34**(7):421–432.

Answers to Self-study Questions

1. Deviation of the chin at opening, disturbed occlusion, nonsymmetric magnitude of laterotrusion.

2. CT scan is an appropriate technique for both detailed information of mandibular fractures and for illustration of displacements, if any, of the segments.

3. The aim on the treatment of condylar fractures is to guide the occlusion back to normal position.

4. Expectation, closed treatment or open surgery.

5. Initially, minor changes of the occlusion can be observed over a few days to find out whether the occlusion will be normalized spontaneously. If the occlusion has to be guided to be normalized, nonrigid or rigid fixation attached to alternatively arch bars, brackets, or intermaxillary fixation screws can be used. Nowadays, major displacement of a fractured condyle resulting in a more disturbed occlusion frequently is reduced and fixated by open surgery, allowing anatomic repositioning and immediate postoperative function of the jaw.

6. In children, open surgery is usually not indicated for treatment of condylar fractures as their capacity to remodel a displaced condyle to normal configuration is excellent.

3

Masticatory Muscle Disorders

Clinical Cases in Orofacial Pain, First Edition. Edited by Malin Ernberg and Per Alstergren.
© 2017 John Wiley & Sons Ltd. Published 2017 by John Wiley & Sons Ltd.

A: Muscle Pain

Case 3.1

Myalgia with Limited Emotional Disturbance

Karina Bendixen and Peter Svensson

A. Demographic Data and Reason for Contact

- A 37-year-old female Caucasian referred from her general dentist due to pain in the jaw and temple.

B. Symptom History

- Pressing, aching, and spreading pain for about 9–10 months in the jaw, the ears, and the temples (Figure 3.1).
- Pain comes and goes.
- Pain 2–3 days per week.
- Pain is worsened when chewing hard foods.
- Pain not affected by stress.
- Pain is described as mild aching and tender. Present pain intensity: 3 (NRS 0–10). Average pain intensity: 4. Worst pain intensity: 6.

C. Medical History

- Healthy – no known medical conditions.
- No other pain complaints.
- No known allergies.
- No previous relevant hospitalizations or surgeries.
- No head trauma.
- Regular check-up at her private general dentist.
- Orthodontic treatment with fixed appliances as adolescent.
- No other major dental treatments.

D. Psychosocial History

- Married, two children.
- Secretary in full-time work.
- Middle socio-economic status.
- Rarely sports or exercise.
- Low disability with low pain intensity (GCPS).
- Limitations in chewing tough foods (JFLS).
- Report of some parafunctional activity during daytime (OBCL).

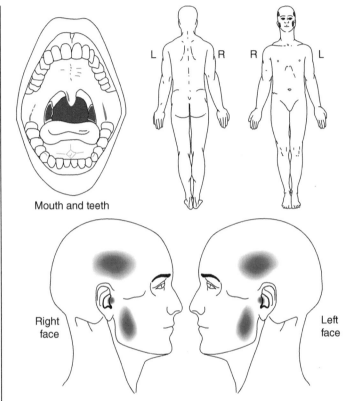

Mouth and teeth

Right face

Left face

Figure 3.1 Pain drawing by patient.

- No symptoms of anxiety, depression, or other physical symptoms (PHQ-9, GAD-7, PHQ-15).

E. Previous Consultations and Treatments

- ENT specialist due to ear pain, but no disorder was detected.
- Medication, analgesics (over the counter): paracetamol (acetaminophen) 2 g three times per week; some pain relief.

- Stabilization splint nighttime use prescribed by general dentist because of bruxism; no effect on pain.

F. Extraoral Status
Face

- Normal appearance and body-mass index (BMI) within normal limits.
- No asymmetries, swelling, or redness.
- No neurological abnormalities upon screening.
- No somatosensory or motor function abnormalities.

Temporomandibular joint

- No noise/sounds on standardized palpation.
- No pain on movements or standardized palpation.

Masticatory muscles

- Bilateral familiar masseter pain on palpation.
- Bilateral familiar temporalis pain on palpation.

Jaw movement capacity

- Open movements: straight. Pain-free opening: 31 mm. Maximum unassisted/assisted opening: 41/43 mm. No pain.
- Lateral movements: right excursion, 10 mm; left excursion, 11 mm. No pain.
- Protrusion: 9 mm. No pain.

Neck and shoulders

- Mild pain on palpation of trapezius muscles.

G. Intraoral Status
Soft tissues

- Moderate tongue scalloping.
- Teeth impressions in buccal mucosa.

Hard tissues and dentition

- Full arch dentition (28 teeth), few composite fillings. Wear grade 1. No dental caries or periodontal disease.
- Neutral sagittal relations. Horizontal overlap: 2 mm. Vertical overlap: 2 mm. No midline deviation.

Occlusion

- Stable.

Saliva

- Normal quantity/quality.
- Good oral hygiene.

H. Additional Examinations and Findings

- Not considered needed.

I. Diagnoses

- Myalgia.
- Subtype local myalgia of masseter and temporalis muscles.

J. Case Assessment

- The physical examination revealed jaw muscle pain and temple headache. The pain is modified by jaw function and fulfills the criteria for the two common pain TMDs: myalgia and headache attributed to TMD. TMD etiology is considered to be multifactorial. Several risk factors are identified, of which in this case the female gender and the age seem to be of main relevance.
- From the history and the physical examination it is apparent that she suffers from a mild type of TMD since the pain level is on average moderate; however, several days a week she has no pain at all. Also, no severe pain comorbidities are present and mild analgesics provides some pain relief. From both physical and psychosocial aspects she is generally healthy.

K. Evidence-based Treatment Plan including Aims

- The overall aims are to eliminate or as a minimum reduce the pain level and numbers of days with pain and also to increase jaw function in a noninvasive manner. This is by low-intensity management and active patient involvement.
- First management steps are information, counselling, and education, including a tailored self-care program and approaches (exercise, awareness of jaw posture, "lips closed – teeth apart," avoid parafunctional activity, etc.). Discontinue oral splint usage, since no effect on pain. Also, instruction in physiotherapy exercises "self-performed" (jaw stretching, relaxation, heat (diathermy), massage).
- If additional management approaches are needed, pharmacotherapy by the use of topical NSAIDs could also be applied on muscles before massage.
- Monitoring systemic analgesia (paracetamol) usage to avoid medication overuse headaches is indicated.

L. Prognosis and Discussion

- Reversible condition with good prognosis; however, good patient cooperation necessary.
- Based on anamnestic information the patient appears to cope well with minimal influence of and consequence for the psychosocial status.

- Tailored self-care program requires monitoring and adjustments as needed.
- Since the headache is attributed to TMD, the prediction is that management of the TMD will also result in headache remission.

Background Information

- TMD prevalence 3–15%. Peak age 20–45 years. TMD pain prevalence 4.6% (ratio women : men, 2 : 1). Myofascial TMD pain most frequent TMD diagnosis (42%). Myofascial TMD common comorbid conditions (e.g., primary headaches – migraine and tension-type headache) (Ballegaard *et al.*, 2008; Schiffman *et al.*, 2014; Speciali and Dach, 2015; Fernández-de-Las-Peñas and Svensson, 2016).
- Etiology and pathology of TMD are unclear but multifactorial, including some degree of peripheral and central sensitization and also involvement of endogenous modulatory systems. Genetical predisposition to some degree cannot be excluded.
- Occlusion and bruxism are considered as minor risk factors (Michelotti and Iodice, 2010; Fernández-de-Las-Peñas and Svensson, 2016).

Diagnostic Criteria

Expanded DC/TMD for **Local myalgia** (Schiffman *et al.*, 2014). Sensitivity and specificity have not been determined.

Pain of muscle origin plus a report of pain localized to the immediate site of tissue stimulation (e.g., localized to the area under the palpating finger). Limitation of mandibular movement(s) secondary to pain may be present.

History. Positive for both of the following:

1. Pain in the jaw, temple, in front of the ear, or in the ear.
   AND
2. Pain modified with jaw movement, function, or parafunction.

Examination. Positive for all of the following, when examining the temporalis or masseter muscles:

1. Confirmation of pain location(s) in the temporalis or masseter muscle(s).
   AND

2. Familiar muscle pain with palpation.
   AND
3. Pain with muscle palpation with pain localized to the immediate site of the palpating finger(s).
   Note: the pain is not better accounted for by another pain diagnosis.

DC/TMD criteria for **Myalgia** (Schiffman *et al.*, 2014), see Case 3.3.

Fundamental Points

- Comprehensive and systematic anamnesis and clinical examination (including the DC/TMD) are essential (Dworkin *et al.*, 2002; Schiffman *et al.*, 2014; Fernández-de-Las-Peñas and Svensson, 2016).
- Management conservative, noninvasive, reversible, low-cost approach and with emphasis on the importance of self-care. Patient involvement in the decision-making since it allows the patient to take responsibility for the management of her condition (Dworkin *et al.*, 2002, List and Axelsson, 2010; Fernández-de-Las-Peñas and Svensson, 2016).

Self-study Questions

1. Does orthodontic treatment cause TMD?
2. Are TMD and primary headaches related?
3. Is imaging relevant in myalgia cases?
4. Discuss the female : male ratio in TMD prevalence in the clinic.

References

Ballegaard V, Thede-Schmidt-Hansen P, Svensson P, Jensen R (2008) Are headache and temporomandibular disorders related? A blinded study. *Cephalalgia* **28**(8):832–841.

Dworkin SF, Huggins KH, Wilson L, et al. (2002) A randomized clinical trial using research diagnostic criteria for temporomandibular disorders–axis II to target clinic cases for a tailored self-care TMD treatment program. *J Orofac Pain* **16**(1):48–63.

Fernández-de-Las-Peñas C, Svensson P (2016) Myofascial temporomandibular disorder. *Curr Rheumatol Rev* **12**:40–54.

List T, Axelsson S (2010) Management of TMD: evidence from systematic reviews and meta-analyses. *J Oral Rehabil* **37**(6):430–451.

Michelotti A, Iodice G (2010) The role of orthodontics in temporomandibular disorders. *J Oral Rehabil* **37**(6):411–429.

Schiffman E, Ohrbach R, Truelove E, et al. (2014) Diagnostic Criteria for Temporomandibular Disorders (DC/TMD) for clinical and research applications: recommendations of the International RDC/TMD Consortium Network and Orofacial Pain Special Interest Group. *J Oral Facial Pain Headache* **28**(1):6–27.

Speciali JG, Dach F (2015) Temporomandibular dysfunction and headache disorder. *Headache* **55**(Suppl 1):72–83.

Answers to Self-study Questions

1. The topic remains controversial; however, no firm evidence exists that orthodontic treatment could have a significant role for TMD development (Michelotti and Iodice, 2010; Fernández-de-Las-Peñas and Svensson, 2016).

2. TMD and primary headaches, such as migraine and tension-type headache, have a comorbidity relationship. The presence of one condition increases the risk of the other condition (Ballegaard *et al.*, 2008; Speciali and Dach, 2015).

3. Imaging is useful in detecting tissue structural differences; however, there is no evidence that imaging is of relevance in myalgia cases.

4. Factors such as neurobiological differences in pain sensitivity, differences in endogenous pain inhibition, impact of sex hormones, and psychological and behavioral aspects are identified.

Case 3.2

Myalgia with Emotional Disturbance

Peter Svensson and Karina Bendixen

A. Demographic Data and Reason for Contact

- A 47-year-old female Caucasian referred from her private general practitioner due to chronic orofacial pain complaints.

B. Symptom History

- Pressing, aching, and intense pain in the jaw and head for more than 6 years (Figure 3.2).
- Pain is always present.
- Pain intensity varies; most days severe pain. Present pain intensity: 8 (NRS 0–10). Average pain intensity: 7. Worst pain intensity: 10 (occurs two or three times per week).
- Pain is worsened when chewing and talking and during emotional stress.
- Pain is worrying and disturbing.

C. Medical History

- Comorbid pain conditions: chronic tension-type headache, neck and shoulder pain, and low back pain diagnoses by her general practitioner.
- Allergies to nickel, perfume, and latex.
- No previous relevant hospitalizations or surgeries.
- No other known medical conditions.
- No head trauma.
- Regular check-up at her private general dentist.
- Third molars complicated extractions 20 years ago.
- No other major dental treatments.

D. Psychosocial History

- Divorced, one child age 18 years old living at home.
- Teacher at a primary school part time.
- At present on sick leave due to the pain.
- Middle socio-economic status.
- No sport activities or exercise.
- Poor sleep quality and quantity.
- Pain is highly disabling, but moderately limiting (GCPS).

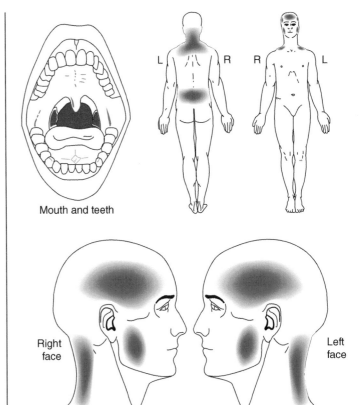

Figure 3.2 Pain drawing showing pain locations.

- Moderate to severe limitations in chewing tough food, hard bread, open wide enough to bite from a whole apple, talk, and sing (JFLS).
- Report of some parafunctional activity during daytime, such as some of the time tense muscles without clenching, place tongue between teeth, hold the jaw in rigid or tense position, and sustained talking (OBCL).
- Moderate symptoms of anxiety (GAD-7), depression (PHQ-9), and physical (PHQ-15).

E. Previous Consultations and Treatments

- Stabilization splint used during sleep with no effect on pain.

- Analgesic medication (over the counter) with paracetamol (acetaminophen) 3 g and ibuprofen 1200 mg 6–7 days per week provided minor pain relief.
- Physiotherapy due to neck and shoulder pain gave partial and temporary pain relief.
- Acupuncture and craniosacral therapy attempted several times, but with only minor pain relief.

F. Extraoral Status

General and face

- Normal appearance and BMI within normal limits.
- No asymmetries, swelling, or redness.

Neurologic findings

- No neurologic abnormalities upon screening.

Somatosensory and motor function

- No somatosensory or motor function abnormalities.

Temporomandibular joint

- No noise/sounds on standardized palpation.
- No pain on movements or standardized palpation.

Masticatory muscles

- Bilateral familiar masseter pain upon palpation with spread within the muscle (but not beyond).
- Bilateral familiar temporalis pain upon palpation, also familiar to her headache.

Jaw movement capacity

- Opening movement: straight. Pain-free opening: 42 mm. Maximum unassisted/assisted opening: 44/46 mm. Bilateral familiar masseter and temporalis pain.
- Lateral movements: right excursion, 12 mm; left excursion, 10 mm. Bilateral familiar masseter and temporalis pain.
- Protrusion: 10 mm. Bilateral familiar masseter and temporalis pain.

Neck and shoulders

- Pain on palpation of bilateral trapezius, splenius, and sternocleidomastoid muscles.

G. Intraoral Status

Soft tissues

- Negative.

Hard tissues and dentition

- Full arch dentition (28 teeth), few restorations, wear grade 1 and 2. No dental caries or periodontal disease.

Occlusion

- Sagittal: neutral. Horizontal overlap 3 mm. Vertical overlap 2 mm. No midline deviation.

Saliva

- Normal quantity and quality.
- Good oral hygiene.

H. Additional Examinations and Findings

- Generalized musculoskeletal pain conditions was ruled out.

I. Diagnosis/Diagnoses

DC/TMD

- Myalgia
  - subtype myofascial pain.
- Headache attributed to TMD.

ICHD-3 beta

- Chronic tension-type headache (Headache Classification Committee of the International Headache Society (IHS), 2013).

J. Case Assessment

- From the history and the physical examination it is revealed that the patient has suffered from chronic pain for several years in the jaw and the head. The pain and headache, which is always present, varies in intensity and is worsened by jaw movements, jaw functions, and jaw parafunctions and thereby fulfills the criteria for the common pain-related TMDs: myalgia and headache attributed to TMD. The pain also spreads to other anatomical structures (myofascial pain). Several comorbid pain conditions exist. The etiology of TMD is multifactorial. Risk factors of relevance in this case are gender and age, but also the comorbid pain conditions, the poor sleep, and psychosocial status, of which there are notably indications of distress.
- Several treatments have been attempted, but with no or minor effect on the pain. Analgesics provide minor pain relief; however, risk of medication-overuse headache exists due to the high intake of paracetamol and ibuprofen.

K. Evidence-based Treatment Plan including Aims

- The overall aims are to reduce the pain level and improve quality of life. Owing to the complexity, multimodal management is required.
- First management steps are information, counselling, and education, including tailored self-care program

and approaches (exercise, sleep hygiene, awareness of jaw posture, etc.), but also instruction and monitoring of physiotherapy exercises self-performed (jaw stretching, relaxation, heat and/or cold (diathermy), and massage). Discontinue oral splint usage since no effect on pain levels.

- Inclusion of psychological therapy and pain support group are highly relevant.
- Pharmacological switch from paracetamol and NSAIDs to low-dose tricyclic antidepressants (TCAs) could also be relevant, this in cooperation with her general practitioner. TCA drugs are secondary analgesics. When a TCA is used in the management of chronic pain it is of great importance that sufficient high doses are used for a sufficient amount of time. If TCA treatment is chosen, monitoring TCA serum levels can be considered due to the individual variations in metabolism and diurnal levels, and so on. Other management options could include topical NSAID and hypnosis.

L. Prognosis and Discussion

- Moderate to good prognosis provided good patient cooperation and high-intensity, multimodal management approaches, including both the physical (Axis I) and the psychosocial (Axis II) factors that must be addressed.
- Tailored self-care program requires monitoring and adjustments as needed.
- The oral splint device does not provide pain relief, and since there are no signs of bruxism discontinuation is recommended.

Background Information

- TMD prevalence is reported to be between 3 and 15% with a peak age of 20–45 years and a women-to-men ratio of 2 : 1. The TMD pain prevalence is 4.6%. Myofascial TMD pain is the most frequent TMD diagnosis, accounting for 42%. Comorbid conditions (e.g., headaches – migraine and tension-type headache) are common.
- Etiology and pathology of TMD are unclear but multifactorial, including some degree of peripheral and central sensitization and involvement of endogenous pain modulatory systems. Genetical predisposition to some degree cannot be excluded.
- Occlusion and bruxism are considered low risk factors.

- Central nervous system changes, such as structural reorganization and neurodegeneration (changes in the white and grey matter volume), are associated with chronic pain conditions.

(Schiffman *et al.*, 2014; Fernández-de-Las-Peñas and Svensson, 2016)

Diagnostic Criteria

DC/TMD criteria for **Myofascial pain** (Schiffman *et al.*, 2014). Sensitivity and specificity have not been established.

Pain of muscle origin plus a report of pain spreading beyond the immediate site of tissue stimulation (e.g., the palpating finger) but within the boundary of the masticatory muscle being examined. Limitation of mandibular movement(s) secondary to pain may be present.

History. Positive for the following:
1. Local myalgia (see Case 3.1).

Examination. Positive for all of the following, when examining the temporalis or masseter muscles:
1. Confirmation of pain location(s) in the temporalis or masseter muscle(s).
   AND
2. Familiar muscle pain with palpation.
   AND
3. Pain with muscle palpation with spreading of the pain beyond the location of the palpating finger(s) but within the boundary of the muscle.

DC/TMD criteria for **Myalgia**, see Case 3.3, and for **Headache attributed to TMD**, see Case 4.1 (Schiffman *et al.*, 2014).

Fundamental Points

- Comprehensive and systematic anamnesis and clinical examination (including the DC/TMD) are essential.
- Addressing the psychosocial (Axis II) issues are of high importance for the treatment outcome.
- Management must be multimodal involving several health-care professionals, but also conservative, noninvasive, reversible, and low cost.
- Tailored self-care program is of uttermost importance, but also patient involvement in the

decision-making since it allows the patient to take responsibility for the management of her condition.

(Dworkin *et al.*, 2002; List and Axelsson, 2010; Schiffman *et al.*, 2014; Fernández-de-Las-Peñas and Svensson 2016)

Self-study Questions

1. Which role does psychological factors play in pain patients?

2. How is medication-overuse headache defined?

3. How does sleep quality affect pain?

References

Dworkin SF, Huggins KH, Wilson L, et al. (2002) A randomized clinical trial using research diagnostic criteria for temporomandibular disorders–axis II to target clinic cases for a tailored self-care TMD treatment program. *J Orofac Pain* **16**(1):48–63.

Fernández-de-Las-Peñas C, Svensson P (2016) Myofascial temporomandibular disorder. *Curr Rheumatol Rev* **12**:40–54.

Finan PH, Goodin BR, Smith MT (2013) The association of sleep and pain: an update and a path forward. *J Pain* **14**(12):1539–1552.

Headache Classification Committee of the International Headache Society (IHS) (2013) The International Classification of Headache Disorders, 3rd edition (beta version). *Cephalalgia* **33**(9):629–808.

List T, Axelsson S (2010) Management of TMD: evidence from systematic reviews and meta-analyses. *J Oral Rehabil* **37**(6):430–451.

Sanders AE, Slade GD, Bair E, et al. (2013) General health status and incidence of first-onset temporomandibular disorder: the OPPERA prospective cohort study. *J Pain* **14**(12 Suppl):T51–T62.

Schiffman E, Ohrbach R, Truelove E, et al. (2014) Diagnostic Criteria for Temporomandibular Disorders (DC/TMD) for clinical and research applications: recommendations of the International RDC/TMD Consortium Network and Orofacial Pain Special Interest Group. *J Oral Facial Pain Headache* **28**(1):6–27.

Answers to Self-study Questions

1. Myofascial TMD patients are associated with higher levels of anxiety, depression, stress, and somatization; however, causal relationships have not been demonstrated. Catastrophizing increases risk of chronic pain development and also the maintenance and/or exaggeration of existing pain (Dworkin *et al.*, 2002, Sanders *et al.*, 2013, Fernández-de-Las-Peñas and Svensson, 2016).

2. Medication overuse headache: according to the IHS Classification/ICHD-3 beta, the risk occurs at intake of analgesics ≥ 15 days per month for >3 months (Headache Classification Committee of the International Headache Society (IHS), 2013).

3. Poor sleep quality is associated with increased pain symptoms (Finan *et al.*, 2013).

Case 3.3

Myalgia in Adolescents

Claudia Restrepo and Ambra Michelotti

A. Demographic Data and Reason for Contact

- Latin American Hispanic female, 14 years old (Figure 3.3).
- Pain in her left side of the face and concerned about the asymmetry of her face.
- Referred to an orofacial pain specialist from her general dental practitioner.

B. Symptom History

- The patient reports pain during rest and function in the left masticatory muscles.
- Pain comes and goes and increases during clenching, chewing, and mandibular movements.
- Pain intensity is 2 (NRS 0–10) at rest but increased to 5 (NRS 0–10) on mouth opening and chewing.
- Pain onset was 2.5 years ago.
- Patient uses chewing gums some of the time and clenches her teeth during the day most of the time (OBCL).
- No functional limitations according to JFLS.
- Mother tells that she and her daughter are concerned about the asymmetry of the daughter's face.
- Patient chews exclusively with the left posterior teeth.

C. Medical History

- Diagnosed with hypermobility syndrome at the age of 8.
- No known allergies to any food or medication.
- No medications, except for occasional NSAIDs for pain.
- Overall health is very good.
- No sleep-related problems.
- No smoking habits, no use of drugs, no use of caffeine or alcohol.
- Surgeries or hospitalizations: negative.
- Trauma: negative.
- Family medical background: no particular information as reported by the patient or her mother.

D. Psychosocial History

- Parents are married.
- Mother does not work and father works full-time outside the home.
- Middle socio-economic status.
- Patient is a student and a professional swimmer.
- Mother is the primary care giver; patient lives with her parents and a sister aged 12.
- When the patient was evaluated using PHQ-4, -9, and -15 and GAD-7, she expressed she was feeling afraid, as if something awful might happen, several days during the last 2 weeks. She reported no problems at all regarding situations that could have affected her at school, her capacity to take care of things at home, and getting along with other people. However, when the patient was asked about the implications of the face asymmetry, she answered she was concerned about her facial morphology, because the swimming team members have bullied her, so her self-esteem is affected both as an adolescent and as an athlete. She expressed also to be affected by the orofacial pain that sometimes is intolerable, especially after swimming. PSS-10 showed severe stress.

E. Previous Consultation and Treatment

- The patient had undergone comprehensive dental visits each 6 months since she was 5 years old.
- A posterior crossbite was corrected with a fixed orthodontic treatment during the primary dentition in another dental center.
- When the patient was 6 years old, the former dentist told her that, according to the panoramic X-ray at that moment, 46, 47, and 48 were congenitally absent.

F. Extraoral Status

Head and neck

- Normal head and neck morphology.

Hypermobility

- Beighton hypermobility score 7.

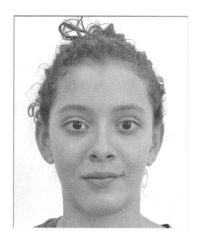 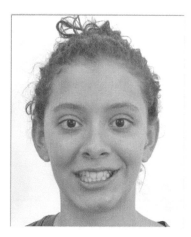 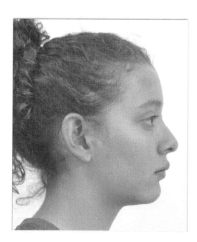

Figure 3.3 Face, frontal, and profile images.

Weight and height
- Normal.
- There are no signs of changes in tissue volume or color.

Neurologic findings
- Normal.

Somatosensory abnormalities
- None detected during standard TMJ examination. No additional examination was considered necessary.

Motor function abnormalities
- None noted.

Temporomandibular joint
- Familiar pain in left TMJ during palpation and lateral movements but not familiar pain during palpation of the right TMJ.

Masticatory muscles
- Familiar palpation pain in masseter and temporalis muscles as well as temporalis insertion, bilaterally. Palpation pain, not familiar, in the submandibular region was also detected during palpation.

Jaw movements
- Opening pattern has uncorrected deviation to the left.
- Pain-free opening 40 mm; maximum unassisted opening 45 mm and maximum assisted opening 48 mm, both with familiar pain from masseter and temporalis muscles bilaterally. Horizontal jaw movements are 8 mm to the right, 11 mm to the left, and 8 mm in protrusion; all were pain free.

Neck
- Cervical hypermobility with local pain on movement and palpation but no pain radiation toward the face.

G. Intraoral Status
Dentition
- Full dentition, except that teeth 18, 28, 38, and 46–48 are missing (Figures 3.4 and 3.5).
- Upper left canine in vestibular position without causing any trauma to soft tissues.
- Overbite 2 mm, overjet 1 mm.
- Left molar class I, right molar class cannot be determined, left canine class I and right canine class II. Transversal and vertical asymmetry and crowding in the upper arch; vertical asymmetry in the lower arch and vertical asymmetry in occlusion were noted (Figure 3.5).

Occlusion
- Bilateral contacts premolars and molars in intercuspal position. Canine and anterior guidance.

H. Additional Examination and Findings
- Class II skeletal relationship found in the lateral cephalic X-ray
- Absence of 46, 47, and 48, found in the panoramic imaging.

I. Diagnosis/Diagnoses
DC/TMD
- Myalgia of masticatory muscles.
- Arthralgia of the left TMJ.

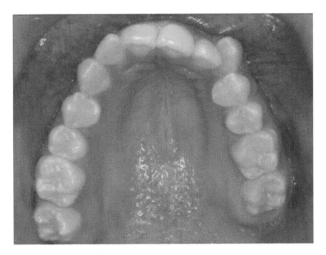
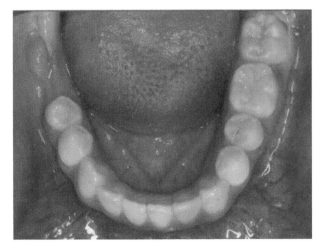

Figure 3.4 Dental arches.

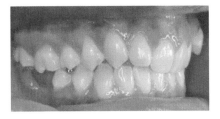
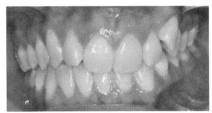
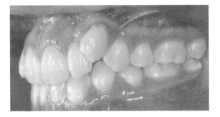

Figure 3.5 Occlusion.

J.   Case Assessment

- Etiology to the myalgia and arthralgia may be a stress-related muscle hyperactivity.
- Based on the history, overload of the masticatory system may have occurred due to the missing 46, 47, and 48 resulting in mainly unilateral chewing.
- Generalized hypermobility is a risk factor for future musculoskeletal problems and has to be considered in the treatment and follow-up planning.
- The patient has a facial asymmetry, but the asymmetry in itself is not considered as a cause of the myalgia and arthralgia.

K.   Evidence-based Treatment Plan including Aims

- Counselling is always the first approach. Provide reassurance regarding the recent state of the disease, explain the nature, the etiology, and the good prognosis of this benign disorder. Thus, detailed information should be given.
- Initial reduction of the pain in the affected muscles with NSAIDs with the aim to put the patient in a better (less pain) position to embrace the coming treatment.

- Reduce repetitive strain of the masticatory system, encourage rest and relaxation, and control the amount of the masticatory activity. Thereafter, ask the patient to undertake stretching exercises for the jaw muscles. In addition, the patient should be instructed to avoid chewing gum and to use the physiological rest position (lips together, teeth apart).
- Exercise therapy is important in the rehabilitation of musculoskeletal disorders, and the model for care is similar wherever the location of the musculoskeletal disease is. The physiotherapy regimen includes "self-management" that facilitates coping for the patient. It has been suggested that these exercises help to relieve musculoskeletal pain and to restore normal function by reducing inflammation, decreasing and coordinating muscle activity, and promoting the repair and regeneration of tissue (Figure 3.6).

L.   Prognosis and Discussion

- The majority of patients respond positively to treatment of myalgia in masticatory muscles and TMJ arthralgia with occlusal splint, massage, exercises,

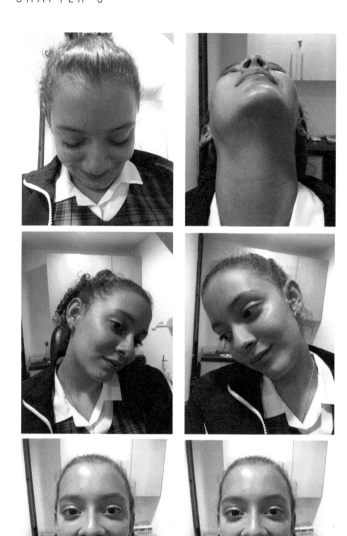

Figure 3.6 Exercises recommended to the patient.

and education to change parafunctional habits, within a short period of time (2–4 weeks).

- After 1 month the patient was pain free. The patient continues to wear the occlusal stabilization splint at nighttime.
- Self-management strategies have been effective and allowed the patient to maintain the results. The patient has been followed up for 8 months and has not reported any TMD sign or symptom.
- Long-term prognosis is good.

Background Information

- Musculoskeletal pain in children and adolescents can be idiopathic or provoked by noninflammatory conditions such as joint hypermobility syndrome. Data from well-controlled epidemiological studies are not available for the prevalence of orofacial myalgia in adolescents, but the available literature reports an estimate of 31%, based on studies in the general population.
- Masticatory myalgia is the most common orofacial pain and is usually accompanied by TMD symptoms. At the same time, TMD is one of the most important causes of pain and disability.

(Yap *et al.*, 2003; Anastassaki and Magnusson, 2004; NICDR, 2014; Romero-Reyes and Uyanik, 2014; Schiffman *et al.*, 2014; Sperotto et al., 2015)

Diagnostic Criteria

DC/TMD criteria for **Myalgia** (Schiffman *et al.*, 2014). Sensitivity 0.90 and specificity 0.99.

Pain of muscle origin affected by jaw movement, function, or parafunction, and replication of this pain with provocation testing of the masticatory muscles. Limitation of mandibular movement(s) secondary to pain may be present. Whilst a diagnosis is made based on examination of the masseter and temporalis muscles, a positive finding with the specified provocation tests when examining the other masticatory muscles can help to corroborate this diagnosis. There are three subclasses of myalgia: local myalgia, myofascial pain, and myofascial pain with referral. When myalgia is further subclassified as local myalgia, myofascial pain, or myofascial pain with referral, the latter diagnoses are based on using only the examination findings from palpation with the palpation pressure being held over the site being palpated for 5 s compared with 2 s for myalgia.

History. Positive for both of the following:
1. Pain in the jaw, temple, in front of the ear, or in the ear.
   AND
2. Pain modified with jaw movement, function, or parafunction.

Examination. Positive for both of the following, when examining the temporalis or masseter muscles:

1. Confirmation of pain location(s) in the temporalis or masseter muscle(s).
AND
2. Report of familiar pain in the temporalis or masseter with at least one of the following provocation tests:
   a. Palpation of the temporalis or masseter muscle(s).
   OR
   b. Maximum unassisted or assisted opening.

Note: the pain is not better accounted for by another pain diagnosis.

Criteria for DC/TMD **Arthralgia** (Schiffman *et al.*, 2014), see Case 2.1.

Fundamental Points

- The treatment protocol is based on considering patient goals, the psychosocial condition of the patient (stress generated by pain in the left hemi-face and decreased self-esteem due to bullying at school), the ongoing condition of the patient (hypermobility syndrome), and the absence of teeth 46 and 47.
- Physical therapy has been used for decades for treating craniomandibular disorders, and is considered the first treatment approach in musculoskeletal problems, although a multidisciplinary health-care approach may be required in more severe cases.
- The goals of physical therapy in the treatment of TMD, including myalgia, myofascial pain with referral, and TMJ arthralgia are to decrease pain, enable muscle relaxation, and reduce muscular and TMJ hyperactivity and to reestablish muscle and joint function. One of the main advantages of physical therapy treatment is that not only is it reversible and noninvasive, but most importantly it provides self-care management to create patient responsibility for their own health.
- Further dental procedures, if needed, such as orthodontic treatment of class II and correction of skeletal asymmetry, should be initiated only after the resolution of myalgia and arthralgia.

- Stress the importance of controlling muscle overuse and be sure that the patient memorizes the suggestion to maintain relaxation.

Self-study Questions

1. According to approved diagnostic criteria, what is the difference between myalgia and myofascial pain with referral?
2. In treating TMD, why is it important to consider any systemic conditions of the patient?
3. Concerning TMD, what is the role of occlusal splints in its treatment?

References

Anastassaki A, Magnusson T (2004) Patients referred to a specialist clinic because of suspected temporomandibular disorders: a survey of 3194 patients in respect of diagnoses, treatments, and treatment outcome. *Acta Odontol Scand* **62**:183–192.

NICDR (2014) *Facial pain.* National Institute of Dental and Craniofacial Research. http://www.nidcr.nih.gov/DataStatistics/FindDataByTopic/FacialPain/ (accessed November 8, 2016).

Romero-Reyes M, Uyanik JM (2014) Orofacial pain management: current perspectives. *J Pain Res* **7**:99–115.

Schiffman E, Ohrbach R, Truelove E, et al. (2014) Diagnostic Criteria for Temporomandibular Disorders (DC/TMD) for clinical and research applications: recommendations of the International RDC/TMD Consortium Network and Orofacial Pain Special Interest Group. *J Oral Facial Pain Headache* **28**(1):6–27.

Sperotto F, Brachi S, Vittadello F, Zulian F (2015) Musculoskeletal pain in schoolchildren across puberty: a 3-year follow-up study. *Pediatr Rheumatol Online J* **13**:16–21.

Yap AU, Dworkin SF, Chua EK, et al. (2003) Prevalence of temporomandibular disorder subtypes, psychologic distress, and psychosocial dysfunction in Asian patients. *J Orofac Pain* **17**:21–28.

Answers to Self-study Questions

1. Myalgia is defined as pain of muscle origin that is affected by jaw movement, function, or parafunction, and replication of this pain occurs with provocation testing of the masticatory muscles. Myofascial pain with referral is a type of myalgia, where referral of pain is beyond the boundary of the muscle being palpated when using the myofascial examination protocol. Spreading pain may also be present.

2. TMJ is anatomically and functionally related to muscular, osseous, articular, nervous, vascular, and connective tissue structures. Systemic conditions affecting any of these structures could generate TMD and have to be known in order to receive adequate treatment.

3. The exact mechanism by which an occlusal splint gives treatment effects is not known. It is most likely a combination of placebo, alteration of sensory input, stabilization of the occlusion, and unloading of masticatory muscles and the TMJ by reducing masticatory forces. Occlusal splints have been shown to have a better effect than no treatment, but it is not certain that a splint is better than placebo for treatment of myalgia.

Case 3.4

Myofascial Pain

Paulo César R Conti

A. Demographic Data and Reason for Contact

- Female, Caucasian, 30 years old, married, no children, dentist and student at postgraduate level, presented with chief complaint of facial and temple pain in the right side (Figures 3.7 and 3.8).
- Patient had orthodontic treatment finished 9 months ago for esthetic reasons.

B. Symptom History

- Current symptoms started 3 months ago, not associated with any life event. The pain is constant, located in the right side of face and spreading to the frontal/temple area, graded 6 in intensity (NRS 0–10). Quality is dull, aching, sometimes burning, and remains for hours.
- The end of the day is the moment when the pain gets worse.
- Stress and concentration make the pain worse, while medication and relaxation are ameliorating factors.
- Awake and sleep bruxism are reported. No other parafunctional activities were reported.

C. Medical History

- No report of any medical problems or regular use of medication, other than a diagnosis of frequent tension-type headache made by a neurologist. Patient also reports the sporadic use of cyclobenzaprine (muscle relaxant), when her pain gets worse.
- No history of facial/head trauma or other accidents.
- No report of any aerobic physical activity.

D. Psychosocial History

- Patient has just got married, working in a private office and finishing writing her PhD thesis. Quality of sleep is good.
- Normal score for depression according to PHQ-9, but mild anxiety according to GAD-7. PHQ-15 showed moderate score for physical symptoms. Moderate level of stress according to PSS-10.
- No smoking or alcohol regular consumption reported.

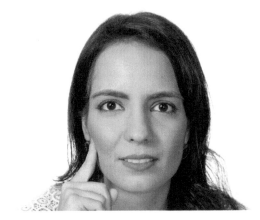

Figure 3.7 Patient's pain location, right masseter muscle.

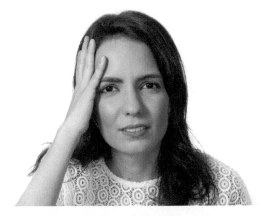

Figure 3.8 Patient showing pain location, right temporalis muscle.

E. Previous Consultations and Treatments

- Patient reported the first episode of facial pain about 6 years ago, accompanied by limited mouth opening, treated with NSAIDs, muscle relaxants, and physiotherapy. She reported mild relief after, but symptoms are recurrent, getting worse in the last 3 months.

F. Extraoral Status
Face
- No asymmetries, swelling, or other abnormality detected.

Mandibular active range of motion
- Jaw opening was straight. Maximum pain-free opening was 32 mm; maximum unassisted and assisted mouth opening was 40 mm with mild familiar pain on the right side of face, reproducing her chief complaint. Lateral and protrusive movements were within normal limits.

Temporomandibular joint
- No joint sound detected under manual inspection.
- Palpation of the both lateral and posterior aspects of the TMJs did not reveal any tenderness.

Masticatory muscle palpation
- Familiar pain on palpation was detected in the body of the right masseter. Pressure was then maintained, eliciting a referral pattern of pain to the frontal and temporal area, reproducing patient's main complaint.
- No significant pain on cervical muscles was detected.

G. Intraoral Status
- Patient has a normal occlusion, wear facets were found in anterior dentition (Figure 3.9), along with bilateral indentation in the buccal mucosa (Figure 3.10). No other significant findings.

H. Additional Examinations and Findings
- Vapor coolant spray was performed over the painful area followed by stretch of the masticatory muscles. Passive opening was increased with partial relief of the baseline pain (de Leeuw and Klasser, 2013).

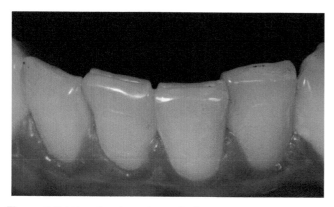

Figure 3.9 Wear facets on lower incisors.

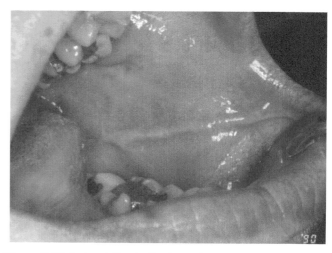

Figure 3.10 Indendation in the buccal mucosa.

I. Diagnosis/Diagnoses
DC/TMD
- Myofascial pain with referral.

ICHD-3
- Frequent tension-type headache.

Other
- Probable bruxism.

J. Case Assessment
- The case presented illustrates a typical manifestation of masticatory myofascial pain, a chronic muscular condition. An association of findings is probably responsible for the recurrence of patient's symptoms. She is aware of sleep/awake bruxism/clenching, which, associated with indentations in the mucosa and dental wear facets, can be considered indicative of sleep/awake bruxism (Lobbezoo *et al.*, 2013). No polysomnography was performed.
- Indeed, patient reported to be in a stressful phase of life, living in a new city, just married, and getting prepared to defend her PhD thesis. She also reported not to have free time to make any sort of aerobic physical activities.
- The reported stress, overload of masticatory muscles, and absence of physical activity are considered risk factors for muscle pain. Physical activity is considered an important method to stimulate pain modulation in chronic pain patients, by increasing the circulating endogenous opioids, and by decreasing pain transmission, among others (Mense and Gerwin, 2010).

- There is no strong scientific evidence for most of the modalities used to manage myofascial pain. Based on that, noninvasive and reversible modalities must be the first choice to manage such chronic conditions. In this case, reduction of muscles overload and increasing of modulatory system activity are fundamental management strategies.

K. Evidence-based Treatment Plan including Aims

- The implementation of a program to decrease the system overload has been demonstrated to be an efficient method to decrease TMD pain and to increase masticatory function (Conti *et al.*, 2012). The self-regulation of the trigeminal system is able to reduce the amount of nociceptive stimuli to the brain, allowing the system to heal.
- Patients need to be carefully instructed about the importance of their participation in the management plan. Improving sleep quality, decreasing exposure to stressful situations, implementing relaxation techniques, decreasing caffeine intake, and avoiding masticatory/cervical muscles overfunction are important steps in this educational program.
- Patient was instructed to implement all these behavioral alterations and to practice home exercises, including biofeedback training to keep "lips together/teeth apart" while awake, decreasing daytime loading. Application of moist heat over the painful area for 15 min, two times a day, to decrease pain and assist muscle relaxation was also suggested. Patient was also encouraged to start practicing regular aerobic exercises and to avoid the use of over-the-counter medication for pain.
- Occlusal splints are one of the most used therapeutic modalities in the management of TMD of all sources, including myofascial pain. Muscle relaxation,

decreasing overload to joints and muscles, reestablishment of an "ideal" occlusion, cognitive and sensorial impulses alterations, and placebo effect are frequently reported as probable mechanisms of action of these intraoral devices.

- Regardless of the mechanism involved, the use of occlusal splints has been supported by systematic reviews (Fricton *et al.*, 2010). A precise occlusal design, the amount of increased vertical dimension of occlusion, and the ideal maxillomandibular position, however, seem not to play an important role in the efficacy of this modality.
- Among many types of devices, the stabilization splint is the most used. It is considered the safest, not leading to significant occlusal alterations, and it is relatively easy to fabricate.
- A flat, hard acrylic stabilization splint was delivered for use during sleep time (Figure 3.11). The splint design included bilateral simultaneous posterior contacts and anterior and canine guidance during excursive movements.

L. Prognosis and Discussion

- Myofascial pain is a relatively common diagnosis in the orofacial region. The phenomenon of referred pain, where the source of pain is different from the pain location, as described in this case, is frequently a common cause of confusion and results in inadequate management strategies. The management must always be directed to the source and not to the site of pain. A positive prognosis is highly dependent upon the patient's adherence and collaboration to follow instructions on home care and exercises.
- The patient also has to be informed that the fundamental goal in the management of chronic pain conditions is to significantly decrease pain/dysfunction and to improve/increase mandibular function, and not necessarily "cure" the disease, considered as fluctuant, cyclic, and frequently associated with stressful life events (de Leeuw and Klasser, 2013).

Background Information

- Neuronal convergence and expansion of receptor fields, associated with peripheral and central sensitization, are probable mechanisms implicated in the phenomenon of referred pain, also known as heterotopic pain, where the source and site of pain are different.

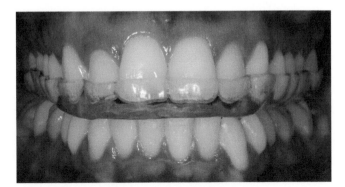

Figure 3.11 Occlusal stabilization appliance.

- In case of pain in the head, it is always important to rule out the presence of a primary headache, which can be the patient's main complaint and/or coexist with masticatory muscle pathologies (Costa *et al.*, 2015).
- Although not required for this diagnosis, taut bands (i.e., contracture of muscle fibers) in the muscles may be present.
- TMJ disorders and pain, as well as systemic conditions (e.g., fibromyalgia), are frequently present in myofascial pain patients and should be considered when treatment is defined.
- The nociceptive information and transmission of the trigeminal system (responsible for masticatory pain sensation) is anatomically correlated with the upper cervical nerves (C1 to C3). Based on that, cervical myofascial pain can cause referred pain in trigeminal-related territories. In other words, one should be aware that cervical muscles are potential source of pain for face and head.
- Chronic and repetitive muscle contraction is frequently associated with myofascial pain. It has been suggested that some muscle fibers become overcontracted, leading to the pain sensation, associated with shortening of the muscle length (Mense and Gerwin, 2010).

Diagnostic Criteria

DC/TMD criteria for **Myofascial pain with referral** (Schiffman *et al.*, 2014). Sensitivity 0.86 and specificity 0.98.

Pain of muscle origin as defined for myalgia (Case 3.3) plus a referral of pain beyond the boundary of the masticatory muscle(s) being palpated, such as to the ear, teeth, or eye. Limitation of mandibular movement(s) secondary to pain may be present. Although not required for this diagnosis, taut bands (i.e., contracture of muscle fibers) in the muscles may be present.

History. Positive for both of the following:
1. Pain in the jaw, temple, ear, or in front of ear. AND
2. Pain modified with jaw movement, function, or parafunction.

Examination. Positive for all of the following:
1. Confirmation of pain location(s) in the temporalis or masseter muscle(s). AND
2. Report of familiar pain with palpation of the temporalis or masseter muscle(s). AND
3. Report of pain at a site beyond the boundary of the muscle being palpated.

ICHD-3 beta criteria for **Frequent tension-type headache** (Headache Classification Committee of the International Headache Society (IHS), 2013). Sensitivity and specificity have not been established.

Frequent episodes of headache, typically bilateral, pressing, or tightening in quality and of mild to moderate intensity, lasting minutes to days. The pain does not worsen with routine physical activity and is not associated with nausea, but photophobia or phonophobia may be present.

A. At least 10 episodes of headache occurring on 1–14 days per month on average for >3 months (≥12 and <180 days per year) and fulfilling criteria B–D.
B. Lasting from 30 min to 7 days.
C. At least two of the following four characteristics:
   1. bilateral location;
   2. pressing or tightening (nonpulsating) quality;
   3. mild or moderate intensity;
   4. not aggravated by routine physical activity, such as walking or climbing stairs.
D. Both of the following:
   1. no nausea or vomiting;
   2. no more than one of photophobia or phonophobia.
E. Not better accounted for by another ICHD-3 diagnosis.

Criteria for **Probable bruxism** (Lobbezoo *et al.*, 2013), see Case 4.11.

Fundamental Points

- As for many of TMD management therapies, most of the modalities for treating masticatory myofascial pain do not meet the scientific evidence-based criteria. So, noninvasive approaches must be the first choice.

- Multidisciplinary management is usually demanded for myofascial pain, and behavioral adjustments are extremely important for long-term success.

- Spray and stretch and trigger-point injections with local anesthetics (Figure 3.12) or dry needling are also recommended. It is not clear if it is the needling per se or the anesthesia of the muscle that relieves pain. Although controversial, the procedure of needling (with or without the injection) is supposed to produce a mechanical disturbance, responsible for creating a transient inflammatory environment, helping the process of taut band relaxation, and may be used as adjunct therapy for myofascial pain.

- The use of a short-lasting, cold stimulus is supposed to act as a counter irritation, stimulating large myelinated fibers, suppressing the pain sensation and allowing the muscle to stretch to its full length. Based on that principle, vapor coolant spray can be applied over the affected area, followed by passive stretching of the elevator masticatory muscles.

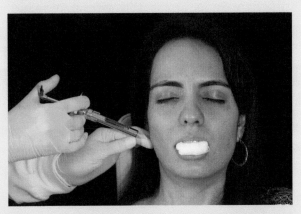

Figure 3.12 Trigger-point injection of the masseter muscle. After a careful palpation and determination of the muscle taut band, a needle is inserted into the muscle and moved around the painful area. This is followed by aspiration and injection of local anesthetic into the muscle.

Self-study Questions

1. Please list the clinical findings characteristics of "myofascial pain with referral" diagnosis.

2. What is the main goal of the spray/stretch technique in cases of myofascial pain?

3. Please list counselling and behavior modifications used in this case.

4. Why was a flat stabilization splint used as part of the management strategies?

References

Conti PC, de Alencar EN, da Mota Correa AS, et al. (2012) Behavioural changes and occlusal splints are effective in the management of masticatory myofascial pain: a short-term evaluation. *J Oral Rehabil* **39**:754–760.

Costa YM, Porporatti AL, Stuginski-Barbosa J, et al. (2015) Headache attributed to masticatory myofascial pain: clinical features and management outcomes. *J Oral Facial Pain Headache* **29**(4):323–330.

De Leeuw R, Klasser GD (eds) (2013) *Orofacial pain: Guidelines for assessment, diagnosis, and management*, 5th edn. Hanover Park, IL: Quintessence Publishing Co. Inc.

Fricton J, Look JO, Wright E, et al. (2010) Systematic review and meta-analysis of randomized controlled trials evaluating intraoral orthopedic appliances for temporomandibular disorders. *J Orofac Pain* **24**:237–254.

Headache Classification Committee of the International Headache Society (IHS) (2013) The International Classification of Headache Disorders, 3rd edition (beta version). *Cephalalgia* **33**(9):629–808.

Lobbezoo F, Ahlberg J, Glaros AG, et al. (2013) Bruxism defined and graded: an international consensus. *J Oral Rehabil* **40**(1):2–4.

Mense S, Gerwin RD (2010) *Muscle pain: understanding the mechanisms*. Berlin: Springer-Verlag.

Schiffman E, Ohrbach R, Truelove E, et al. (2014) Diagnostic Criteria for Temporomandibular Disorders (DC/TMD) for clinical and research applications: recommendations of the International RDC/TMD Consortium Network and Orofacial Pain Special Interest Group. *J Oral Facial Pain Headache* **28**(1):6–27.

Answers to Self-study Questions

1. Confirmation of pain location(s) in the temporalis or masseter muscles AND report of familiar pain with palpation of the temporalis or masseter muscle(s); AND report of pain at a site beyond the boundary of the muscle being palpated.

2. The use of a short-lasting cold stimuli, such as vapocoolant spray, is supposed to act as a counter irritation, stimulating large myelinated fibers, suppressing the pain sensation, and allowing the muscle to stretch to its full length.

3. Improve sleep quality, decrease exposure to stressful situations, implement relaxation

techniques, decrease caffeine intake, and avoid masticatory/cervical muscles over function. To practice home exercises, and to apply moist heat over the painful area for 15 min, two times a day, were also suggested. Patient was also encouraged to initiate regular aerobic exercises and to avoid the use of over-the-counter medication for pain.

4. Because it is considered the safest, not leading to significant occlusal alterations and it is relatively easy to fabricate. Muscle relaxation, decreasing overload to muscles, reestablishment of an "ideal" occlusion, cognitive and sensorial impulses alterations, and placebo effect are possible mechanisms of action.

Case 3.5

Temporalis Tendonitis

Ambra Michelotti

A. Demographic Data and Reason for Contact

- Italian female, 36 years old, unable to open her mouth as wide as previously, complaining of facial pain on the left side (Figure 3.13).

B. Symptom History

- Eight months prior, she began to experience facial pain on the left side. Pain was reported in the area of the cheek, the zygomatic arch, and the temple.
- From the same time she was complaining of pain also at the left upper dental arch. Periodically, she reported a burning pain inside the mouth at left cheek and gingiva, close to teeth 27–28.
- Present pain localized to the left masseter and temporalis region and intraorally on the left side.
- At present she reports a moderate pain with a characteristic pain intensity of 43 (NRS 0–100).
- At the same time started complaining of headache located in the temporalis area, two or three times per week.
- Both facial pain and headache were modified and worsened when chewing and when opening wider.
- No history of joint sounds and no previous limitation in mouth opening were reported.

C. Medical History

- Review of systems for eyes, ears, sinus, and teeth is negative.
- Cervical mobility is without complaint.
- No medications.
- Overall health is very good.
- No sleep-related problems.
- No smoking habit, minimal use of caffeine and alcohol.

D. Psychosocial History

- The patient is a shopkeeper with a medium socio-economic status. She is married and lives with her husband and two children.

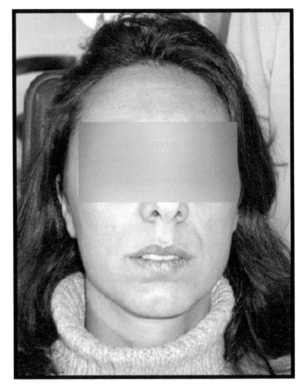

Figure 3.13 Italian female, 36 years old.

- She takes care of her body by doing gym exercises and yoga twice a week.
- Standardized testing indicates the following: low pain intensity and no pain-related disability (GCPS). Reported functional limitation especially in mastication and in movement (JFLS). High parafunction (OBCL), few physical symptoms (PHQ-15), no anxiety (GAD-7), but mild depression (PHQ-9).

E. Previous Consultations and Treatments

- Had previously visited three dentists; one made a diagnosis of aphthous stomatitis and prescribed topical medication, the second prescribed anti-inflammatory drugs, and the third hypothesized burning mouth syndrome. She also consulted a maxillofacial surgeon, who suggested extraction of the upper left third molar.

F. Extraoral Status

Asymmetries

- The maxilla and mandible were symmetrical.

Swelling or redness

- There was evidence of slight changes in tissue volume in the area of the left cheek.

Neurologic findings

- None noted.

Somatosensory abnormalities

- None detected during standard TMD examination. Special testing not performed.

Motor function abnormalities

- Bilateral masseter muscles exhibited normal contraction on requested clench, accompanied by pain. Tapping sounds of the teeth were singular and moderate in intensity.

Temporomandibular joint

- No TMJ noises were present during opening, closing, lateral, and protrusive movements. There was no pain on palpation. It was not possible to do TMJ manual translation because of intraoral pain.

Masticatory muscles

- Replication of familiar pain during palpation of left masseter muscle; replication of familiar pain and familiar headache during palpation of left temporalis muscle; replication of familiar pain during palpation of left temporalis tendon (Figure 3.14).

Jaw movement capacity

- The opening pattern is straight. Pain-free opening 14 mm; maximum unassisted opening 19 mm with familiar pain in left masseter, familiar pain in the zygomatic area, and temporalis pain familiar to the headache. Maximum assisted opening 21 mm, with the same familiar pain and familiar headache. Horizontal jaw movements 8 mm to the right, 9 mm to the left, and 6 mm in protrusion without notable deviation; all were pain free.

Neck

- Cervical mobility is normal for flexion, extension, bilateral rotation, and bilateral side-bend.

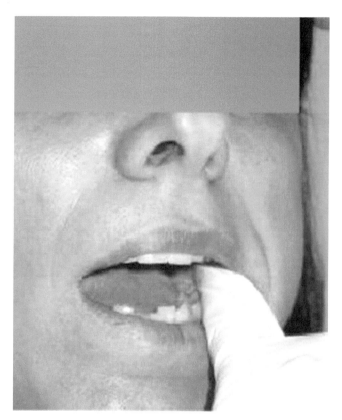

Figure 3.14 Palpation of left temporal tendon.

G. Intraoral Status

- Overbite 4 mm; overjet 3 mm; no deviation of midlines.
- Decubitus ulcer in buccal mucosa left side close to upper third molar.
- Swelling and redness in the gingiva and mucosa around the third upper left molar.

Occlusion

- Stable.

H. Additional Examinations and Findings

- None.

I. Diagnosis/Diagnoses

Expanded DC/TMD

- Tendonitis of left temporalis muscle.

DC/TMD

- Myalgia.
- Headache attributed to TMD.

J. Case Assessment

- The tendonitis of the temporalis muscle is secondary to overloading of the muscle tendon, consequent to parafunctional habits such as clenching. The consequence is severe pain and stiffness for the reduced elasticity of the tendon. Tendon stiffness leads to muscle pain and tightness. The therapy has to be started as soon as possible in order to avoid chronic tendonitis or tendinosis with tendon degeneration and loss of elasticity.

- Pain of the masticatory muscles during palpation and mandibular movements replicates the pain reported by the patient, allowing the diagnoses of myalgia of the left masseter and temporalis muscles and headache attributed to TMD (Schiffman et al., 2014; Schiffman and Ohrbach, 2016). These diagnoses are related to the same cause as tendonitis, meaning overloading of the masticatory muscles due to clenching.

- Limited mobility is a common TMD complaint with many possible causes. One possible cause could be disc displacement without reduction with limited opening. This is improbable for the following reasons: there was no history of joint sounds, no joint pain, no uncorrected deviation of opening pattern, lateral movements within normal limits and symmetric. On the contrary, a limited mobility due to muscular problems is characterized by a progressive limitation of mandibular opening and lateral movements within normal limits. A diagnosis of tendonitis requires that overall symptoms need to be considered in terms of identifying initial etiology and progression.

- Headache reported by the patient in the temporalis area was diagnosed as headache attributed to TMD as a consequence of the tendonitis. A differential diagnosis with migraine is necessary. However, the characteristic of the reported headache (not throbbing), the onset contemporary to the tendonitis, the headache located in the temple area and affected by jaw movement, function, or parafunction, and the replication of the headache with provocation testing (jaw movements and palpation of the temporalis muscle) fulfill the diagnostic criteria.

K. Evidence-based Treatment Plan including Aims

- Counselling is always a first approach. Provide reassurance regarding the recent state of the disease, explain the nature, the etiology, and the good prognosis of this benign disorder. Consider that the patient consulted different doctors without receiving a clear explanation. Reduce the inflammation of the tendon with NSAIDs. Reduce repetitive strain of the masticatory system, encourage rest and relaxation,

and control the amount of the masticatory activity. Thereafter, ask the patient to undertake stretching exercises for the jaw muscles. In order to stretch the muscles, the patient is asked to slowly open the mouth until she experiences an initial pain sensation. Then, she is invited to open the mouth a little bit more, positioning thumbs on the upper arch approximately on the premolar area and index fingers on the lower arch always on the premolar area (Michelotti et al., 2005; Armjio-Olivo et al., 2016).

- Start the treatment protocol for masticatory muscle pain and limited mouth opening. Exercise therapy is the cornerstone of rehabilitation of all regional musculoskeletal disorders, and the model for care is similar wherever the location of the musculoskeletal disease. The physiotherapy regimen includes several exercises with "self-management" that ameliorate coping for the patient. It has been suggested that these exercises help to relieve musculoskeletal pain and to restore normal function by reducing inflammation, decreasing and coordinating muscle activity, and promoting the repair and regeneration of tissue.
  - Stretching exercises to promote elasticity in contracted tendon and for reeducation of functional jaw movement.
  - Self-massage to the painful or tense masseter and temporalis muscles to prepare for movement reeducation.
  - Coordination exercises and postural reeducation to promote balanced structures as jaw muscles and neck muscles show a co-activity.
  - Superficial moist heat combined with ice can be used as palliative therapy.

L. Prognosis and Discussion

- Long-term prognosis is good for maintaining the functional opening slightly reduced for the coronoid process, and for muscular pain management.

- Self-management strategies have been effective and allowed the patient to maintain the results. The patient was followed up for 5 years (because her children had orthodontic treatment) and did not report any TMD sign or symptom.

- After 2 months the patient was pain free and showed increased mouth opening capacity from pain-free opening 14 mm before to pain free opening 43 mm at follow-up. The possible use of an occlusal stabilization splint to be worn during the night has been discussed with the patient in case of relapse of symptoms.

Background Information

- Temporalis tendonitis is a disorder of the fibrous insertion of the temporalis muscle tendons on the coronoid process of the mandible characterized by both inflammation and degeneration. It is often initiated by trauma and is often associated with TMJ and dental pathologies (Ernest *et al.*, 1991; Dupont and Brown, 2012). The temporalis tendonitis occurs at a lower rate compared with shoulder, elbow, or patella, and can be misdiagnosed with intracapsular TMJ disorders.
- Tendonitis is usually painful. Pain of tendon origin is affected by jaw movement, function, or parafunction, and is replicated with provocation testing of the masticatory tendon (palpation or mandibular movements). Limitation of mandibular movement(s) secondary to pain may be present. The temporalis tendon may be a common site of tendonitis and refer pain to the teeth and other nearby structures. Among masticatory muscles, tendonitis of the temporalis muscle is more commonly reported.
- Tendonitis is most commonly associated with an acute injury. Tendonitis injuries are more frequent in the shoulder and the elbow or at the Achilles and patellar tendons, with an estimated prevalence of 7%. They are related to specific sports or overuse. The patient reports pain, local stiffness, and a burning sensation due to inflammation.
- The history often show progressive loss of range of motion. The examination is positive for limited unassisted and assisted jaw movements, and opening will exhibit pain, sometimes severe.

Diagnostic Criteria

Expanded DC/TMD criteria for **Tendonitis** (Peck *et al.*, 2014). Sensitivity and specificity have not been established.

Pain of tendon origin affected by jaw movement, function, or parafunction, and replication of this pain with provocation testing of the masticatory tendon. Limitation of mandibular movement(s) secondary to pain may be present. The temporalis tendon may be a common site of tendonitis and refer pain to the teeth and other nearby structures. Tendonitis could also apply to other masticatory muscles' tendons.

History. Positive for the following:
1. Myalgia.

Examination. Positive for the following:
1. Myalgia in any tendon in the masticatory muscles, including the temporalis tendon.

Note: the pain is not better accounted for by another pain diagnosis.

DC/TMD criteria for **Myalgia**, see Case 3.3, and for **Headache attributed to TMD**, see Case 4.1 (Schiffman *et al.*, 2014).

Fundamental Points

Diagnosis

- Tendonitis is part of a musculoskeletal problem; therefore, all orthopedic principles should be utilized, including palpation, dynamic tests, and provocation tests, and evaluation of the end-feel that may be indicative of a muscle/tendon restriction.
- Assessment should include the following: within the masticatory system, altered length or hypertonicity of primary masticatory muscles. The temporalis muscle should be checked for the headache, and temporalis tendon has to be palpated for differential diagnosis. In this case, the diagnoses of tendonitis, myalgia, and headache attributed to TMD are the consequence of the same initiating factor: TMJ accessory motions and joint capsule mobility.

Treatment plan

- The treatment protocol is based on considering patient goals and duration of the disease. In this case the pain was relatively recent and the patient had a positive coping without particular psychosocial distress. Physical therapy has been used for decades for treating TMDs, and is considered the first treatment approach in musculoskeletal problems, although a multidisciplinary health-care approach may be required.
- The goals of physical therapy in the treatment of TMD, including tendonitis, are to decrease pain, enable muscle relaxation, reduce muscular hyperactivity and tendon stiffness, and

reestablish muscle function and joint mobility. One of the main advantages of physical therapy treatment is that not only is it reversible and noninvasive, but most importantly provides self-care management in an environment to create patient responsibility for their own health.

- Handing written instructions only is not correct. In good communication, it is advised to address the patient's experiences and expectations, build a partnership, present recommendations, and check for understanding and agreement. Further dental procedures should be avoided.

Management

- The stretch can be executed in a more dynamic hold–relax strategy or in a static stretch. The patient can also use a number of tongue depressors piled together, as a reference for the amount of jaw opening, by positioning the tongue depressors between arches without touching them with teeth; the patient is invited to add one tongue depressor a day to verify the increased mouth opening.
- Not all tendonitis will respond favorably to manual therapy, and there is the risk of chronicity and tendinosis. If necessary, it should be given a program of physical therapy (laser, ultrasound).
- Successful treatment of tendonitis should be constantly reevaluated across time, and changes should be made accordingly.
- Stress the importance of controlling muscle overuse and be sure that the patient memorizes the suggestion to maintain relaxation.
- Teach the patient to monitor range of motion and perform exercises when needed.
- Suggest a possible application of an occlusal stabilization splint for addressing exacerbations.

Self-study Questions

1. What are the main characteristics to differentiate between limited mouth opening due to skeletal problems, TMJ problems and muscular problems, tendinopathies?

2. What are the main characteristics to distinguish between headache attributed to TMD and migraine?

3. Acute pain patients differ importantly from chronic pain patients. What is the importance of the Axis II evaluation?

References

Armijo-Olivo S, Pitance L, Singh V, et al. (2016) Effectiveness of manual therapy and therapeutic exercise for temporomandibular disorders: systematic review and meta-analysis. *Phys Ther* **96**:9–25.

Dupont JS, Jr, Brown CE (2012) The concurrence of temporal tendinitis with TMD. *Cranio* **30**:131–135.

Ernest EA, III, Martinez ME, Rydzewski DB, Salter EG (1991) Photomicrographic evidence of insertion tendinosis: the etiologic factor in pain for temporal tendonitis. *J Prosthet Dent* **65**:127–131.

Michelotti A, de Wijer A, Steenks M, Farella M (2005) Home-exercise regimes for the management of non-specific temporomandibular disorders. *J Oral Rehabil* **32**:779–785.

Peck CC, Goulet JP, Lobbezoo F, et al. (2014) Expanding the taxonomy of the diagnostic criteria for temporomandibular disorders. *J Oral Rehabil* **41**:2–23.

Schiffman E, Ohrbach R, Truelove E, et al. (2014) Diagnostic Criteria for Temporomandibular Disorders (DC/TMD) for clinical and research applications: recommendations of the International RDC/TMD Consortium Network and Orofacial Pain Special Interest Group. *J Oral Facial Pain Headache* **28**(1):6–27.

Schiffman E, Ohrbach R (2016) Executive summary of the Diagnostic Criteria for Temporomandibular Disorders for clinical and research applications. *J Am Dent Assoc* **147**(6):438–445.

Answers to Self-study Questions

1. Myalgia with limited opening and tendonitis are characterized by muscular or tendon pain, progressive limitation of mandibular opening, and lateral movements within normal limits, end-feel elastic. Disc displacement without reduction with limited opening is characterized by joint pain (arthralgia), sudden reduced mouth opening, deviation of the mandible to the affected side during opening (if unilateral), limitation of contralateral movements (if unilateral), disappearance of the joint sound (if previously present).

2. The more commonly reported types of headache are tension-type headache and migraine. Tension-type headache is usually described as a pain that feels like a tight hat round the forehead or a weight on top of the head. Usually, the pain is moderate, bilateral, and is not aggravated by movements. Conversely, migraine presents a throbbing pain, with a severe intensity, disabling, and inhibits the movements of the body. Another type of headache is the headache attributed to TMD that is related to, and aggravate by TMDs. The headache must be located in the temple area, affected by jaw movement, function, or parafunction, and replicated by provocation testing of

the masticatory system. A diagnosis of pain-related TMD also has to be present.

3. According to the bio-psychosocial model, the Axis II evaluation is necessary mainly in chronic pain patients because pain involves both sensory and emotional domains. Thus, it is important to assess also the cognitive, psychosocial and behavioral factors that can contribute to chronicity and influence the treatment outcome.

Case 3.6

Masticatory Muscle Myositis

Malin Ernberg

A. Demographic Data and Reason for Contact
- Female, 37 years old.
- New patient presenting as an emergency because of pain and swelling left cheek (Figure 3.15).

B. Symptom History
- Continuous, dull, aching pain in left cheek since 3 months ago.
- Pain worsens with function (jaw opening, chewing).
- Limitations in jaw opening and chewing.
- Can only eat soup and mashed food due to inability to open mouth wide and muscle weakness upon chewing.
- Unaware of body temperature; does not think it is elevated.
- Patient recalls that the pain started a few days after uncomplicated treatment of left upper molar (filling) under local infiltration anesthesia.
- Characteristic pain intensity 57 (NRS 0–100), current pain intensity 5 NRS (0–10), no pain-related disability. Pain localized to left masseter muscle region (Figure 3.16). JFLS revealed severe limitation in chewing tough food, moderate in chewing chicken, crackers, and soft food, and severe limitation to open wide enough to bite into a whole apple and into a sandwich as well as to yawn. Reports no oral parafunctions (OBCL-21).

C. Medical History
- Previously healthy, no allergies. Paracetamol 500 mg gives short-lasting pain relief.
- Neck and shoulder muscles feel tense and ache at times (Figure 3.16). She believes this is attributed to her work as a cleaner.

D. Psychosocial History
- Born in Poland, living in Sweden for 15 years.
- Married, no children, lives in an apartment in a suburb of Stockholm. Satisfied with home situation.
- Work as a cleaner. Low income. Moderately satisfied with work situation.

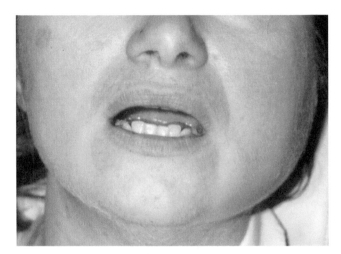

Figure 3.15 Facial photograph of patient.

- Describes herself as normally a quite calm person. At present resigned mood with low grade of depression according to PHQ-9, but no anxiety according to GAD-7. No physical symptoms according to PHQ-15. Low grade of stress according to PSS-10. Moderate sleep quality (PSQI).
- Nonsmoker and does not drink alcohol.

E. Previous Consultations and Treatments
- Sought her dentist a week after the treatment, who recommended expectation.
- After 2 weeks she received an occlusal appliance and instructed in jaw exercises. Her experience of jaw exercises was that they were too painful and did not do them. The occlusal appliance had no effect on symptoms.
- She was then referred to an oral and maxillofacial surgeon who gave intramuscular injections with local anesthetics and performed jaw stretching. No effect.

F. Extraoral Status
Face
- Edema and erythema left cheek.
- Increased skin temperature over left cheek.
- Glassy eyes.

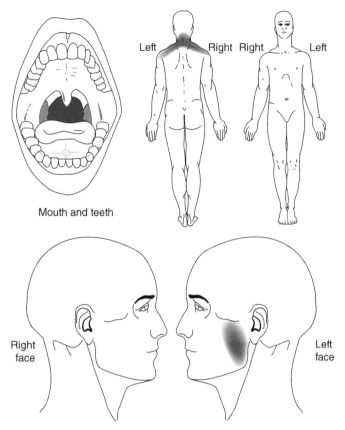

Figure 3.16 Pain drawing by patient.

Temporomandibular joint

- No joint sounds.
- No pain on palpation.

Masticatory muscles

- Left masseter feels firm and hard upon palpation.
- Familiar pain on palpation of masseter left side.
- Familiar pain in left masseter when clenching.
- No pain on palpation of other jaw muscles.

Jaw movement capacity

- Maximum unassisted and assisted jaw opening 11 mm. Familiar pain in left masseter at jaw opening.
- Reduced translatory movements due to pain, with slight deviation to the left side during protrusion.

Neck

- Normal movement capacity neck; no movement-evoked pain.
- Familiar bilateral pain upon palpation of the trapezius muscles.

G. Intraoral Status

Soft tissues

- Mild gingivitis in general, mucosa and tongue normal appearance, normal salivary flow from parotid ducts.

Hard tissues

- Full dentition except mandibular first molars (36, 46). Moderately restored teeth (amalgam/composite). Slight attrition canines. Vertical overbite 3 mm, horizontal overjet 2 mm. Normal sagittal relations.

Occlusion

- Bilateral contacts premolars and molars in intercuspal position. Canine and anterior guidance. Mediotrusive contact bilaterally second molars.

H. Additional Examinations and Findings

- In this case the glossy eyes lead the examiner to suspect an infection, but the patient did not think she had a fever. A venous blood sample was taken for analysis of CRP level and ESR. As she appeared at the clinic late in the afternoon it was decided that she should come back the next morning when the blood sample was analyzed and she had taken her morning temperature.
- Body temperature measurement revealed slight fever (morning temperature 37.9 °C).
- Serologic test revealed increased CRP (62 mg/L) and ESR (47 mm/h).

I. Diagnosis/Diagnoses

Expanded DC/TMD

- Myositis left masseter muscle.

DC/TMD

- Myalgia.

J. Case Assessment

- The cause of the infection could have been related to the dental treatment, perhaps due to hematoma from the injection in the vestibular region, spreading to the masseter muscle (Gallagher and Marley, 2003), but it might also have been spontaneous and just happened to coincide with the dental treatment.
- Medically the patient is healthy, and apart from occasional work-related neck–shoulder pain she has no other pains. The mild depressive symptoms are most probably a result of the chronic pain and the accompanied feeling of resignation.
- Differential diagnoses that should be considered include parotitis or tumors. Also, TMD myalgia of masticatory muscles may be considered.

K. Evidence-based Treatment Plan including Aims

Treatment goals

- To cure infection/inflammation and hence to relieve pain and restore jaw function.

Management

- As the myositis in this case was caused by an infection with affected general well-being, she received intravenous antibiotics for 1 week and then oral antibiotics for another week. The infection responded well to the treatment and after 1 week she was pain free and the swelling had declined. She was then recommended jaw stretch. After about 1 month the trismus had totally resolved.

L.   Prognosis and Discussion

- For localized myositis due to trauma or infection the prognosis is good. In the case presented the infection resolved after a few days of intravenous antibiotic treatment, and the inflammation and pain subsequently declined. In this case the patient had a minor influence of psychosocial symptoms on pain that were regarded as the result of the unsuccessful previous treatments leading to a chronic situation.

Thus, there was no need to specifically address this, but she was reassured that the treatment would relieve pain and that jaw function would be expected to be totally restored with time.

- The patient had visited several other clinics that had treated her as having myofascial pain or TMD myalgia. This had delayed proper treatment. Local myalgia of masticatory muscles sometimes may resemble myositis with pain and limited jaw opening, especially in early stages when swelling and erythema may be minor. However, in patients with myositis, usually the whole muscle is firm and hard upon palpation, whereas in local myalgia and myofascial pain the muscle may be tense, but not firm and hard with focal tenderness.
- It is important also to rule out parotitis and tumors as etiologic factors. These often show similar symptoms; that is, a firm, non-fluctuant swelling of the cheek and trismus, but usually are relatively painless (Jones *et al.*, 2003).

Background Information

- Localized myositis of masticatory muscles is a rare condition with only case reports presented in the literature (Conner and Duffy, 2008). The clinical characteristics include common signs of inflammation, such as swelling, erythema, and increased temperature over the affected muscle. Additional symptoms are pain at rest that worsens with function, and restrictions in jaw movements secondary to pain. The muscle often is tender and feels hard and firm upon palpation (Jones *et al.*, 2003).
- The etiology to myositis includes trauma, either macro or micro, infection, or systemic autoimmune disease, such as polymyositis and dermatomyositis. Sometimes calcification of the muscle can occur, so-called myositis ossificans.
- Myositis ossificans is described most frequently in male young athletes, most often in muscles susceptible to trauma, such as the flexor muscles of the upper arm, the quadriceps femoris, and the abductor muscles of the thigh (Demirkol *et al.*, 2015). Myositis ossificans of jaw muscles is rarer, mostly reported in the masseter muscle, but also the temporalis and medial pterygoid muscles may be affected. In up to 75% of cases of myositis ossificans in jaw muscles blunt trauma to the face is reported. A few cases are also reported after extraction or anesthetic injection (Conner and Duffy, 2008). CT/MRI scans reveal calcified tissue within the muscle.
- Another cause to myositis is a submasseteric abscess (Figure 3.17). This is a chronic localized infection between the muscle and the mandible, in a bare area or loose attachment between the layers of the deep and middle portions of the muscle (Jones *et al.*, 2003). The suggested most common causes for the infection are pericoronitis, mandibular third molar surgery, misdirected local anesthetics, osteomyelitis, and fractures, but it is also reported after extraction of a noninfected maxillary third molar (Gallagher and Marley, 2003).
- Myositis may also be secondary to systemic diseases, such as polymyositis and dermatomyositis, infections, or cancer. Polymyositis and dermatomyositis can occur at any age, from childhood to late adult life, and present with generalized muscle weakness, stiffness, and pain. In dermatomyositis there is also typically an erythematous skin rash over the joints co-joined with the other symptoms. Histological sections typically show that the muscle fibers are surrounded and invaded by mononuclear cells (Figure 3.18). Jaw muscles are rarely affected, but a few cases of trismus in patients with polymyositis and in children with dermatomyositis are described in the literature (Singer *et al.*, 1985; Singh *et al.*, 1997).

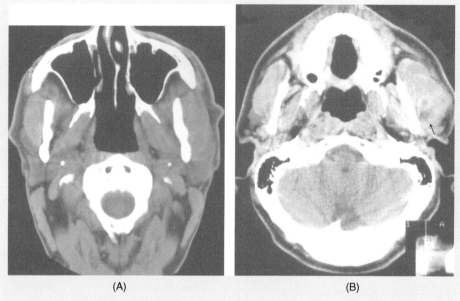

(A)   (B)

Figure 3.17 Submasseteric abscess of the left masseter muscle: (a) 6 months after lower left third molar extraction myositis of the masseter muscle is noted on CT; (b) 1 year after extraction the submasseteric abscess is visible on the radiograph (arrow). Incision and drainage yielded purulent material. *Source:* Jones *et al.* (2003). Reproduced with the permission of American Society of Neuroradiology.

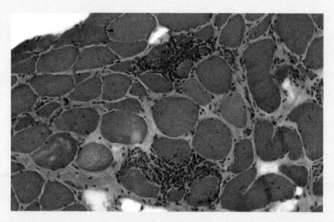

Figure 3.18 Histological biopsy section of a muscle affected by polymyositis. The muscle fibers are surrounded and invaded by mononuclear cells. *Source:* https://upload.wikimedia.org/wikipedia/commons/a/a2/Polymyositis_HE.jpg

Diagnostic Criteria

Expanded DC/TMD criteria for **Myositis** (Peck *et al.*, 2014). Sensitivity and specificity have not been established.

Pain of muscle origin with clinical characteristics of inflammation or infection: edema, erythema, and/or increased temperature. It generally arises acutely following direct trauma of the muscle or from infection, or chronically with autoimmune disease. Limitation of unassisted mandibular movements secondary to pain is often present. Calcification of the muscle can occur (i.e., myositis ossificans).

History.   Positive for the following:

1. Local myalgia.

Examination. Positive for both of the following, when examining the temporalis or masseter muscles:

1. Local myalgia.
AND
2. Presence of edema, erythema, and/or increased temperature over the muscle.

Laboratory testing.

1. Serologic tests may reveal elevated enzyme levels (e.g., creatine kinase), markers of inflammation, and the presence of autoimmune diseases.

Note: the pain is not better accounted for by another pain diagnosis.

DC/TMD criteria for **Local myalgia**, see Case 3.1 (Schiffman *et al.*, 2014).

Fundamental Points

- In most cases myositis is unilateral, which may guide diagnosis, although bilateral affection is reported in the literature.
- The reader should be reminded that the diagnostic criteria for myositis have not been validated. Therefore, to increase diagnostic accuracy, additional diagnostic tests are recommended.
- CT or MRI scans may show edema (Figure 3.17) and calcification (myositis ossificans) of the affected muscle.
- Serologic testing may reveal inflammatory markers such as elevated acute phase reactants, increased neutrophil count (if infection is present), and elevated enzyme levels such as creatine kinase, as well as autoimmune disease.
- The treatment should be directed toward the cause of the myositis in the individual case. If caused by an infection, the first goal should be to resolve this. Then management should be directed toward pain relief and restored function.
- For noninfectious myositis there are no evidence-based treatments. Treatment of myositis is therefore based on general recommendations for inflammations. Owing to its anti-inflammmatory effect, an NSAID (e.g., naproxen 250–500 mg × 2 for 2 weeks) is recommended for pain relief in the literature and

should be described. If the patient has gastric problems NSAIDs could be combined with a proton pump inhibitor (e.g., omeprazole). The patient is usually recommended rest, to avoid using the jaw, physical therapy (cold), and a soft diet until the swelling has resolved. Then jaw exercises, especially jaw stretch, are recommended to restore function (de Leeuw and Klasse, 2013).

- When the myositis is caused by submasseteric abscesses, incision and drainage is often needed. Antibiotics are recommended if the patient's general well-being is affected, bearing in mind that oral antibiotics may contribute to chronification of the infection (Jones *et al.*, 2003). In patients with myositis ossificans, surgery to remove calcified tissue is often needed to restore function.
- For patients with trismus due to polymyositis or dermatomyositis, corticosteroids (prednisolone) are reported to resolve trismus in most cases. However, about 20% do not respond to corticosteroids. For these patients methotrexate may be effective (Singer *et al.*, 1985; Singh *et al.*, 1997).

Self-study Questions

1. Discuss different possible causes of masticatory muscle myositis reflected in the literature.
2. Myositis may be mistaken as local TMD myalgia/myofascial pain. What are the clinical similarities and differences that may aid you to a correct diagnosis?
3. How can blood levels of creatine kinase be of help in diagnosing myositis?
4. Discuss the benefit of jaw exercises in the management of myositis?

References

Conner GA, Duffy M (2009) Myositis ossificans: a case report of multiple recurrences following third molar extractions and review of the literature. *J Oral Maxillofac Surg* **67**:920–926.

De Leeuw R, Klasser GD (eds) (2013) *Orofacial pain: Guidelines for assessment, diagnosis, and management*, 5th edn. Hanover Park, IL: Quintessence Publishing Co. Inc.

Demirkol M, Aras MH, Tutar E (2015) Myositis ossificans circumscripta in the masseter muscle mimicking phleboliths. *J Craniofac Surg* **26**:2020–2021.

Gallagher J, Marley J (2003) Infratemporal and submasseteric infection following extraction of a non-infected maxillary third molar. *Br Dent J* **194**:307–309.

Jones KC, Silver J, Millar WS, Mandel L (2003) Chronic submasseteric abscess: anatomic, radiologic, and pathological features. *AJNR Am J Neuroradiol* **24**(6):1159–1163.

Peck CC, Goulet JP, Lobbezoo F, et al. (2014) Expanding the taxonomy of the diagnostic criteria for temporomandibular disorders. *J Oral Rehabil* **41**:2–23.

Schiffman E, Ohrbach R, Truelove E, et al. (2014) Diagnostic Criteria for Temporomandibular Disorders (DC/TMD) for clinical and research applications: recommendations of the International RDC/TMD Consortium Network and Orofacial Pain Special Interest Group. *J Oral Facial Pain Headache* **28**(1):6–27.

Singer PA, Chikarmane A, Festoff BW, Ziegler DK (1985) Trismus. An unusual sign in polymyositis. *Arch Neurol* **42**:1116–1118.

Singh S, Kumar L, Shankar KR (1997) Juvenile dermatomyositis in north India. *Indian Pediatr* **34**:193–198.

Answers to Self-study Questions

1. The most common causes to masticatory myositis reported in the literature are blunt trauma to the face, third molar surgery, and pericoronitis, causing spreading infection to the masseter, medial pterygoid muscle, and/or temporalis muscle. Another probable cause is intramuscular bleeding from local anesthetic injections causing an encapsulated hematoma. Also, tumors and autoimmune diseases, such as polymyositis, dermatomyositis, SLE, may involve jaw muscles.

2. Both TMD myalgia and myositis present with familiar pain on palpation of masticatory muscles and both may show reduced jaw opening. In fact, according to the suggested diagnostic criteria (Peck *et al.*, 2014), a diagnosis of myalgia must be present also in myositis. Even muscle swelling may be present in myalgia, but then caused by muscle hypertrophy. To differentiate between them, signs of infections (fever) and inflammation (erythema, increased temperature) are not seen in TMD myalgia. In myositis, often the whole muscle feels hard and firm and is tender upon palpation, whereas in myalgia the tenderness is more focal. Finally, in myositis the trismus is more severe and it is often not possible to regain normal jaw opening, even during assisted opening.

3. Creatine kinase catalyzes the conversion of creatine and adenosine triphosphate (ATP) to phosphocreatine and adenosine diphosphate. Tissues with high metabolic activity (i.e., that rapidly consume ATP), such as muscle, are rich in phosphocreatine, which serves as an energy reservoir. Creatine kinase is a sensitive measure of muscle damage (i.e., necrosis, degeneration, and regeneration) as it leaks from damaged cells. Thus, in myositis, elevated levels of creatine kinase are often seen. The most common cause of elevated creatine kinase levels, however, is exercise.

4. Physical exercise is shown to be effective in the treatment of myositis, including poly- and dermatomyositis. It is therefore probable that jaw exercises are effective also in the treatment of myositis in masticatory muscles, even if evidence for this is lacking in the literature. It is important to restore function as muscle damage due to myositis otherwise may lead to contracture with more or less permanent restriction of jaw opening (see also Case 3.7).

B: Other Masticatory Muscle Disorders

Case 3.7

Contracture

Richard Ohrbach and Dorothy Foigelman-Holland

A. Demographic Data and Reason for Contact

- Female, 60 years old, unable to open her mouth as wide as previously (Figure 3.19).

B. Symptom History

- Thirty-five years prior, she was the passenger in a car involved in a motor vehicle collision; her car was hit from behind at the same time as her head was turned to the side window and she had a whiplash trauma. Within a month, she began to experience facial pain and mechanical problems of the jaw and was no longer able to open as wide. Functionally, she could no longer bite into a whole apple.
- Three years later the right TMJ received a silastic implant and the left TMJ received a disc repair. New symptoms emerged in the right TMJ, and the silastic implant was removed; residual scar tissue was allowed to replace the disc.
- Following implant removal, chewing triggered minor pain and some limitation, but otherwise her jaw condition was self-managed well.
- About 2 months prior to this consultation, a fractured mandibular tooth underlying a loose crown was extracted as part of a long dental appointment, and postoperative jaw opening was limited to a few millimeters; this gradually improved over about 6 weeks, during which her symptoms were affected by chewing, opening, and other jaw activities. Now her jaw opening has returned to her "normal."

C. Medical History

- Occipital headaches, attributed to cervical spine arthritis. Previous 10-year history of bad headaches following the motor vehicle collision 35 years ago.
- Review of systems for eyes, ears, sinus, and teeth is negative.
- Cervical mobility is without complaint, though left upper extremity paresthesias occur on occasion, attributed to the cervical arthritis.
- Acid reflux well-managed with Prilosec®.

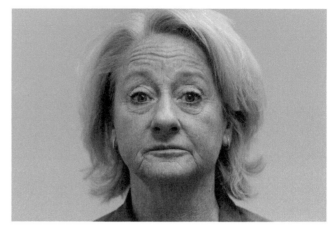

Figure 3.19 Slight facial asymmetry with prominence of chin deviated to patient's left. There was no functional or symptom history significance to this asymmetry, and the asymmetry was judged to be within normal range.

- No other medications.
- Overall health is "great."
- Sleep onset is immediate, and sleep is maintained well; however, sleep is never restorative.
- One caffeinated beverage daily and minimal alcohol.

D. Psychosocial History

- Following the motor vehicle collision 35 years prior, she coped with the consequences and continued to function at a high level.
- Mood is excellent.
- She presently owns and manages a dance studio, which is very challenging as a business, but she reports that this is very positive.
- Standardized testing indicates the following: low characteristic pain intensity and no pain-related disability (GCPS); pain localized solely to the left preauricular region, including both TMJ and masseter inferior to the joint (pain manikin); severe limitation with chewing tough food, but no limitation from chicken, crackers, or soft food, and severe limitation to open wide enough to bite into a whole apple and

moderate limitation with opening wide enough to bite into a sandwich, and no opening limitation otherwise (JFLS); no parafunctional behaviors other than leaning jaw on the hand some of the time, unilateral chewing all of the time, and singing most of the time (OBCL); mild physical symptoms (PHQ-15); normal for anxiety (GAD-7) and depressive symptoms (PHQ-9).

E.   Previous Consultations and Treatments
- No other treatments for her jaw are reported.

F.   Extraoral Status
Asymmetries
- Slight facial asymmetry with prominence of chin deviated to patient's left. There was no functional or symptom history significance to this asymmetry, and the asymmetry was judged to be within normal range (Figure 3.19).

Swelling or redness
- There is no evidence of changes in tissue volume or tone, and skin color is uniform across the distribution of the trigeminal system.

Neurologic findings
- Bilateral masseter muscles exhibit normal contraction on requested clench. Tapping sounds of the teeth are singular and moderate in intensity.

Somatosensory abnormalities
- None detected during standard TMD examination. Special testing not performed.

Motor function abnormalities
- None noted.

Temporomandibular joint
- TMJ noises are present in the left TMJ during opening, closing, and horizontal movements, without pain. There is no pain from palpation. TMJ translation is resistant to traction on the right side but is normal on the left side.

Masticatory muscles
- No masticatory muscles exhibit pain from palpation.

Jaw movement capacity
- Pain-free opening 35 mm, maximum unassisted opening 38 mm with left masseter pain replicating pain of recent post-dental treatment complication, and maximal assisted opening 40 mm that was

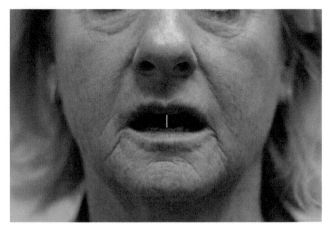

Figure 3.20 Mouth slightly open, displaying alignment of dental midlines (white solid line).

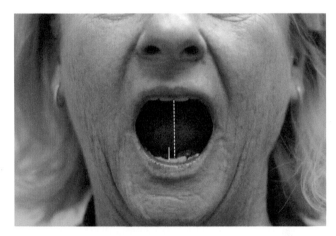

Figure 3.21 Maximal unassisted opening, with mandible deviated to the patient's right. Note solid white line positioned at dental midline, relative to the dashed reference line in the mid-sagittal plane extending from the incisal embrasure of the maxillary central incisors.

terminated by patient due to concern, with slightly yielding end-feel and without pain. Deviation of 5 mm to the right on maximal opening (Figures 3.20 and 3.21). Horizontal jaw movements are 10 mm to the right, 5 mm to the left, and 3 mm in protrusive without notable deviation; all are pain free.

Neck
- Cervical mobility is normal for flexion, extension, bilateral rotation, and bilateral side-bend.

G.   Intraoral Status
Soft tissues and hard tissues
- Unremarkable.

Occlusion
- Unremarkable.

Saliva
- Not evaluated.

H. Additional Examinations and Findings
Physical therapy consultation was requested in order to assess for any other treatment options. Evaluation revealed the following:
- Normal seated and standing postural curves. Negative cervical spine segmental screen for somatic dysfunction.
- Symmetrical hypertonic cervical extensors with full cervical spine active and passive range of motion.
- Palpation pain present in the submandibular muscles on the left, as examined intraorally, adjacent to the prior tooth extraction site, and in the symmetrical cervical extensors. Palpation pain and tightness absent in the sublingual muscles. Palpation tightness and pain in the medial aspect of the bilateral masseter muscles.
- Inferior and anterior glide of the TMJ resistant to passive mobilization on the right side.
- Initial maneuvers of grade 1–3 inferior and inferior–anterior mandibular glides until accessory motion was restored resulted in short-term reduction in resistance to the mobilizations, with gain of 2–3 mm in jaw opening with less deviation, demonstrating viability of possible improvement in opening.

I. Diagnosis/Diagnoses
Expanded DC/TMD
- Bilateral masseter contracture.

Other
- Right TMJ capsular contracture.

J. Case Assessment
- The contracture of the masseter muscles and right TMJ capsule are secondary to prolonged limitation in opening which was a consequence of the TMJ mechanical disc problems associated with an motor vehicle collision 35 years previously and not addressed at that time. Because of the 3 year period during which the mechanical disc problems continued, loss of normal resting length of the masseter muscles would have likely occurred; the limitation in opening due to contracture versus the limitation in opening due to the mechanical disc problems can be very challenging to distinguish, and given the history of the whiplash trauma (see Case 3.10) and the clear history of mechanical disc problems, treatment was focused primarily on the disc problems, and the contracture was not addressed.
- The left TMJ sounds at present meet the criteria for disc displacement with reduction; however, those sounds are not relevant in terms of chief complaint or functional status, given the absence of mechanical locking, and therefore this diagnosis is set aside and further investigation via MRI is not recommended.
- The contracture is presently stable but is also responsive to guarding behaviors, evident on examination and supported by history, resulting in nonsymmetrical restriction on opening.
- History of recent trismus was secondary to a dental treatment visit; possible causes include injection trauma by the anesthesia, prolonged mouth opening, force on the mandible during extraction, and exacerbation of factors associated with perpetuating the chronic contracture. The relatively fast recovery was in part due to her self-management skills and determination to return to her prior level of functioning.
- Medically and psychosocially, she is doing extremely well, and there are no identified major risk factors at this time for active contribution to the contracture; therefore, the contracture is regarded as stable.
- While the patient would like to open her mouth wider, she is realistic and would rather remain with the current restrictions and mild symptoms that she effectively self-manages than risk aggravating the condition with new treatment that may not yield substantial benefits.

K. Evidence-based Treatment Plan including Aims
- Provide reassurance regarding the temporary state of the recent trismus and the continued stability of the contracture in the absence of any further treatment.
- Describe, as part of patient education, possible treatment as follows, recognizing that the model for care is based on that which has been developed for adhesive capsulitis of the shoulder (see later):
  - Manual therapy to promote elasticity in contracted capsule and ligaments.
  - Massage to hypertonic muscles to prepare for movement reeducation.
  - Postural reeducation to promote balanced structures and optimal muscle length and strength.

- Exercise for reeducation of functional jaw movement.
- Stretching to tolerance to retain or gain motion.

L. Prognosis and Discussion

- Patient has adapted to limited opening due to chronic contractures and she experienced a loss of jaw opening following a recent dental procedure; it is likely that the chronic contracture contributed to the development of the trismus, first via restricted opening that hindered normal dental procedures (e.g., more strain was placed on the mandible for sufficient intraoral access), and second via loss of normal soft tissue elasticity, such that the tissues did not recover normally from any prolonged stretch during the dental procedure.
- Long-term prognosis remains favorable for retaining a functional opening and restoring any remaining lost mobility following the recent dental procedures.
- Self-management strategies have been effective and include gradual stretching and awareness of posture, and maintaining cervical spine mobility and elasticity of masticatory and cervical soft tissues.

Background Information

- The most dramatic form of musculoskeletal contracture depicts arms and legs unable to straighten, stuck in bent angles with minimal hope of returning to normal. In contrast, we focus here on musculoskeletal contracture that involves the abnormal shortening of muscle and which may also include the associated tendons as well as joint ligaments and capsule. Most such contractures are not dramatic but rather are often inadequately identified.
- Contractures are most commonly associated with prior trauma and prolonged immobilization. One of the most common non-trauma etiologies, and for which good data exist, is adhesive capsulitis of the shoulder ("frozen shoulder"), which has estimated prevalence of 2–5% of the general population (Reeves, 1975). Masticatory system contractures probably occur at a much lower rate.
- Loss of mobility within the masticatory system can occur without rapid detection because most individuals have greater jaw mobility than required for typical functional demands of food ingestion; by one study, 95% of the US adult population exhibit a maximal nonassisted jaw opening of 39 mm or greater, more than sufficient for food ingestion (Ohrbach et al., 2011).

- An initial loss of jaw mobility is readily compensated by adaptive movements permitted by the bilateral joint system. Because initial mobility losses are often undetected, an insidious development of contractures in muscle and associated connective tissues may occur. Within the masticatory muscles, the prevalence of contracture is unknown but believed to be much lower than the prevalence of masticatory muscle myalgia, for example. Challenges in both diagnosis and treatment accompany this condition.
- There are no published data regarding demonstrated etiologic pathways for masticatory muscle contracture. Extrapolating from other joints for which mechanisms have been established, the available evidence suggests the following as contracture mechanisms of the masticatory system: altered biomechanics likely predispose the TMJ to develop contractures, and altered mandibular posture (a deviation from anatomic neutral which alters muscle length–strength relationships) likely sets the stage for contractures.
- If the primary mechanism of contracture in the jaw targets the masticatory muscles, then such contractures most certainly lead to altered biomechanics of the TMJ, thereby establishing a positive feedback loop leading to yet further worsening of a muscle contracture.
- Time is the major factor affecting contracture severity: the longer a muscle or joint tissue is maintained in a shortened position, the more likely that reduced mobility will become permanent and have repercussions throughout that system and adjacent musculoskeletal system.

Diagnostic Criteria

Expanded DC/TMD criteria for **Contracture** (Peck et al., 2014). Sensitivity and specificity have not been established.

The shortening of a muscle due to fibrosis of tendons, ligaments, or muscle fibers. It is usually not painful unless the muscle is overextended. A history of radiation therapy, trauma, or infection is often present. It is more commonly seen in the masseter or medial pterygoid muscle.

History. Positive for the following:

1. Progressive loss of range of motion.

Examination. Positive for the following:

1. Unassisted and assisted jaw movements are limited (i.e., for jaw closing muscles, opening will be limited to an assisted opening of <40 mm and assisted opening will demonstrate a hard end-feel (firm, unyielding resistance to assisted movements).

Fundamental Points

Diagnosis

- Contracture is defined as a shortening of a muscle fiber due to fibrosis of tendons, ligaments, or muscle fibers.
- Contracture is usually not painful unless the muscle is overextended. A history of radiation therapy, trauma, or infection is often present. Among masticatory structures, contracture is more commonly seen in the masseter or medial pterygoid muscle.
- While limited mobility may be the most common TMD complaint, a diagnosis of contracture requires that overall system functioning needs to be considered in terms of identifying initial etiology and progression. Consequently, assessment must extend beyond the identified problem; however, current diagnostic frameworks are inadequate to address all possible considerations and critical problem-solving of the following elements should be considered.
- Utilizing established orthopedic principles (Rocabado and Iglarsh, 1991), a thorough evaluation of the masticatory system recognizes it as part of a dynamic musculoskeletal complex, influenced by posture, kinesthetic awareness, and proprioceptive skill.
- Assessment should include the following: within the masticatory system, altered length or hypertonicity of primary masticatory muscles and accessory muscles of the throat and hyoid, TMJ accessory motions and joint capsule mobility; and within the cervical system, muscle length, cervical spine mobility, posture, and segmental joint motion.
- A yielding end-feel may be indicative of a contracture that may respond favorably to treatment (Wong *et al.*, 2015). Gentle palpation of sublingual, submandibular, suprahyoid, and infrahyoid muscles to detect imbalance, restrictions, guarding, and pain leads to additional treatment options.
- Taut fibrous bands, spasm, and areas of pain referral should be considered within both systems as possible indicators of altered biomechanics of resting position, speech, and eating, recognizing that existing data indicate that these findings are less reliable due to poor operationalization of evaluation methods.
- Differential diagnosis of contracture includes trismus and avoidance (guarding) due to pain; both are distinguished by history and examination. Trismus is described earlier. Deviated opening to one side may be an obvious clinical indicator of contracture, or it may indicate avoidance of stretch-induced pain associated with the affected masseter during attempted straight opening. The latter condition is quite common amongst patients with TMD, often detected only by careful observation of the mandibular pattern on opening and where detection is facilitated by slowing the rate of the opening movement. That the muscle can distend normally precludes this condition from being classified as a contracture; however, we bring attention to this clinical observation because we believe that, if not directly addressed, over time this avoidance pattern can lead to a contracture of the affected muscle and ipsilateral joint capsule.

Treatment plan

- Decision-making is based on consideration of patient goals, needs, and duration of contracture. Each individual's ability to tolerate short-term discomfort will dictate future decisions to move forward. The pain of aggressive therapeutic stretching continues until soft tissue has been sufficiently reorganized. The shoulder model of adhesive capsulitis also informs the approach outlined here (Johnson *et al.*, 2007; Neviaser and Hannafin, 2010).

- The evidence for treating masticatory system contractures is limited to a small number of anecdotal reports. Consequently, our recommendations for treatment rely on our understanding of all mechanisms underlying muscle facilitation, which in turn lead to a logical and effective approach to treat contractures of the masticatory system (Steindler, 1935; Rocabado and Iglarsh, 1991).
- Treatments for contracture include doing nothing, physical therapy by self or therapist, intraarticular corticosteroid injections when the joint is inflamed, closed manipulation, and arthroscopic capsular release (Hannafin and Chiaia, 2000).
- Goals of physical therapy-based treatment for soft tissues affected by contracture are (1) increase extensibility of the affected muscle and capsule, (2) use symptom-based pain management techniques during active treatment, (3) restore normal functional patterns of the affected system, (4) identify barriers to progress during treatment, (5) identify risk factors for exacerbations and relapse, and (6) insure adherence to any self-management program.

Management
- Treatment to increase the extensibility of contracted soft tissues can include the following: (1) Therapist application of manual pressure in the forms of active range of motion, contract–relax techniques, gentle overpressure, and soft tissue massage. Fibrous muscle bands respond to stroking (in the direction of) or strumming (across the direction of) muscle fibers. (2) Pain-free mobilizations of the TMJ can lengthen non-contractile tissues of the joint capsule and thereby restore accessory motion and reduce resistance to active and passive stretch of the muscles. (3) Regular heat applications. (4) Restore functional mandibular opening while avoiding inflammation-inducing strain on the joint and muscles (Hammer, 2007; Johnson *et al.*, 2007; Neviaser and Hannafin, 2010).
- Neutral or optimal head and neck alignment is attempted during joint mobilization and all exercises in order to foster balanced integration of new movement patterns.

- Risk factors, such as future dental procedures or stress reactivity, as well as patient education for managing a recurrence of pain and increased limitation, must be addressed.
- Neuromuscular reeducation for symmetrical opening can use slow movement and visual feedback from a mirror so that reeducation and awareness of movement are achieved.
- Not all contractures will respond favorably to manual intervention, but if manual therapy to the joint capsule is applied properly (pain-free graduated forces) then observable gains can generally be accomplished.
- Self-managed exercises are a required adjunct to manual therapy and at times the only intervention required if the contracture is not too long-standing. Observation of exercise quality to avoid pain and asymmetry is paramount to achieving goals.
- Successful treatment of contractures requires small corrections persistently made across time.

Relapse prevention
- Correlating history with physical findings to develop a working hypothesis on how this came to be helps unravel it.
- Implement patient-based method for monitoring range of motion in order to maintain full extensibility of the muscle affected by contracture.
- Develop a rescue plan for addressing exacerbations.

Self-study Questions

1. Under what circumstances would a unilateral muscle contracture, as per the diagnostic criteria from Peck *et al.* (2014), be regarded as an isolated problem?

2. How should a clinician proceed with a broader, "system" assessment when there are no firm guidelines in place for conducting a reliable and valid examination at that system-level, and the diagnostic interpretations as presented here are not yet validated?

3. Does the persistence of a contracture in either masticatory muscles or TMJ act as a risk factor for other problems affecting the masticatory system?

4. A patient with chronic contracture is functioning adequately but not without some symptoms that

every so often become exacerbated into significant bouts of pain and limited function; the patient is concerned that in the absence of treatment, such flare-ups will continue. Given the concern about system integration for healthy adaptive functioning, should the patient be treated?

References

Hammer WI (2007) *Functional soft-tissue examination and treatment by manual methods*, 3rd edn. Burlington, MA: Jones & Bartlett Learning.

Hannafin JA, Chiaia TA (2000) Adhesive capsulitis: a treatment approach. *Clin Orthop Relat Res* **372**:95–109.

Johnson AJ, Godges JJ, Zimmerman GJ, Ounanian LL (2007) The effect of anterior versus posterior glide joint mobilization on external rotation range of motion in patients with shoulder adhesive capsulitis. *J Orthop Sports Phys Ther* **37**(3):88–99.

Neviaser AS, Hannafin JA (2010) Adhesive capsulitis: a review of current treatment. *Am J Sports Med* **38**(11):2346–2356.

Ohrbach R, Fillingim RB, Mulkey F, et al. (2011) Clinical findings and pain symptoms as potential risk factors for chronic TMD: descriptive data and empirically identified domains from the OPPERA case–control study. *J Pain* **12**(11, Supplement 3):T27–T45.

Peck CC, Goulet J-P, Lobbezoo F, et al. (2014) Expanding the taxonomy of the diagnostic criteria for temporomandibular disorders. *J Oral Rehabil* **41**(1):2–23.

Reeves B (1975) The natural history of the frozen shoulder syndrome. *Scand J Rheumatol* **4**(4):193–196.

Rocabado M, Iglarsh ZA (1991) *The musculoskeletal approach to maxillofacial pain*. Philadelphia, PA: Lippincott Williams and Wilkins.

Steindler A (1935) *Mechanics of normal and pathological locomotion in man*. Baltimore, MD: Charles C Thomas.

Wong K, Trudel G, Laneuville O (2015) Noninflammatory Joint contractures arising from immobility: animal models to future treatments. *Biomed Res Int* **2015**:848290.

Answers to Self-study Questions

1. Muscle contracture, while identified as a specific problem associated with a given tissue, should be first considered to be the observable part of a larger system problem, and only after evaluating the system as a whole should a given contracture be considered an isolated result and managed as such; otherwise, the system should be treated.

2. The art of clinical medicine always requires finding a balance between generalized knowledge, specialized knowledge that emerges from experience but not yet codified by research, and the particular array of findings within the specific history of a given patient. Using methods with either poor or no evidence for validity, when such methods are the only ones available for use with a given patient's complaint, should be done with the full awareness of the limitations inherent in such methods; in other words, the clinician must be careful to not overinterpret such findings.

3. Because contractures are part of a system, their persistence can affect overall functioning, even in the individual who has adapted well to the limitation imposed by the contracture, and such adaptations are themselves factors that can increase risk for further problems.

4. Exploration of other risk factors that may account for the recurrent flare-ups is an essential step before concluding that alteration of the contracture is considered. TMD seldom occurs in response to a single risk factor.

Case 3.8

Masticatory Muscle Hypertrophy

Malin Ernberg

A. Demographic Data and Reason for Contact

- Male, 21 years old.
- Referred to specialist clinic because of mild pain and swelling left cheek (Figure 3.22).

B. Symptom History

- Gradually increasing swelling right cheek last year.
- Intermittent mild, aching pain right cheek.
- Pain worsens with chewing.
- Mild tenderness right cheek.
- Characteristic pain intensity 13 (NRS 0–100), current pain intensity 0 (NRS 0–10), no pain-related disability. Pain primarily localized to right masseter muscle and TMJ, but mild pain eventually occurs also left masseter region, especially in morning. JFLS reveals no limitation in jaw function. No frequent gum chewing, but reports grinding and clenching a few nights per week (girlfriend has noticed) and daytime grinding and clenching, as well as press, touch, or hold teeth together other than while eating and to hold or jut jaw to the side frequently while studying and some other daytime parafunctions (OBCL).

C. Medical History

- Previously healthy, allergic to pollen, cats, dogs, and horses.
- Broke his left arm when cycling as a child and has had some blows to the body during floorball play, but no severe hits and no fractures.
- Frequent headache localized to forehead, temples, and back of head. Headache is sometimes present at awakening, but may also develop throughout the day. Neck and shoulder muscles often feel sore. Otherwise no pains.

D. Psychosocial History

- Single, no children, lives in an apartment in Stockholm. Satisfied with home situation.
- Studying second year at Stockholm University (mathematics); plans for a master's degree. Very

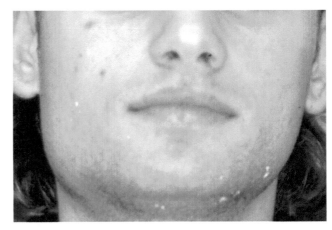

Figure 3.22 Facial photograph of patient.

satisfied with school situation. Frequent computer work.
- Exercises regularly at a gym and plays floorball once per week.
- Describes himself as a calm person, but with high current stress level due to demanding studies. He felt a little lacking in energy, but has no depression according to PHQ-9 and no anxiety according to GAD-7 No physical symptoms according to PHQ-15. Low grade of stress according to PSS-10. Moderately good sleep quality.
- Nonsmoker, moderate alcohol consumption.

E. Previous Consultations and Treatment

- Patient noticed the swelling on the cheek and consulted a general physician.
- Referred to hospital for further examination to rule out tumor by a CT scan. No tumor was found.

F. Extraoral Status

Face

- Facial asymmetry with a single, large swelling of approximately 4 cm in diameter in anterior–posterior direction present on the right angle area of the mandible (Figure 3.22).

Temporomandibular joint

- Left-side clicking at opening and closing movement.
- No pain on palpation.

Masticatory muscles

- Right masseter feels firm and hard upon palpation.
- Familiar pain on palpation masseter and temporalis muscle right side (familiar to his headache) and left lateral pterygoid muscle. No referred pain on palpation.
- No pain on palpation of other jaw muscles.

Jaw movement capacity

- Maximum unassisted jaw opening 55 mm; maximum assisted jaw opening 57 mm. No pain.
- Laterotrusion to the right 10 mm, left 11 mm; protrusion 8 mm. No pain.

Neck

- Normal movement capacity neck; no movement-evoked pain.
- No pain to palpation neck muscles (trapezius, sternocleidomastoideus).

G. Intraoral status

Soft tissues

- Bilateral mucosal ridging buccal mucosa. No tongue scalloping. Normal salivary flow.

Hard tissues

- Full dentition except mandibular third molars. Few restorations (occlusal composite fillings first mandibular molars). Slight attrition canines, more evident wear right side where active bruxism facets were noted. Vertical overbite 2 mm; horizontal overjet 2 mm. Normal sagittal relations.

Occlusion

- Bilateral contacts premolars and molars in intercuspal position. Canine and anterior guidance. Mediotrusive contact tooth 27, no laterotrusive or protrusive interferences.

H. Additional Examinations and Findings

- CT scan revealed an enlarged masseter muscle right side, but with otherwise normal appearance (Figure 3.23).

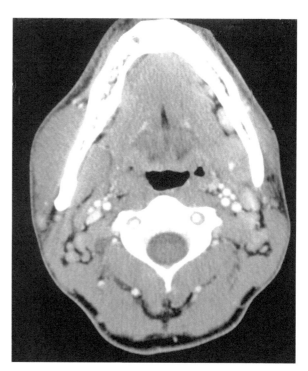

Figure 3.23 CT showing right side masseter (and pterygoid muscle) hypertrophy.

I. Diagnosis/Diagnoses

Expanded DC/TMD

- Hypertrophy right masseter muscle.

DC/TMD

- Myalgia.
- Headache attributed to TMD.
- Disc displacement with reduction left TMJ.

J. Case Assessment

- From the OBCL it was apparent that the patient was aware of frequent day- and nighttime parafunctions, and when questioned in detail about it he recalled that he frequently was grinding the canines on the right side when studying (Figure 3.24). This had started as a bad habit, but now he did not think so much about it. He had noted that his jaw muscle pain and headache worsened when he was more stressed, such as before exams.
- The signs of attrition and bruxism facets on the right canines supported that the hypertrophy was due to unilateral tooth grinding.
- Medically the patient was healthy. Neck–shoulder pain and headache deemed to be work- and stress-related. Because of the demanding studies he felt stressed but said that the stress was under control.
- There were no signs of dental infections and no suspicion of parotitis or myositis. To rule out the

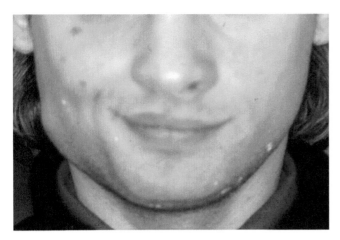

Figure 3.24 Patient showing how he grinds his teeth at the right side. The hypertrophic masseter is clearly visible.

suspicion of tumor he was referred for a CT examination.

K. Evidence-based Treatment Plan including Aims

Treatment goals

- To reduce muscle hyperactivity and relieve pain.

Management

- The patient was informed about the nonmalignant condition and the cause of the muscle enlargement. He was also informed about the relation between psychosocial stress and bruxism and of "work hygiene" during computer work and studies and instructed in relaxation techniques. To avoid daytime grinding he was recommended visual feedback, and an occlusal appliance was made to reduce nighttime muscle activity. He was followed for 3 months, during which time the jaw muscle pain and morning headache totally disappeared. He still eventually had headache in the daytime, but much less frequent. The muscle hypertrophy was still there but did not bother him.

L. Prognosis and Discussion

- As masticatory muscle hypertrophy is a benign condition the prognosis is good and treatment is often not needed. Case studies have shown reduction in muscle size with time. In this case the patient was satisfied with the information he received that the swelling would probably normalize with time. The most important factor for normalization of muscle size was to discontinue the daytime parafunction with grinding of the right canines. This may be difficult as

Table 3.1 Differential diagnoses to unilateral masticatory muscle hypertrophy

---

I **Reactive hypertrophy**

II **Nonreactive hypertrophy**

  A Genetic or possible genetic

  B Congenital

  C Masticatory muscle myopathy (hypertrophic branchial myopathy)

  D Vascular (intramuscular cavernous hemangioma)

  E Inflammatory and infective processes

    Focal myositis

    Eosinophilic fasciitis

    Necrotizing fasciitis due to odontogenic infection

    Idiopathic inflammatory myopathy

    Parotitis

    Submasseteric abscess

  F Neoplasm

    Benign

      Lipoma

    Malignant

      Intramuscular lymphoma

      Granulocytic sarcoma

      Liposarcoma

      Rhabdomyosarcoma

      Metastatic tumors (carcinoma, melanoma, sarcoma)

Source: adapted after Katsetos *et al.* (2014).

the patient is usually unaware of the parafunction. Visual feedback is a type of biofeedback that instead of technical devices relies on the eye, such as by posting colored stickers at different places/devices that the individual sees/uses every day (e.g., the cell phone) to remind the individual about the parafunction. Because of his intermittent pain from jaw muscles and the suspicion of nocturnal bruxism the patient also received a stabilization appliance to reduce masticatory muscle load. As he experienced a stressful life situation he was informed about its relation to bruxism and instructed in relaxation techniques and to take pauses during computer work.

- It is important also to rule out parotitis and tumors as etiologic factors. These often show similar symptoms; that is, a firm, non-fluctuant swelling of the cheek and are usually relatively painless (Table 3.1).

Background Information

- Enlargement of masticatory muscles is considered a relatively rare finding, and the literature mostly consists of case presentations.

It is often not associated with pain, although occasionally some individuals may complain of pain. Masticatory muscle hypertrophy occurs most frequently in Pacific Asians, is associated with ethnic characteristics and dietary habits, is more common in younger individuals, and is slightly more prevalent in men (Sannomya *et al.*, 2006; Fedorowicz *et al.*, 2013).

- The hypertrophy is mostly bilateral, and unilateral cases seem rarer. Most cases presented involve the masseter muscle, but it may also affect the temporalis and pterygoid muscles, or combinations of them (Albuquerque *et al.*, 2012; Katsetos *et al.*, 2014).
- Masticatory muscle hypertrophy is divided into acquired and congenital forms. The etiology is controversial and includes muscle hyperfunction (bruxism, gum or betel chewing) and/or chronic tension of the muscles, unilateral chewing (unilateral cases), imbalance in the extrapyramidal neurotransmitters, HIV infection, use of anabolic steroids, mandibular retrognathia, and genetic factors (Albuquerque *et al.*, 2012; Katsetos *et al.*, 2014; Peck *et al.*, 2014).
- Studies that have examined muscle fiber composition in hypertrophic jaw muscles show enlarged fibers with otherwise normal appearance, but varying results in fiber type distribution, frequency, and diameter. Histologically, muscle hypertrophy is often divided into reactive and nonreactive forms. In reactive masseter muscle hypertrophy due to excessive workload, progressive enlargement of the diameter of type II fibers with peripheral position of the nucleus is typically seen (Rokadiya and Malden, 2006). However, in a patient with temporalis muscle hypertrophy with a history of bruxism both type I and type II fibers were enlarged (>50 μm), but there was a predominance of type I fibers (Katsetos *et al.*, 2014). In a patient with bilateral masseter hypertrophy, a decreased frequency of type I fibers, loss of type IIB, and increased frequency of type IIC, IIA, and IM were noted (Satoh *et al.*, 2001). The authors of that study suggested that these changes were not caused by excessive workload, but rather were a result of compensatory enlargement due to lack of high-tetanus-tension type IIB fibers in this specific patient.

Diagnostic Criteria

Expanded DC/TMD criteria for **Hypertrophy** (Peck *et al.*, 2014). Sensitivity and specificity have not been established.

Enlargement of one or more masticatory muscles. Usually not associated with pain. Can be secondary to overuse and/or chronic tensing of the muscle(s). Some cases are familial or genetic in origin. Diagnosis is based on clinician assessment of muscle size, and needs consideration of craniofacial morphology and ethnicity.

History. Positive for the following:
1. Enlargement of one or more masticatory muscles as evidenced from photographs or previous records.

Examination. Positive for the following:
1. Enlargement of one or more masticatory muscles.

DC/TMD criteria for **Myalgia**, see Case 3.3, for **Disc displacement with reduction**, see Case 2.3, and for **Headache attributed to TMD**, see Case 4.1 (Schiffman *et al.*, 2014).

Fundamental Points

- The diagnostic criteria for masticatory muscle hypertrophy have not been validated. Therefore, to increase diagnostic accuracy, additional diagnostic tests are recommended.
- CT or MRI scans are considered gold standard for diagnosis and should show enlargement of the affected muscle. Mandibular angle prominence and bone spurs may also be present (Figure 3.24). Ultrasound may also be used for diagnostics.
- Histochemical analyses may reveal hypertrophic fibers, but with normal appearance. As few studies have investigated fiber composition in hypertrophic masticatory muscles and only in single cases, it is unknown if there are any general changes in fiber-type composition. It is possible that changes in fiber-type composition

vary depending on etiology (Katsetos et al., 2014).

- If bruxism or other muscle hyperfunction is suspected electromyography (EMG) might show increased nocturnal and/or diurnal activity.
- Especially for unilateral cases it is important to rule out other causes of the muscle enlargement. Differential diagnoses include infections (e.g., parotitis), inflammatory lesions (e.g., myositis), as well as benign and malignant tumors in muscle, parotis, mandible, and vascular system.
- In most cases myositis is unilateral, which may guide diagnosis, although bilateral affection is reported in the literature.
- In many cases no treatment is needed, as the hypertrophy is benign in nature. If the change in facial appearance causes a stigma to an individual, then treatment may be indicated.
- As there are mostly case presentations in the literature, there is no evidence-based treatment for muscle hypertrophy, but management should preferably be reversible. The individual should be informed about the benign nature of the swelling and to avoid parafunctions. An occlusal appliance may be used to reduce muscle tension due to nocturnal bruxism (Manfredini et al., 2015). In many cases this is enough and satisfactory for the individual. If the parafunctions can be controlled, the enlarged muscle may normalize with time (Albuquerque et al., 2010).
- For some individuals the muscle swelling is cosmetically disfiguring, which is why other treatment options have been suggested. These range from pharmacologic treatment with muscle relaxants to more or less invasive surgical procedures.
- The use of botulinum toxin is considered less invasive and has been the subject of an increasing interest for treatment of jaw muscle hypertrophy. However, a systematic review that identified 683 published studies regarding the use of botulinum toxin for masseter muscle hypertrophy found 660 to be nonapplicable, and all the remaining studies were excluded, as they did not meet the inclusion criteria. The authors concluded that at present the therapeutic benefits of botulinum toxin for management of masseter muscle hypertrophy are unclear and that clinicians should carefully consider not only its benefits, but also any potential harms with their patients (Fedorowicz et al., 2013).

- Although surgical muscle reduction of masseter muscle hypertrophy is sometimes used, it is mostly not needed and should only be used occasionally because of its invasive nature and potential side effects; for example, trismus, fibrosis, and decreased range of motion (Katsetos et al., 2014). However, in some cases surgical reduction of the bone spurs from the mandibular angle may be done (Sannomya et al., 2006).

Self-study Questions

1. Discuss different possible causes of idiopathic masticatory muscle hypertrophy as reflected in the literature.

2. Given that the suggested criteria for masticatory muscle hypertrophy in the expanded taxonomy for TMD are not validated, which additional tests may aid confirmation of diagnostic accuracy?

3. Describe the normal fiber structure of masticatory muscles and the alterations that are reported in muscle hypertrophy.

4. Discuss the mechanism and benefit of botulinum toxin in the management of masticatory muscle hypertrophy.

References

Albuquerque CE, Prado R, Pereira-Stabile CL, Filho AM (2012) Conservative treatment of bilateral temporalis muscle hypertrophy in a pregnant woman. *J Craniofac Surg* **23**(1):e20–e22.

Fedorowicz Z, van Zuuren EJ, Schoones J (2013) Botulinum toxin for masseter hypertrophy. *Cochrane Database Syst Rev* (**9**):CD007510.

Katsetos CD, Bianchi MA, Jaffery F, et al. (2014) Painful unilateral temporalis muscle enlargement: reactive masticatory muscle hypertrophy. *Head Neck Pathol* **8**:187–193.

Manfredini D, Ahlberg J, Winocur E, Lobbezoo F (2015) Management of sleep bruxism in adults: a qualitative systematic literature review. *J Oral Rehabil* **42**(11):862–874.

Peck CC, Goulet JP, Lobbezoo F, et al. (2014) Expanding the taxonomy of the diagnostic criteria for temporomandibular disorders. *J Oral Rehabil* **41**:2–23.

Rokadiya S, Malden NJ (2006) Variable presentation of temporalis hypertrophy – a case report with literature review. *Br Dent J* **201**:153–155.

Sannomya EK, Gonçalves M, Cavalcanti MP (2006) Masseter muscle hypertrophy: case report. *Braz Dent J* **17**:347–350.

Satoh K, Yamaguchi T, Komatsu K, et al. (2001) Analyses of muscular activity, energy metabolism, and muscle fiber type composition in a patient with bilateral masseteric hypertrophy. *Cranio* **19**(4):294–301.

Schiffman E, Ohrbach R, Truelove E, et al. (2014) Diagnostic Criteria for Temporomandibular Disorders (DC/TMD) for clinical and research applications: recommendations of the International RDC/TMD Consortium Network and Orofacial Pain Special Interest Group. *J Oral Facial Pain Headache* **28**(1):6–27.

Answers to Self-study Questions

1. The most common cause of idiopathic masticatory hypertrophy reported in the literature is muscle hyperactivity, such as nighttime bruxism and daytime parafunctions (e.g., tooth clenching, gum or betel chewing). Other causes discussed are compensatory contralateral hyperactivity, premature occlusal contacts and malocclusion, genetic factors, mandibular retrognathia, and HIV infection.

2. CT and MRI scans are considered gold standard. Ultrasound, EMG, muscle biopsy, and morphometric analyses are also recommended.

3. In normal masticatory muscles, type I (slow-twitch/oxidative), type II (fast-twitch/glycolytic), and intermediate (IM) fibers are present. Normally, type II fibers have a smaller diameter than type I fibers. Type II fibers are further divided into IIA, IIB, and IIC fibers. There is no consensus from the literature regarding the histochemical alterations in muscle fiber size and types. In reactive masseter hypertrophy, a predominance of type I fibers has been reported, whereas in nonreactive hypertrophy type II fibers are mostly reported.

4. Botulinum toxin reduces muscle activity by inhibiting the release of acetylcholine from the motor-end plate by chemical denervation. The effect is reversible, and due to sprouting of nerve fibers new connections form, which takes approximately 3 months. During the effective time of the drug the muscle is weakened and thus muscle activity is reduced. Botulinum toxin has therefore gained a huge interest for the treatment of muscle hypertrophy. However, there is a lack of high-quality randomized controlled studies regarding its effect. In addition, the long-term effect can be questioned due to formation of antibodies.

C: Masticatory Muscle Pain Attributed to Regional/Generalized Pain Disorders

Case 3.9

Jaw and Neck Pain

Annemiek Rollman

A. Demographics Data and Reason for Contact

- Female, 68 years old.
- The patient was referred to a TMD and orofacial pain clinic due to pain in the jaw and neck.
- An additional examination was performed by the attending physical therapist, resulting in the following details.

B. Symptom History

- Main complaint: increasing pain in the right TMJ and cheek area accompanied by neck pain, especially on the right side (Figure 3.25).
- Pain of the jaw increases during eating.
- Current pain intensity: 6 (NRS 0–10); characteristic pain intensity 34 (NRS 0–100).
- Pain started about 1 year ago.
- Pain aggravates during the day.
- Jaw pain aggravates during eating and wide opening of the mouth.
- Neck pain aggravates while looking over the shoulder to the left.
- Headache, almost daily, located in temple (right side) and back of head. Temple headache changes with jaw function.

C. Medical History

- No other health issues.

D. Psychosocial History

- Patient studied physical therapy years ago but was never active in this profession.
- She and her husband lived abroad for years and returned to the home country 1 year ago (when the pain complaints started).
- Her daily activities are housekeeping, spending time with her family and working with the computer.
- Patient specific complaint: pain is interfering in her daily life: 55 (VAS 0–100).

- Patient reports moderate stress, especially since the move (PSS-10).
- Moderate pain-related disability (Grade II; GCPS).
- Mild anxiety (GAD-7).
- Mild depression (PHQ-9).
- Parafunctions: lip-biting (OBCL).
- Bruxism: not aware of clenching or grinding (OBCL).

E. Previous Consultations and Treatments

- None.

F. Extraoral Status

- No asymmetries.
- Jaw movement capacity: normal mandibular movements, no pain on movement.
- TMJ: no palpation pain, no noises.
- Palpation: familiar pain with palpation of the right masseter and temporalis muscles; for the temporal muscle the pain was familiar to the headache.
- Dynamic: static provocation tests of the jaw. All static tests (opening, closing and protrusion) gave familiar pain from the right masseter muscle, while the dynamic tests gave familiar pain from both masseter and temporalis muscles on the right side.

G. Intraoral Status

- Tooth indentations in the cheek and lips, tongue scalloping.
- Full dentition except wisdom teeth.
- Stable occlusion.

H. Additional Examinations and Findings

- Neck movement: limited range of motion on rotation with radiating pain to the right ear and jaw.
- Palpation of the right sternocleidomastoid and trapezius muscles gave familiar pain.
- The static provocation tests of the neck flexion, rotation to the left, lateroflexion to the left, were positive and provoked jaw pain on the right side.
- The dynamic neck tests were negative.

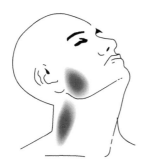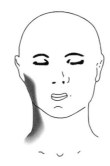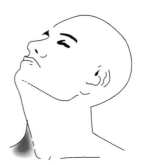

Figure 3.25 Pain location as reported by the patient.

I. Diagnosis/Diagnoses
DC/TMD
- Myalgia in masticatory muscles.
- Headache attributed to TMD.

ICHD-3 beta
- Headache attributed to cervical myofascial pain.

Other
- Cervical spinal pain, myalgia spreading to orofacial region.

J. Case Assessment
- Clenching (suspicion based on the intraoral examination) and psychosocial aspects (stress) in combination with tightening shoulders, especially while working at the computer, are likely background factors to the masticatory muscle and neck pain and headache.
- The onset of pain complaints was at the same time as moving to the home country.
- Returning to live in the home country as well as concerns about children and grandchildren that adds to her total stress level seem to play a role in experiencing increased muscle tension, as well as concerns about the pain complaint itself. This could be considered a risk factor, as her concerns might influence a good outcome negatively.

K. Evidence-based Treatment including Aims
- The main aim of the treatment plan is to substantially reduce the interference by the jaw and neck pain on her daily life.
- The physical therapy is focused on offering tools such as counselling, exercises and insight in the complaints to the patient so that she can manage her pain in such a way that it does not interfere with her daily life.
- As the patient reports that her pain mainly increases during the day, the first choice of treatment is physical therapy (a splint is mainly indicated for night-time bruxism and is therefore less likely to be beneficial in this case).
- If necessary, re-evaluate after 4 months for more extensive treatment with splint and behavioural therapy.

L. Prognosis and Discussion
- The prognosis for physiotherapy as described in this case is good since physiotherapy can provide a coordinated therapy for neck and jaw pain.

Background Information
- TMD patients four times more often show neck pain than persons without TMD.
- Patients with both TMD and neck pain report higher psychological and stress scores than patients with only TMD pain. (Visscher *et al.*, 2001).

Diagnostic Criteria
ICHD-3 beta criteria for **Headache attributed to cervical myofascial pain** (Headache Classification Committee of the International Headache Society (IHS), 2013). Sensitivity and specificity have not been established.
A. Head and/or neck pain fulfilling criterion C.
B. A source of myofascial pain in the muscles of the neck, including reproducible trigger points, has been demonstrated.
C. Evidence of causation demonstrated by at least two of the following:
   1. Either or both of the following: (a) pain has developed in temporal relation to onset of the cervical myofascial pain disorder; (b) pain has significantly improved in parallel

with improvement in the cervical myofascial pain disorder.

2. Significant pressure-tenderness is elicited in cervical muscles corresponding to the pain perceived by the patient.

3. Pain is temporarily abolished by local anaesthetic injections into trigger points, or by trigger-point massage.

D. Not better accounted for by any other ICDH-3 diagnosis.

DC/TMD criteria for **Myalgia**, see Case 3.3, for **Headache attributed to TMD**, see Case 4.1 (Schiffman *et al.*, 2014).

Fundamental Points

- Literature suggest that for patients with persisting pain the treatment should focus on coping with the pain. This case study presents a practical approach to guide such patients.
- A good therapeutic relationship is a prerequisite to gain information about the (chronic) pain experience in order to set an adequate treatment.
- A patient with chronic TMD and neck pain serves as an example on providing guidance on how to stimulate a patient in changing the way of coping with pain in their life.
- Three perspectives on the functioning of the clinician in this are: medical focus, focus on pain education and a focus on combined expertise.
- These three perspectives are all valuable with subtle but considerable differences on the relation between the patient and clinician and, in the long run, on compliance and treatment outcome (Table 3.2).
- Dynamic/static tests imitate joint and muscle function. During dynamic tests, the joint structures are tested for pain on articulation and the muscles are slightly loaded. During static tests the muscles are tested for pain on isometric contraction (Figure 3.26; Visscher *et al.*, 2000).
- Positive findings on static tests point in the direction of myalgia.
- Positive findings on dynamic test point in the direction of arthralgia.

Table 3.2 Aligning the relation between clinician and health-care provider that is not influenced by a biomedical focus can bring balance in the relation between the patient and the clinician

Perspective	Clinician expertise	Patient expertise
Medical focus	++	−
Focus on pain education	++	+
Focus on combined expertise	++	++

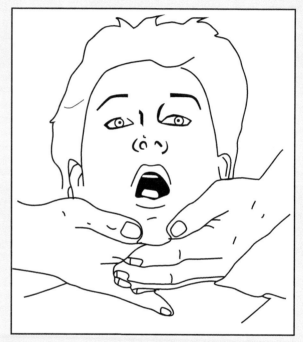

Figure 3.26 An example of the dynamic opening test for the masticatory system.

Patient–Therapist Interaction

In this part, fragments of the first visit of the patient to the physical therapist are presented, in which the physical therapist will give exercises to relax the jaw and neck and give instructions for auto-massage.

Perspective 1: medical focus

The first perspective focuses on the biomedical point of view in which the expertise of the clinician is leading. This perspective demonstrates the diagnostics, the treatment plan and evaluations. If this were the only focus, a relational tension can occur, as the goals of the patient might be conflicting to those of the clinician. Such a conflict can lead to less compliance.

Patient (P): But she did say that in the picture the TMJ was flattened.

Clinician (Cl): Yes.

P: When I asked "Is that because of osteoarthritis (…)?" she said yes, but there is nothing you can do about it.

Cl: OK, would you like me to say something about that?

P: Yes, please, I would like to know what is going on!

Cl: I read here in your file that there is some flattening of the TMJ that could indicate arthrosis in the joint. But when looking at our tests that are testing the structure that is related to your pain, they indicate that especially the muscles are painful, and not the joint.

P: Oh, so it has to do with the muscles

In this fragment the patient discusses the results with the physical therapist that were presented to her after the clinical examination. There seems to be a misunderstanding about the origin of the pain complaints. The patient's idea of the origin of the complaints:

P: My jaw and neck pain is caused by arthrosis of the TMJ.

The explanation of the physical therapist is focused on a better understanding of the patient of the clinical findings. There is a dominance of the expertise of the clinician.

Perspective 2: focus on pain education

- The persistence of the pain cannot merely be explained as the consequence of an obvious tissue damage (Nijs *et al.*, 2011).
- Often patients suspect their pain is caused by tissue damage, and believe that movement will only make it worse.
- To reduce the discrepancy between beliefs of the patient and scientific knowledge of the clinician:
  - The first step is (if necessary) to help the patient to examine the possibility of other causes of the complaints, besides their current beliefs.
  - The second step is that the clinician presents an aetiology by which the patient can develop another relation to the complaints. That is by creating images in which the pain interferes less in daily life.
- In this fragment the clinician provides a further explanation of the patient of the role of overloading the jaw muscles as a possible aetiology for the pain complaints.
- By introducing an experiment, the patient's curiosity is triggered to look for other explanation.

Cl: Would you like to investigate how much your jaw and neck are relaxed?

P: Yes.

Cl: Maybe it helps you if we introduce some sort of scale that measures the tension of the jaw muscle.

P: Ok.

Cl: In this scale, "0" is no muscle tension, and "10" is your maximal muscle tension. I would like to ask you to clench as much as you can, and then completely let go of the jaw and drop your shoulders. …

When it was completely tensed, what would the score then be?

P: 7.

CL: And after you released?

P: 4.

Cl: Ah 4, could you relax even more?

P: Yes, I think so (focuses on breathing) …

… Now it's 3.

Cl: Do you often feel that the jaw and neck are this relaxed?

P: Not often …

- As muscle tension can play a role in the continuation of pain, to examine the relaxation of the jaw (and neck) can give some new insights in daily habits, which helps breaking the pattern.
- Also in this perspective there is a dominance of the expertise of the clinician. However, it allows the patient to express their experience.

Perspective 3: focus on combined expertise

- In the third perspective the focus will be on the impact of pain in the daily life of the patient and the possibility of diminishing it and regaining their autonomy over pain.

- A combined expertise in which both patient and clinician co-create a future plan of how to deal with daily situations leads to an optimum treatment.
- The following fragment is a part from the second session. In the time between the two sessions the patient monitored if there was tension in her jaw or neck in her daily life.

CI: Do you have an idea of the kind of moments in which more tension occurs?

P: Yes, when I get behind the laptop, I usually sit on the couch. But then my shoulders get really tensed!

CI: Shall we use this situation as an example of how you could relax more regularly?

P: Yeah, yeah.

P: I should sit somewhere else, not on the couch, but at the table.

P: Yes, this week I will really do this differently.

CI: And then?

P: I have to lower my shoulders … And my jaw.

CI: You love to write, and then you focus only on that, you just said, how could you remind yourself?

P: If I feel pain.

CI: Emm, that seems to be too late, right? Shall we search for another reminder?

P: I have a picture of my grandson on my desktop. I see it a lot.

CI: That sounds like an appropriate reminder, I'm wondering if that will work for you.

P: Certainly.

In this combined expertise the patient and the clinician are looking for a way how to integrate the relaxation into the daily life.

Self-study Questions

1. Which aspects of oral history taking that are not directly related to the diagnosis are especially important in patients with persistent pain jaw and neck pain complaints?

2. Could you describe why in the first fragment the question "OK, would you like me to say something about that?" is labelled as "the medical focus"?

3. Could you describe why in the second fragment the question "Would you like to investigate how much

your jaw and neck are relaxed?" is labelled as "focus on pain education"?

4. Could you describe why in the third fragment the question "Do you have an idea of the kind of moments in which more tension occurs?" is labelled as "focus on combined expertise"?

5. In your daily practice, what type of questions do you most often use (A: medical diagnostic focus; B: pain education; C: combined expertise)?

6. How could you practise with questions that focus on a combined expertise?

Acknowledgements

I would like to especially thank Q Merkies for his contributions to this writing.

References

Headache Classification Committee of the International Headache Society (IHS) (2013) The International Classification of Headache Disorders, 3rd edition (beta version). *Cephalalgia* **33**(9):629–808.

Nijs J, van Wilgen P, van Oosterwijck J, et al. (2011) How to explain central sensitization to patients with 'unexplained' chronic musculoskeletal pain: practice guidelines. *Man Ther* **16**:413–418.

Schiffman E, Ohrbach R, Truelove E, et al. (2014) Diagnostic Criteria for Temporomandibular Disorders (DC/TMD) for clinical and research applications: recommendations of the International RDC/TMD Consortium Network and Orofacial Pain Special Interest Group. *J Oral Facial Pain Headache* **28**(1):6–27.

Visscher CM, Lobbezoo F, de Boer W, et al. (2000) Clinical tests in distinguishing between persons with or without craniomandibular or cervical spinal pain complaints *Eur J Oral Sci* **108**:475–483.

Visscher CM, Lobbezoo F, de Boer W, et al. (2001) Prevalence of cervical spinal pain in craniomandibular pain patients. *Eur J Oral Sci* **109**(2):76–80.

Answers to Self-study Questions

1. Especially in patients with persisting (and spreading) pain, it is important to identify non-helping beliefs about the pain, such as fear of (further) tissue damage. Furthermore, it is important to identify stressors and life events during or around the time of the start of the pain complaints or current.

2. With this question, the clinician gives information about the content; that is, background information of the diagnosis.

3. Now the physical therapist shows a new perspectives on pain sources.

4. The physical therapist here asks about the integration of the exercises in the daily life of the patient.

5. *A recommendation.* To get insight in the types of questions you ask, you could audio-record your treatment session (with permission of your patient of course). Together with a colleague you can listen to the recording and order your questions in the categories: medical focus, focus on pain education and a focus on combined expertise.

6. *A recommendation.* As a continuation of the previous recommendation, you could retrospectively look for moments in the interaction with your patient that a question with a focus on the combined expertise would be more appropriate, and then retrospectively rephrase your question in such a way. By doing this frequently, you will become more familiar with asking questions from this perspective.

Case 3.10

Whiplash-Associated Disorders

Birgitta Häggman-Henrikson and Richard Ohrbach

A. Demographic Data and Reason for Contact

- Male, 49 years old, referred by physician at pain rehabilitation clinic due to post-traumatic neck pain following whiplash trauma, teeth grinding during sleep, and headache on awakening (Figure 3.27).

B. Symptom History

- Primary complaints are pain in face, neck, and shoulder region following whiplash trauma associated with a motor vehicle collision 2 years previously, and headache on awakening.
- The neck pain began immediately after the accident, whereas jaw pain developed 2–3 months after. Since the accident, the neck pain has remained at high intensity, whereas the jaw pain, which was initially of low intensity, has gradually worsened.
- Characteristic pain intensity for the jaw is now 77 (NRS 0–100).
- The facial pain improves with rest. Headache is worsened by jaw function.
- Patient is aware of teeth grinding during sleep and teeth clenching during the waking hours.

C. Medical History

- Diabetes type II.
- Post-traumatic neck pain after whiplash trauma
- Medication: metformin, tramadol, Saroten®, paracetamol, Lyrica®.
- No allergies.

D. Psychosocial History

- Married, no children, and works full time as an electrician. He enjoys his home life and work, but is finding work activities increasingly difficult because lifting arms above shoulder height provokes the neck pain, which leads to substantial job frustration and mood change.
- Sleep quality is poor due to the neck pain.
- Standardized Axis II assessment, pain intensity and pain-related disability (GCPS): high pain intensity, low

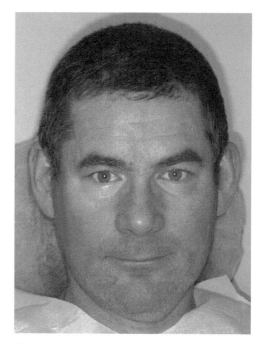

Figure 3.27 Facial photograph of patient.

pain-related disability. Mild depression (PHQ-9), moderate anxiety (GAD-7), many physical symptoms (PHQ-15). Frequent and multiple parafunctions (OBCL), moderate jaw functional limitation (JFLS-20), and pain drawing (Figure 3.28) indicates pain in the head, neck, right shoulder, and both hands. In addition to the DC/TMD Axis II assessment instruments, the following were also assessed: severe stress (PSS-10) and clinically relevant catastrophizing (PCS).

E. Previous Consultations and Treatments

- Recently referred by his general practitioner to the pain rehabilitation clinic, where initial assessment has been conducted but treatment has not yet begun.

F. Extraoral Status

Face

- No asymmetries, swelling, or redness.

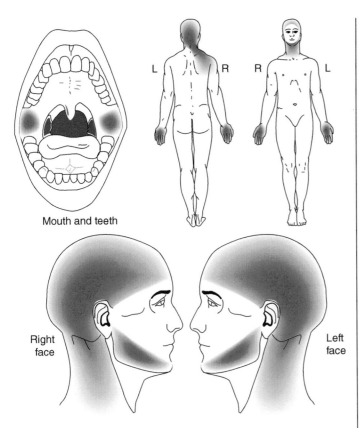

Mouth and teeth

Right face

Left face

Figure 3.28 Pain drawing.

Neurologic function and motor function
- Within normal limits.

Somatosensory abnormalities
- Trigeminal nerve on the right side to:
  (i) touch – hyperesthesia third branch;
  (ii) cold – hypoesthesia second branch and hyperesthesia third branch; (iii) pinprick – hypoalgesia second branch and hyperalgesia third branch. Wind-up on repeated pinprick third branch: 2 to 4 (NRS 0–10).

Temporomandibular joint
- No detectable joint sounds or catching/locking. There was no pain on palpation of the TMJs.

Masticatory muscles
- Familiar pain was elicited on palpation bilaterally in the masseter muscles with referred pain toward the ear on the right side. Bilateral familiar pain was elicited on palpation of the temporal muscles, which also produced familiar headache.

Jaw movement capacity
- Maximal unassisted jaw opening of 46 mm provoked familiar and bilateral pain in the masseter muscles.

Neck examination
- Range of movement in all directions (flexion, extension, rotation, and side-bending) was reduced and provoked pain in the sternocleidomastoid and trapezius muscles. Pain on palpation was elicited bilaterally in the sternocleidomastoid and trapezius muscles with pain referral to the right side of the face.

G. Intraoral Status
- Soft tissues: scalloped tongue bilaterally.
- Hard tissues and dentition: normal dentition, stable occlusion with bilateral molar support. (Figure 3.29).

H. Additional Examinations and Findings
- None.

I. Diagnosis/Diagnoses
DC/TMD
- Myofascial pain with referral.
- Headache attributed to TMD.

ICHD-3 beta
- Persistent headache related to whiplash.

Other
- Post-traumatic neck pain.

J. Case Assessment
- Jaw muscle pain and headache were likely initiated from spread of pain from the neck region within 3 months following whiplash trauma, and have since been maintained by (1) persistent oral parafunction during both waking and sleeping hours, resulting in increased regional muscle tension, and (2) general stress reactivity, both of which collectively contribute to chronicity.
- Central sensitization is suggested by the spread of both neck and jaw pain, as shown on the pain drawing (Figure 3.28), as well as the somatosensory disturbances, although the wind-up on repetitive pinprick was minor.

K. Evidence-based Treatment Plan including Aims
- Patient information. Goal: increase the patient's understanding of the relevant pain mechanisms and to have realistic expectations regarding what can be achieved with proposed treatment.
- Self-management consisting of: (i) jaw relaxation – avoid tooth contact and relax lower jaw during the day and facilitated by use of

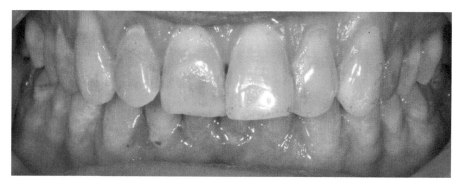

Figure 3.29 Dental occlusion.

person-specific cues, which can be visual, auditory, or kinesthetic; (ii) jaw exercises twice a day incorporating postural training of head–neck, jaw opening–closing, and horizontal jaw movements to improve mobility of jaw muscles. Goal: reduce muscle tension, increase blood flow, and reduce pain.

- Stabilization splint for use during sleep. Goal: reduce muscle pain associated with sleep bruxism.
- This treatment plan is combined with treatment carried out at the pain rehabilitation clinic, which will include further psychological assessment, CBT, and physiotherapy. Goals: acceptance of current limitations in order to work within them, and improve neck mobility and reduce neck–shoulder pain.

L. Prognosis and Discussion

- Guarded at present due to the widespread pain and psychosocial consequences.
- Important to address severe stress, role expectations with his employment, and clinically relevant catastrophizing.
- After discussions with the pain rehabilitation team, the patient will reduce his work hours to 30 h/week in order to reduce stress and allow for sufficient time to attend the pain school program. This decision reflects acceptance of his current situation and willingness to actively work to improve his pain situation.
- Patient responded well to treatment with jaw relaxation training and jaw exercises in combination with a flat plane splint.
- The main treatment outcome was reduced jaw pain intensity and jaw muscles feeling more relaxed on wakening.

Background Information

- The term whiplash describes a soft-tissue injury due to hyperextension–flexion movement of the neck. The incidence is about 1 per 1000 inhabitants, mostly from motor vehicle collisions, but it can also occur from other causes. Most individuals will recover from a whiplash injury, although about one in three individuals will develop persistent problems with post-traumatic neck pain and associated symptoms. The term whiplash-associated disorders (WADs) was proposed to encompass this symptom range.
- Although in some cases the mandible can also sustain trauma at the same time as the whiplash of the neck, it is more likely that a cervical whiplash will indirectly affect the jaw system, thereby acting as a contributing factor to TMD, with TMD onset ranging from days up to 6 months as attributable to the WAD. This timeframe for delayed onset is based on opinion, given the absence of firm evidence.
- The symptoms following whiplash trauma are heterogeneous, and common symptoms include neck pain, impaired cervical mobility, and headache. These symptoms relate to multiple mechanisms: mechanical injury to the neck, pain sensitization, psychological and behavioral factors, and social factors. In addition, catastrophizing and fear of movement or reinjury can maintain and perpetuate pain and dysfunction as well as account for spread of the problem from the initial WAD to include the jaw system.
- The prevalence of TMD in individuals with post-traumatic neck pain has been reported to be more than 20%, suggesting that whiplash trauma can be a risk factor for TMD.
- The treatment outcome for individuals with both TMD and post-traumatic neck pain is poorer

compared with individuals with TMD but without a history of neck injury. This suggests that TMD pain after whiplash trauma may be influenced by any of the following: (1) a different pathophysiology, related to spread of pain between the neck and jaw regions, or related to functional compensations between cervical–head posture and mastication; (2) part of a regional or generalized pain syndrome caused by sensitization mechanisms; (3) pre-morbid behavioral and psychological factors affecting response to injury as well as post-onset changes in those factors; or (4) social factors related to work and role expectations.

(Sessle *et al.*, 1986; Haggman-Henrikson *et al.*, 2002, 2013; Sale and Isberg, 2007)

Diagnostic Criteria

ICHD-3 beta criteria for **Persistent headache related to whiplash** (Headache Classification Committee of the International Headache Society (IHS), 2013). Sensitivity and specificity have not been established.

Headache of greater than 3 months' duration caused by whiplash.

Criteria

A. Any headache fulfilling criteria C and D.
B. Whiplash, associated at the time with neck pain and/or headache, has occurred.
C. Headache has developed within 7 days after the whiplash.
D. Headache persists for >3 months after the whiplash.
E. Not better accounted for by another ICHD-3 diagnosis.

Note: whiplash is defined as sudden and inadequately restrained acceleration/deceleration movements of the head with flexion/extension of the neck. Whiplash may occur after either high- or low-impact forces.

DC/TMD criteria for **Myofascial pain with referral**, see Case 3.4, and for **Headache attributed to TMD**, see Case 4.1 (Schiffman *et al.*, 2014).

Fundamental Points

Treatment plan

- In addition to the DC/TMD examination, which includes a pain drawing and the number and location of additional pain sites (e.g., neck, shoulders, back), it is important to assess other signs of spread of pain and central sensitization. This can include a somatosensory examination and a neck examination. TMD is seldom the result of a single cause; consequently, the interaction of multiple processes should always be considered for evaluation.
- The case history together with findings of referred pain to the face during neck movements or from palpation of neck muscles demonstrates the regional interaction of pain from the neck to the jaw region.

(Slade *et al.*, 2013)

- The treatment plan related to TMD and any factors identified in the Axis II assessment should be planned and coordinated with the treatment provided by other care givers; for example, pain rehabilitation teams including physicians, physiotherapists, and psychologists. Issues identified in the Axis II assessment, such as depression and stress, may need to be addressed before the treatment specifically aimed at TMD can be started if the patient is unable to adhere adequately to self-managed treatment for the jaw; on the other hand, if the patient can adhere at this time to the self-management treatment for the jaw, doing so and achieving positive results can greatly enhance their overall confidence and commitment to further self-management.

Management

- A multidisciplinary multimodal rehabilitation program is advocated for patients with post-traumatic neck pain.
- Litigation or worker's compensation issues warrant additional attention from psychology or vocational counsellors respectively.
- The treatment plan should be tailored in order to address all of the factors identified. For pain intensity the patient may need pharmacological management. For patients with neck pain, caution is advised with regard to the design of

the jaw exercise program. For example, if jaw exercises are carried out against resistance, this will require more neck muscle activity to stabilize the head and may subsequently exacerbate the neck pain.

(Sutton *et al.*, 2014)

Relapse prevention

- For patients with TMD in combination with chronic post-traumatic neck pain, the self-management program initially provided is shaped over time based on patient response and in particular in relation to flare-ups whilst in treatment, thereby identifying the components of a long-term program.
- For a majority of patients, post-traumatic neck pain will resolve within the first year after the trauma. The strongest prognostic factor for persistent symptoms is high intensity of neck pain immediately after the trauma. Individuals who do not recover may always be at risk for developing pain at other body sites, and specifically at risk for recurrence of TMD.

(Berglund *et al.*, 2006; Walton *et al.*, 2013)

Self-study Questions

1. What aspects of the case history are important to incorporate when assessing a patient with TMD combined with WADs?

2. Are there any specific areas of examination that you should include?

3. How will the post-traumatic neck pain affect your treatment plan and prognosis for the treatment?

4. Which mechanical and neurological mechanisms may explain the relationship between WADs and TMD?

References

Berglund A, Bodin L, Jensen I, *et al.* (2006) The influence of prognostic factors on neck pain intensity, disability, anxiety and depression over a 2-year period in subjects with acute whiplash injury. *Pain* **125**:244–256.

Haggman-Henrikson B, Zafar H, Eriksson PO (2002) Disturbed jaw behavior in whiplash-associated disorders during rhythmic jaw movements. *J Dent Res* **81**:747–751.

Haggman-Henrikson B, List T, Westergren HT, Axelsson SH (2013) Temporomandibular disorder pain after whiplash trauma: a systematic review. *J Orofac Pain* **27**:217–226.

Headache Classification Committee of the International Headache Society (IHS) (2013) The International Classification of Headache Disorders, 3rd edition (beta version). *Cephalalgia* **33**(9):629–808.

Sale H, Isberg A (2007) Delayed temporomandibular joint pain and dysfunction induced by whiplash trauma: a controlled prospective study. *JADA* **138**:1084–1091.

Schiffman E, Ohrbach R, Truelove E, *et al.* (2014) Diagnostic Criteria for Temporomandibular Disorders (DC/TMD) for clinical and research applications: recommendations of the International RDC/TMD Consortium Network and Orofacial Pain Special Interest Group. *J Oral Facial Pain Headache* **28**(1):6–27.

Sessle BJ, Hu JW, Amano N, Zhong G (1986) Convergence of cutaneous, tooth pulp, visceral, neck and muscle afferents onto nociceptive and non-nociceptive neurones in trigeminal subnucleus caudalis (medullary dorsal horn) and its implications for referred pain. *Pain* **27**:219–235.

Slade GD, Fillingim RB, Sanders AE, *et al.* (2013) Summary of findings from the OPPERA prospective cohort study of incidence of first-onset temporomandibular disorder: implications and future directions. *J Pain* **14**:T116–T124.

Sutton DA, Côté P, Wong JJ, *et al.* (2014) Is multimodal care effective for the management of patients with whiplash-associated disorders or neck pain and associated disorders? A systematic review by the Ontario Protocol for Traffic Injury Management (OPTIMa) Collaboration. *Spine J.* doi: 10.1016/j.spinee.2014.06.019.

Walton DM, MacDermid JC, Giorgianni AA, *et al.* (2013) Risk factors for persistent problems following acute whiplash injury: update of a systematic review and meta-analysis. *J Orthop Sports Phys Ther* **43**:31–43.

Answers to Self-Study Questions

1. Type of trauma; development of symptoms over time; relationship between trauma, neck pain onset, and jaw pain onset. Psychosocial status according to both standard Axis II measures as well as patient-specific measures; inquiry via history into role of other factors (e.g., financial difficulties following serious injury) exacerbating symptoms.

2. In addition to the DC/TMD, a cervical examination for mobility, abnormal posture, and pain on palpation; sensory examination to assess signs of central sensitization.

3. Liaise with other professionals such as physicians, rehabilitation team, psychologist, and physical therapist, in order to customize treatment to meet the patient's capacity and limitations, taking Axis II into consideration

4. During function such as chewing, the cervical muscles necessarily compensate for powerful contractions of masticatory closing muscles, and it is possible that when cervical structures are inflamed

or dysfunctional due to injury, this may lead to ongoing and progressive compensations between cervical–head posture and mastication. Sensitization, due to persistent nociception from the cervical region can lead to a generalized pain syndrome that includes the masticatory region due to shared neural connections between cervical dorsal horn regions and nucleus caudalis of the trigeminal nerve. Pre-morbid behavioral and psychological factors affecting response to injury to the cervical region can also affect the masticatory system.

Case 3.11

Fibromyalgia

Juliana Stuginski-Barbosa

A. Demographic Data and Reason for Contact

- Female, Caucasian, 40 years old, married, two children, cleaner (Figure 3.30).
- Complaint: bilateral facial and head pain (Figure 3.31).

B. Symptom History

- Pain is constant and moderate: 6 (NRS 0–10).
- Quality is dull, tight; and chewing hard food or opening mouth, and stress make pain worse. Medication and relaxation are ameliorating factors.
- Awake bruxism is reported (OBCL).
- First episode of facial and head pain 2 years ago treated with sporadic use of muscle relaxant (cyclobenzaprine) and NSAIDs.
- Pain is getting worse since the first episode.
- No report of facial/head trauma, closed or opening locking of the jaw.

C. Medical History

- Patient has hypertension, diabetes type 2, migraine, and polycystic ovaries. She has been treated with propanol and metformin 550 mg.
- Presence of continuous body pain (Figure 3.32), unrelenting fatigue, and sleep disturbances for a year. The pain is widespread, involving both sides of the body. It is aggravated by emotional stress and weather changes. She reported fairly bad sleep quality and she often awoke in the morning without feeling fully rested and with a sensation of muscle fatigue.
- Levels of thyroid hormone, blood calcium, cholesterol and vitamin D are normal.
- Patient did not report any aerobic physical activity.

D. Psychosocial History

- Patient reported loss of energy and reduced ability to concentrate in daily activities. She is under psychological treatment for anxiety disorder.
- GCPS revealed severe pain-related disability.
- PHQ-15 revealed a high number of physical symptoms.

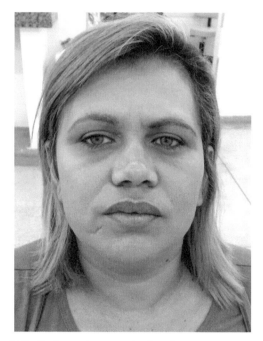

Figure 3.30 En-face photograph of patient.

- Fibromyalgia Symptom Scale was completed. The Widespread Pain Index (WPI) and Symptom Severity Score (SS) indicated that patient had fibromyalgia.

E. Previous Consultations and Treatments

- She visited a dentist 2 years ago. The diagnosis was TMJ arthralgia.
- She used a stabilization splint for a year without pain improvement.
- She is under orthodontic treatment.

F. Extraoral Status

Jaw movement capacity

- Straight with pain-free opening of 24 mm, maximum unassisted opening 31 mm, and maximum assisted opening 41 mm, including overbite.
- In opening movements, familiar pain was presented in bilateral temporalis, masseter, and TMJ.

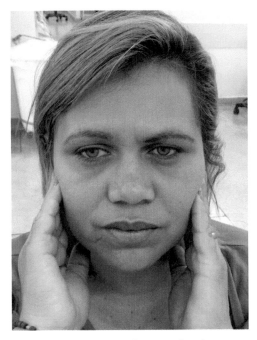

Figure 3.31 Orofacial pain locations confined to masseter muscles.

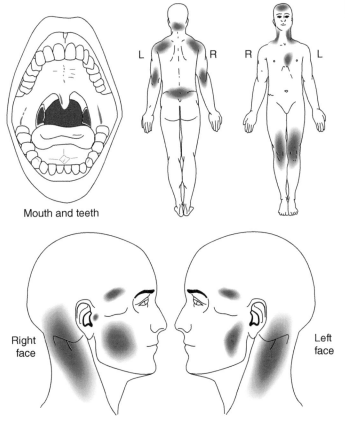

Mouth and teeth

L   R   R   L

Right face

Left face

Figure 3.32 Pain drawing by patient.

- No restrictions or pain were observed in lateral and protrusive movements.

Temporomandibular joint

- No joint sound detected under manual inspection or reported by patient.
- TMJ palpation revealed familiar pain only in the right side.

Jaw muscles

- On the right side, the patient reported familiar pain with temporalis and masseter muscle palpation.
- On the left side, patient reported familiar pain with anterior temporalis and masseter (origin and body) palpation. Pain was also presented in middle and posterior temporalis.
- In bilateral masseter muscle, pressure, when maintained, elicited a referral pattern of pain to frontal and temporal area, reproducing the patient's pain complaint.

Neck examination

- Familiar and referred pain to temporal and frontal areas when sternocleidomastoideus muscle was under sustained pressure.

G.   Intraoral Status

- Teeth with braces. She presented an Angle Class I malocclusion with misalignment of the teeth.
- Wear facets were found in bilateral incisors and molars, along with indentation in tongue and buccal mucosa.
- No other significant findings.

H.   Additional Examinations and Findings

- Patient was referred to a rheumatologist, who confirmed the diagnosis of fibromyalgia.

I.   Diagnosis/Diagnoses
DC/TMD

- Myofascial pain with referral.
- Right TMJ arthralgia.

Expanded taxonomy for TMD

- Fibromyalgia.

Other

- Possible awake bruxism.

J.   Case Assessment

- Patient fulfilled DC/TMD criteria for myofascial pain with referral. From the pain drawing it was evident that she had widespread pain, which is why she was asked to complete the WPI and SS. These indicated fibromyalgia, which was confirmed by a rheumatologist.

- The cause of the jaw pain could be muscle overload as daytime clenching was present, but was more likely a consequence of the generalized pain presenting also in jaw muscles.

- High psychological distress is commonly seen in fibromyalgia, and lack of energy and sleep disturbances are among the key symptoms.

- The high pain intensity in combination with the severe pain-related disability and psychological distress impair the prognosis, which is why multimodal and multidisciplinary treatment is recommended.

K. Evidence-based Treatment Plan including Aims

Patient education and self-management

- To improve symptoms and reduce disability levels and also manage expectations, information about diagnosis, treatment, and prognosis were given.

- Self management included:
  - Visual reminders, like small stickers, strategically placed at home and at work and an application for smartphone (No Clenching app).
  - Heat stimulation to improve pain by stimulation of muscle relaxation and vascular perfusion.
  - Aerobic exercise (e.g., walking), to improve physical function, quality of life, and reduce pain. The "start low, go slow" strategy for any physical exercise program must be advised, which should limit adverse events and better assure adherence.
  - Sleep hygiene (e.g., make sleep routine a priority, optimize relaxing sleep environment, provide advice on diet and exercise) was advised to improve sleep quality, pain scores, and mental well-being.
  - To avoid the use of over-the-counter medication for pain; the overuse of these medications could contribute to pain chronification.

Pharmacologic management

- To reduce pain, naproxen 550 mg, two times a day was prescribed for 10 days. Naproxen was reported as effective for the treatment of painful TMJ.

- Amitriptyline 25 mg/day (once a day at bedtime) was prescribed for 30 days. After this period, dosage increased to 50 mg/day. Data from studies indicate that low doses (10–75 mg/day) of amitriptyline are effective for the treatment of fibromyalgia and also it is beneficial for chronic TMD pain. The analgesic effect of TCAs is thought to be independent of antidepressant effect and it should be related to their ability to increased efficacy of pain modulation, increasing the availability of serotonin and norepinephrine at the synaptic junction. Pain modulation seems to be compromised not only in fibromyalgia, but also in masticatory myofascial pain patients.

Jaw movement rehabilitation

- To improve jaw function, coordination exercises with her tongue behind the upper incisors were recommended as they can decrease pain and increase range of motion.

L. Prognosis and Discussion

- A number of health-care specialists (physical therapist, rheumatologist, and psychologist) were required to collaborate on the patient's care. The step-by-step approach is an important way, rather than trying to solve everything at once.

- More frequent visits may be useful to emphasize the important role of multimodal treatment and to help the management of early treatment's adverse effects, which could improve patient's engagement in all therapies.

- The questionnaires and assessment tools, like VAS and Axis II DC/TMD criteria, must be used to assess the impact of pain across multiple domains (sleep, physical, and emotional symptoms) during follow-up sessions and to develop and prioritize treatment goals with a focus on the symptoms and domains most affected.

- Amitriptyline can improve symptoms and function; however, if necessary, it could be substituted in follow-up visits by others medications with different action to influence transmission of sensory signals via central nociceptive pathways.

- Informing patients with TMD and fibromyalgia of the limitations of treatments as well as potential benefits could be helpful. For example, medications will help to reduce symptoms but may not eliminate them altogether. However, a reduction in symptoms may allow the patient to engage in self-management and exercises.

Background Information

- Fibromyalgia is a dysfunctional syndrome with a prevalence of 2% in the general population, more frequently in females, increasing with age (Clauw, 2009).
- Patients with fibromyalgia present with chronic widespread pain and a variety of physical symptoms, including sleep disturbance, fatigue, decrements in physical functioning, and disruptions in psychological functioning such as memory problems, mood disturbances, and concentration difficulties (Clauw, 2015).
- Fibromyalgia has been shown to be very familial/genetic coupled, and environmental factors (e.g., early life trauma, physical trauma, some infections, emotional stress) may play a prominent role in triggering the development. Fibromyalgia is characterized by central disturbance with dysfunction in endogenous noxious inhibition systems, amplification in pain processing, sleep disturbance, and dysautonomia (Woolf, 2011).
- The classification of fibromyalgia according to the American College of Rheumatism (ACR; Wolfe *et al.*, 1990) has for long been the most used for diagnosis (Fundamental points 2). New clinical criteria for the diagnosis of fibromyalgia have recently been proposed (Wolfe *et al.*, 2011). These criteria involve WPI and SS, but exclude counting tender points as previously required by the criteria from the ACR (Fundamental points 2). There is, however, no consensus regarding which criteria should be used (Staud *et al.*, 2010).

Diagnostic Criteria

Expanded DC/TMD criteria for **Fibromyalgia** (Peck *et al.*, 2014). Sensitivity and specificity have not been established.

Widespread pain with concurrent masticatory muscle pain

History.   Positive for both of the following:
1. A rheumatologic-based diagnosis of fibromyalgia.
   AND
2. Myalgia (see Case 3.3).
   Examination.   Positive for both of the following:

1. A rheumatologic-based diagnosis of fibromyalgia.
   AND
2. Myalgia (see Case 3.3).
   DC/TMD criteria for **Myofascial pain with referral**, see Case 3.4, and for **Arthralgia**, see Case 2.1 (Schiffman *et al.*, 2014). Criteria for **Possible awake bruxism**, see Case 4.10 (Lobbezoo *et al.*, 2013).

Fundamental Points

Classification

- Accoding to the ACR 1990 criteria (Wolfe *et al.*, 1990) a diagnosis of fibromyalgia is fulfilled if the patient has (1) widespread pain (axial plus upper and lower segment plus left- and right-sided pain) more than 3 months and (2) ≥11 of 18 bilateral tender point sites (4 kg pressure).
- The tender points assessed include (1) the neck muscles at the base of the skull and (2) halfway between the shoulder and neck, (3) shoulder blades, (4) lower neck, front area, (5) edge of upper breast bone, (6) 2 cm below the elbow bone, (7) upper area of buttocks, (8) hip bone, and (9) just above the knee on the inside.
- A patient satisfies modified ACR fibromyalgia diagnostic criteria (Wolfe *et al.*, 2011) if the following three conditions are met: (1) WPI ≥ 7 and SS ≥ 5 or WPI between 3 and 6 and SS ≥ 9. (2) Symptoms have been present at a similar level for at least 3 months. (3) The patient does not have a disorder that would otherwise sufficiently explain the pain.
- WPI is the number areas in which the patient has had pain over the last week. These include seven bilateral locations (shoulder girdles, upper arms, lower arms, hips (buttock, trochanter), upper legs, lower legs, jaws) and five unilateral locations (chest, abdomen, upper back, lower back, and neck). The final score is between 0 and 19.
- The SS is the sum of the severity (0–3) of three symptoms (fatigue, waking unrefreshed, and cognitive symptoms) plus the sum of the number of three symptoms occurring during the previous 6 months (headaches, pain or cramps

in lower abdomen, and depression). The final score is between 0 and 12.

Management

- A comprehensive multimodal treatment plan is recommended, integrating (1) ongoing patient education, (2) pharmacotherapy, and (3) nonpharmacological therapies.
- The US Food and Drug Administration (FDA) has approved three medications for fibromyalgia (pregabalin, duloxetine, and milnacipran). Other medications, such as tricyclic medications, cyclobenzaprine, gabapentin, tramadol, fluoxetine, and sodium oxybate, are also used for symptomatic management. It is recommend choosing the most appropriate treatments for each individual patient, according to their clinical history and presentation.
- Among the nonpharmacological approaches that have demonstrated efficacy are aerobic exercise, sleep hygiene, some forms of CBT, and ongoing patient education (Clauw, 2015).

Fibromyalgia and temporomandibular disorder

- Both fibromyalgia and TMD are frequently associated with other pain syndromes (e.g., chronic fatigue syndrome, chronic headache, irritable bowel syndrome) as comorbid conditions characterized by a complaint of pain as well as a mosaic of abnormalities in motor function, autonomic balance, neuroendocrine function, and sleep. The overlap between symptom-based conditions leads the reasons to consider them as "functional pain syndromes."
- The common mechanisms of functional pain syndromes may relate to central sensitization and it may be influenced by the autonomic nervous system and genetic polymorphisms.
- Although fibromyalgia and TMD are comorbid conditions, the relationship between these may be confined to chronic TMD conditions as 35–97% of patients with fibromyalgia met TMD diagnosis criteria, whereas 10–52% of patients with TMD met fibromyalgia criteria (Lim *et al.*, 2011). In people with TMD, the presence of fibromyalgia is associated with an increased TMD pain and disability.

- When comorbidity is known, the parsimony principle (one disease should explain all symptoms) does not apply.
- Management of these patients includes a correct diagnosis, appropriate investigation for associated conditions, adequate treatment, and considering the therapeutic opportunities and limitations the comorbid disorders may impose.

Self-study Questions

1. What are the common symptoms reported by a patient who could have fibromyalgia?
2. Is manual palpation needed for fibromyalgia diagnosis?
3. Almost 75% of fibromyalgia patients met TMD diagnosis criteria. Why is the presence of TMD common in fibromyalgia patients?
4. What are the objectives and the best strategy for TMD and fibromyalgia patients?

References

Clauw DJ (2009) Fibromyalgia: an overview. *Am J Med* **122**(12 Suppl):S3–S13.

Clauw DJ (2015) Diagnosing and treating chronic musculoskeletal pain based on the underlying mechanism(s). *Best Pract Res Clin Rheumatol* **29**(1):6–19.

Lim PF, Maixner W, Khan AA (2011) Temporomandibular disorder and comorbid pain conditions. *J Am Dent Assoc* **142**(12):1365–1367.

Lobbezoo F, Ahlberg J, Glaros AG, et al. (2013) Bruxism defined and graded: an international consensus. *J Oral Rehabil* **40**(1):2–4.

Peck CC, Goulet JP, Lobbezoo F, et al. (2014) Expanding the taxonomy of the diagnostic criteria for temporomandibular disorders. *J Oral Rehabil* **41**:2–23.

Schiffman E, Ohrbach R, Truelove E, et al. (2014) Diagnostic Criteria for Temporomandibular Disorders (DC/TMD) for clinical and research applications: recommendations of the International RDC/TMD Consortium Network and Orofacial Pain Special Interest Group. *J Oral Facial Pain Headache* **28**(1):6–27.

Staud R, Price DD, Robinson ME (2010) The provisional diagnostic criteria for fibromyalgia: one step forward, two steps back: comment on the article by Wolfe et al. *Arthritis Care Res (Hoboken)* **62**(11):1675–1676.

Woolf CJ (2011) Central sensitization: implications for the diagnosis and treatment of pain. *Pain* **152**(3 Suppl):S2–S15.

Wolfe F, Smythe HA, Yunus MB, et al. (1990) The American College of Rheumatology 1990 Criteria for the Classification of Fibromyalgia. Report of the Multicenter Criteria Committee. *Arthritis Rheum* **33**(2):160–172.

Wolfe F, Clauw DJ, Fitzcharles M-A, et al. (2011) Fibromyalgia criteria and severity scales for clinical and epidemiological studies: a modification of the ACR Preliminary Diagnostic Criteria for Fibromyalgia. *J Rheumatol* **38**(6):1113–1122.

Answers to Self study Questions

1. Fibromyalgia common symptoms include widespread pain for at least 3 months, fatigue, sleep disturbances, decrements in physical functioning, and disruptions in psychological functioning such as memory problems, mood disturbances, concentration difficulties, anxiety, and depression.

2. New diagnosis criteria for fibromyalgia recently excluded manual palpation for counting tender points as previously required by ACR diagnosis criteria. The fibromyalgia diagnosis criteria observed symptoms that have been present at a similar level for at least 3 months and results of WPI and SS. The patient does not have a disorder that would otherwise explain the pain.

3. The mechanisms of the comorbidity between fibromyalgia and TMD are still poorly understood and may relate to central sensitization. Indeed, fibromyalgia is a chronic form of pain itself and it is intuitive to consider that the same lack of inhibitory control that happens in fibromyalgia facilitates widespread pain and the occurrence of masticatory myofascial pain.

4. The management goals for patients with TMD are similar to those for fibromyalgia: decreased pain, restoration of function, and improvement in normal daily actives. A number of health-care specialists may be required to collaborate on the patient's care, including the patient taking responsibility for self-management and adherence to all aspects of the treatment plan. A "start low, go slow" strategy is preferred for both pharmacotherapy and any physical therapy program, which should limit adverse events and better assure adherence to any treatment regimen.

4

Other Orofacial Pains

Clinical Cases in Orofacial Pain, First Edition. Edited by Malin Ernberg and Per Alstergren.
© 2017 John Wiley & Sons Ltd. Published 2017 by John Wiley & Sons Ltd.

A: Headache

Case 4.1

Headache Attributed to Temporomandibular Disorders

Daniela AG Gonçalves

A. Demographic Data and Reason for Contact

- Female, 31 years old, married, no children.
- Profession: professor in a nurse school.
- Reports simultaneous attacks of facial pain and headache.

B. Symptom History

- Complaint of facial pain and headache (Figures 4.1 and 4.2).
- The symptoms started 15 years ago but have worsened over the last 5 years.
- The pain starts in the face (masseter, temporalis. and TMJ regions) and progressively intensifies until it embraces the whole face and head.
- The pain is described as a generalized pressure pain in the face, and the headache as a pressing, moderate pain that started bilaterally in the temporal region and later became holocranial. Both jaw pain and headache are aggravated by mastication, jaw movements, and parafunctional habits.
- Pain and headache are always present with moments of increased intensity.

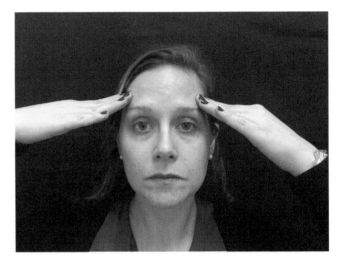

Figure 4.2 Patient pointing to the principal area of her headache.

- Current pain intensity 9 (NRS 0–10). Characteristic pain intensity 78 (NRS 0–100).
- Severe pain-related disability (GCPS).
- Emotional stress, mastication, jaw movements, parafunctional habits (as awake bruxism), and other jaw activities (talking, kissing, yawning) aggravate the facial pain.
- Patient reports presence of fatigue and pain in the face and teeth upon waking and is aware of daytime clenching (OBCL).
- She reports TMJ noises bilaterally during jaw movements, but no history of closed or open locking of the jaw.

C. Medical History

- Hypertension.
- Report of frequent poor digestion. She sought medical attention but did not reach a specific diagnosis.
- Irritable bowel syndrome.
- Recurrent urinary tract infection.

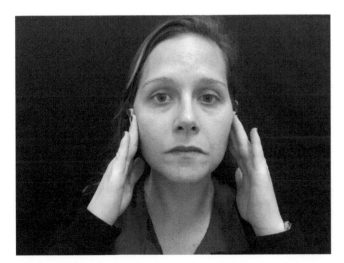

Figure 4.1 Patient pointing to the principal area of her facial pain.

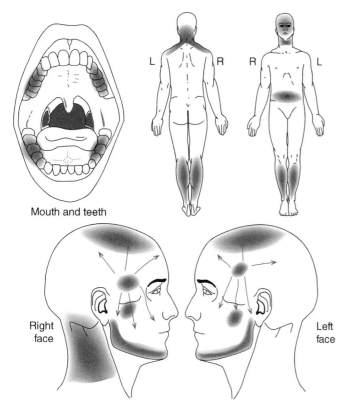

Figure 4.3 Pain drawing.

- Presence of frequent cervicalgia, abdominal and leg pain (Figure 4.3).
- She is using clonazepam and sertraline.
- She reported light and restless sleep but has never undergone polysomnography.
- She reports presence of varicose veins and intermittent edema in her legs.

D. Psychosocial History

- She works as a nurse and as a teacher, giving classes in a school of nursing.
- She has been practicing physical activities, three times per week (gym and walking), for the last 3 months. Before that, she defines herself as sedentary. She started the physical activities aiming to relax, to improve general health, and for weight reduction.
- Grade IV (GCPS); that is, high disability, severely limiting.
- Severe depression and anxiety according to PHQ-9 and GAD-7.
- PHQ-15 shows moderate level of physical symptoms (stomach pain, back pain, chest pain, dizziness, fainting spells, tachycardia, constipation, nausea, feeling tired, poor sleep).

- Frequent emotional stress during the last 5 years, moderate stress during last month (PSS-10).
- Restricted social life because of pain.
- She is undergoing individual psychotherapy.

E. Previous Consultations and Treatments

- She recently started homeopathic treatment for her facial pain and headache, but with no improvement so far.
- A neurologist prescribed clonazepam, which improved her sleep, but had no effect on pain.

F. Extraoral Status
General

- Height 1.57 m; weight 59.8 kg; BMI 24.26 kg/m^2 (BMI: health); total fat percentage (assessed by bioimpedanciometry): 31.2%.

Head and face

- Within normal limits.

TMJ

- No TMJ sounds during the clinical examination.
- Bilateral familiar pain laterally in TMJs.

Masticatory muscles

- Bilateral familiar pain on palpation of temporalis and masseter.
- Familiar headache during palpation of left temporalis muscle.

Jaw movement capacity

- Straight jaw opening pattern.
- Maximum pain-free opening 12 mm, maximum unassisted opening 20 mm, and maximum assisted opening 33 mm with familiar pain bilaterally in masseter, temporalis, and TMJs.

Somatosensory abnormalities

- She reports a slightly reduced hearing since her facial pain increased. Although, the clinical examination did not show any abnormalities related to the cranial nerves.

Neck

- Stiffness, pain, and difficulty in movement.

G. Intraoral Status

She reports previous orthodontic treatment for esthetic purposes.

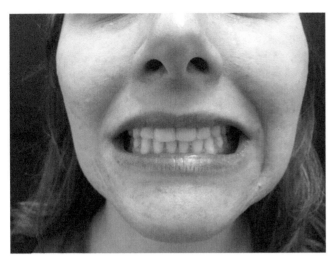

Figure 4.4 Dental occlusion.

Soft tissues

- Within normal limits.

Hard tissues and dentition

- No carious lesions or periodontal problems.
- History of dental fracture (right mandibular first molar, free of carious lesion) and presence of tooth wear (the four canines).
- No abfractions.

Occlusion

- Within normal limits (Figure 4.4).

H. Additional Examinations and Findings

- None performed.

I. Diagnosis/Diagnoses
DC/TMD

- Headache attributed to TMD.
- Myalgia.
- Arthralgia (bilateral).

Other

- Probable sleep bruxism.

J. Case Assessment

- This patient presented a complex case of myalgia and arthralgia, headache attributed to TMD, painful comorbidities (cervicalgia, abdominal, urinary tract infection, body pain), and psychosocial conditions.
- Self-report of fatigue and pain in the face and teeth upon waking, plus the presence of teeth wear observed during the intraoral examination indicate a diagnosis of probable bruxism (Lobbezoo *et al.*, 2013).

- The psychosocial aspect is very relevant, with a high level of depression, anxiety, and somatization. Stress is relevant and plays a role initiating, exacerbating, and perpetuating pain. She also presents a significant impairment of her social life associated with the pain.
- Therefore, it is also important to refer the patient to other health professionals.
- A multimodal treatment plan, as well as counselling aimed for behavioral change, is crucial for the general condition.

K. Evidence-based Treatment Plan including Aims

- To control the TMD signs and symptoms, the management plan for the present patient included: (1) a self-care program for TMD including automassage, thermal therapy and stretching exercises to increase the jaw range of motion; (2) an educational approach making the patient aware of the parafunctional habits; (3) pharmacotherapy (cyclobenzaprine 5 mg – one tablet before sleep).
- We also suggested a substitution of sertraline (serotonin selective reuptake inhibitors – SSRI) by amitriptyline (a TCA), which will be evaluated by the psychiatrist. It is well known that amitriptyline has better analgesic properties than sertraline.
- Additionally, because sertraline is a SSRI, it can exacerbate or initiate sleep bruxism; (4) splint for use during sleep because of sleep bruxism; (5) application of transcutaneous electrical nerve stimulation aiming to control the pain.
- The patient recently started treatment with a psychiatrist and a psychologist (psychotherapy) because of the depression and anxiety.

L. Prognosis and Discussion

- Based on the history and clinical examination, this patient presents a complex case of chronic pain, suggesting an uncertain prognosis. The evidence-based factors indicating a poor prognosis and chronicity include increased mood disorders and somatization, fatigue and sleep disturbances, high pain intensity, generalized pain or other pain conditions, and decreased function of the pain inhibitory system, among others. The patient presented some of the cited factors, such as the long-lasting pain condition, mood disorders (depression and anxiety), complaint of sleep disturbances, high pain intensity, and the presence of painful (widespread body pain, cervicalgia, persistent abdominal pain, urinary tract infection) and nonpainful comorbidities (hypertension).

- The patient reports that she started different treatments but did not follow as recommended by the health-care providers, pointing to a possible limited compliance with previous interventions. This suggests that she needs frequent contact with the professionals and intense motivation approach.

Background Information

- Headaches can be a symptom of a wide variety of diseases (secondary headache), or they can be the disease itself (primary headache) (Headache Classification Committee of the International Headache Society (IHS), 2013).
- TMD and headaches are painful conditions involving the trigeminal system. Both of them are highly prevalent worldwide, and frequently occur in the same individuals simultaneously (Sessle, 2005; Jensen and Stovner, 2008; de Leeuw and Klasser, 2013; Headache Classification Committee of the International Headache Society (IHS), 2013).
- TMD and headache can interact in different ways: (a) painful TMD is comorbid with some types of primary headaches, such as migraine; (b) the pain associated with TMD can be a risk factor for primary headaches chronification; (c) TMD (myalgia) can cause headaches. According to the DC/TMD criteria, the diagnostic of the "Headache attributed to TMD" depends on the presence of the myalgia (Cady, 2007; Gonçalves et al., 2011; Schiffman et al., 2014).
- The treatment options recommended by the AAOP include patient education and self-management, biobehavioral therapy, pharmacologic management, physical therapy, orthopedic appliance, occlusal therapy, and surgery. Considering the increasing evidence and the AAOP recommendation, TMDs are best managed with conservative, reversible treatment (de Leeuw and Klasser, 2013).

Diagnostic Criteria

DC/TMD criteria for **Headache attributed to TMD** (Schiffman et al., 2014). Sensitivity 0.89 and specificity 0.87.

Headaches that are related to, and aggravate, TMDs. Headache in the temple area secondary to pain-related TMD (derived using valid diagnostic criteria) that is affected by jaw movement, function, or parafunction, and replication of this headache occurs with provocation testing of the masticatory system.

History. Positive for both of the following:
1. Headache of any type in the temple.
   AND
2. Headache modified with jaw movement, function, or parafunction.

Examination. Positive for both of the following:
1. Confirmation of headache location in the area of the temporalis muscle(s).
   AND
2. Report of familiar headache in the temple area with at least one of the following provocation tests:
   a. Palpation of the temporalis muscle(s).
      OR
   b. Maximum unassisted or assisted opening, right or left lateral movements, or protrusive movements.

The headache is not better accounted for by another pain diagnosis.

Note: a diagnosis of pain-related TMD (e.g., myalgia or TMJ arthralgia) must be present and is established using valid diagnostic criteria.

DC/TMD criteria for DC/TMD **Myalgia**, see Case 3.3, and for **Arthralgia**, see Case 2.1 (Schiffman et al., 2014). Criteria for **Probable sleep bruxism**, see Case 4.10 (Lobbezoo et al., 2013).

Fundamental Points

- In the presence of TMD and headaches simultaneously, the clinical features can be not so evident to enable the differential diagnosis. Therefore, these cases can be a challenge for neurologists and dentists.
- Individuals presenting TMD, especially the chronic form, can also present painful and nonpainful comorbidities, including psychosocial disorders such as depression, anxiety, and somatization.

- While an efficient treatment requires a multidisciplinary team, each professional should be prepared to identify and diagnose different painful syndromes considering the presence of comorbidity.
- An important aspect to identify a headache attributed to TMD is the temporal relationship between the two conditions. Moreover, the headache should be replicated by the jaw functions, and palpation or functional tests of the TMJs and masticatory muscles.
- Dentists should also be prepared to identify the presence of a primary headache, concomitant with the TMD and the secondary headache. In these cases, patients should be referred to a neurologist to receive a specific treatment for the primary headache.
- Another important fact to observe in clinical practice is the treatment response. If TMD causes a headache, an efficient control for the former should eliminate the latter.

Self-study Questions

1. Which aspects should a dentist consider, beyond the TMD signs and symptoms, when evaluating a patient with chronic pain?

2. How can the TMD and headaches be related in the same patient?

3. Which are the essential criteria for a headache attributed to TMD?

4. In the presence of comorbidity, which points should be addressed in an adequate treatment plan?

References

Cady RK (2007) The convergence hypothesis. *Headache* **47**(Suppl 1):S44–S51.

De Leeuw R, Klasser GD (eds) (2013) *Orofacial pain: Guidelines for assessment, diagnosis, and management*, 5th edn. Hanover Park, IL: Quintessence Publishing Co. Inc.

Gonçalves DAG, Camparis CM, Speciali JG, et al. (2011) Temporomandibular disorders are differentially associated with headache diagnoses: a controlled study. *Clin J Pain* **27**(7):611–615.

Headache Classification Committee of the International Headache Society (IHS) (2013) The International Classification of Headache Disorders, 3rd edition (beta version). *Cephalalgia* **33**(9):629–808.

Jensen R, Stovner LJ (2008) Epidemiology and comorbidity of headache. *Lancet Neurol* **7**(4):354–361.

Lobbezoo F, Ahlberg J, Glaros AG, et al. (2013) Bruxism defined and graded: an international consensus. *J Oral Rehabil* **40**(1):2–4.

Sessle BJ (2005) Peripheral and central mechanisms of orofacial pain and their clinical correlates. *Minerva Anestesiol* **71**(4):117–136.

Schiffman E, Ohrbach R, Truelove E, et al. (2014) Diagnostic Criteria for Temporomandibular Disorders (DC/TMD) for clinical and research applications: recommendations of the International RDC/TMD Consortium Network and Orofacial Pain Special Interest Group. *J Oral Facial Pain Headache* **28**(1):6–27.

Answers to Self-study Questions

1. Dentists, as well other health professionals, should conduct a comprehensive anamnesis to identify painful and nonpainful comorbidities. Chronic pain is frequently associated with psychosocial conditions such as depression, anxiety, and somatization. Also, in the presence of chronic pain, central sensitization can be present, which implicates central approaches (i.e., pharmacology) and not only peripheral procedures. Finally, to be able to identify other conditions, dentists have to be familiar with the diagnostic criteria of the major TMD comorbidities.

2. TMD and headache can be comorbid; TMD can be a risk factor for primary headaches chronification; and TMD can cause headaches (secondary headaches). Dentists should be familiar with the ICHD-3 to be able to identify the presence of different headaches, and to offer appropriate treatment as well to refer the patient to a neurologist when necessary.

3. The presence of a close temporal relation between the TMD signs and symptoms and to a headache first onset. The headache, located in the temporal area, is affected by jaw movement, palpation, function, or parafunction involving the temporomandibular structures (joint and muscles).

4. In these cases, it is important to address all the conditions concomitant with the dental approaches, preferably by a multidisciplinary team. The presence of peripheral and central sensitization should be considered when choosing the treatment modalities. Also, it is important to aggregate an education approach to stimulate behavioral change. Finally, the psychosocial aspects and the sleep features would be evaluated and addressed in an efficient treatment plan.

B: Neuropathic Pain

Case 4.2

Trigeminal Neuralgia

Joanna Zakrzewska

A. Demographic Data and Reason for Contact
- Female, 69 years old, presented with a 10-month history of severe episodic right-sided facial pain.

B. Symptom History
- Patient describes an intermittent unilateral episodic pain for last 10 months, which had not responded to dental treatment.
- The pain starts in the right maxillary area and then radiates to the mandibular area. It is felt both extraorally and intraorally. Presents in the same place each time.
- Each episode comes and goes suddenly and lasts from seconds to 2 min, with more than 10 attacks per day; there can be months of no pain.
- Pain is characterized as an electric shock; uses the metaphor of a drill going into her face and giving her shocks (Figure 4.5). From the McGill Pain Questionnaire, she chooses the following words: shooting, drilling, stabbing, lacerating, searing, exhausting, terrifying, vicious, unbearable, piercing and torturing.

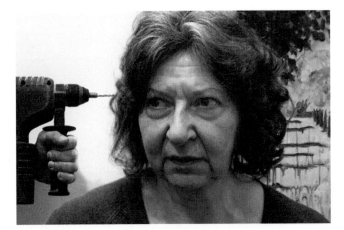

Figure 4.5 Patient, who co-created this image of herself with an artist. © Deborah Padfield and AE from the series *Face2face*.

- Pain severity varies between 0 for least pain and 10 for worst pain (0–10 NRS).
- Pain is provoked by talking, eating, brushing the teeth, washing the face, vibrations and bending; relieved by gabapentin 1200 mg daily.
- Nil associated factors; no eye, nose or ear symptoms.

C. Medical History
- Hernia operation, hypertension.

D. Psychosocial History
- Married with one son. Graphic designer, writer, paints. No significant life events.
- Experiences fatigue, occasionally wakes at night; when severe, pain episodes impact on activities of daily living. No anxiety or depression when pain is controlled.

E. Previous Consultations and Treatments
- First episode: pain in the upper right quadrant while eating. It was thought to be related to an old crown. She had endodontics and then extraction of the tooth, none of which relieved the pain. Everything settled after about 11 days.
- Second episode: 8 months later, pain same location; opioids, diazepam and third molar extraction, no help.
- Nine months later a diagnosis of trigeminal neuralgia (TN) was made and gabapentin started, which reduced the pain. The patient was referred to the facial pain unit.

F. Extraoral Status
- No gross neurological abnormality.
- No TMJ sounds and no TMJ or masticatory muscle pain on palpation. Jaw movement capacity is within normal ranges.

G. Intraoral Status
- Dentate with an extensively restored dentition.

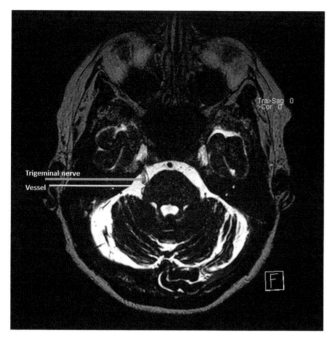

Figure 4.6 MRI showing trigeminal nerve in contact with a vessel.

H. Additional Examinations and Findings

- MRI scan shows neurovascular compression of the trigeminal nerve in the region of the root entry zone on the right side (Figure 4.6).

I. Diagnosis/Diagnoses
ICDH-3 beta
- Classical TN right side.

J. Case Assessment

- This is a typical case of classical TN affecting the maxillary and mandibular branches of the trigeminal nerve. Pain is provoked by oral behaviours such as talking, eating, brushing the teeth and washing the face and is recurring in episodes with full remission in between.
- Although she has classical TN, the major problem is the fear of return of severe pain and how she would cope with it.

K. Evidence-based Treatment Plan including Aims

- As gabapentin had not been effective it is important to use one of recommended drugs, and international guidelines suggest either carbamazepine or oxcarbazepine. She was started on oxcarbazepine, as this drug has improved tolerability.

- She was provided with information leaflets and details of patient support group (www.tna.org.uk) and had a joint consultation with a neurosurgeon and physician to discuss possible surgical options. Recent studies have suggested that fear, lack of confidence and isolation play a role in this condition, so she participated in a psychology pain management group programme with other patients with TN.

L. Prognosis and Discussion

- The patient was pain free 13 months later; low-dose drug only.
- Fourth episode 24 months later, return of pain; used oxcarbazepine for control and stopped when pain free (Figure 4.7).
- Fifth episode 35 months later – recurrence, Brief Pain Inventory showed pain intensity 10/10, quality of life severely affected, anxiety and depression on Hospital Anxiety and Depression scale. On high-dose oxcarbazepine developed hyponatraemia. Unable to control pain medically (Figure 4.8).
- Microvascular decompression to decompress nerve 36 months later and now 1 year on is pain free and off medications.
- One of the main questions posed by patients relates to their prognosis, especially when they are first diagnosed. A systematic review of the epidemiology and diagnosis of this condition shows that there are no studies that provide data on the long-term prognosis. TN is well known to result in natural periods of pain remission, and these seem to be extremely variable in length (Rothman and Monson, 1973). Not all patients require surgery, and some can be managed medically for many years.
- How patients make decisions about treatments is difficult to understand and is compounded by the lack of high-quality evidence. A recent study suggested that surgical management is preferred to medical.

Background Information

Epidemiology
- Older studies have estimate that the prevalence of TN ranges between 0.3% and 4.9% in the general population, with an annual incidence of 2.1 to 4.7 new cases per 100 000 persons, but this is thought to be higher. Females are slightly more frequently affected by TN compared with

Feb 2014 4th Episode	PAIN 0 - 10	DETAIL	ACTIVITY 0 - 10	SIDE EFFECTS 0 - 10	DOSAGE
1/2/2014	.5	1 x spontaneous	Ignore might go		
2/2	1	1 x eating & washing	Ignore might go		
3/2	1	2 x touching side of nose	bit concerned	Phoned Jillie suggested cranial osteopath, she thinks helpful	1 x 150 oxc
4/2	2	3 x touching face Not going away		hope meds will be prophylactic	1 x 150
5/2	2	2 x "	Cranial osteopathy	depressed	1 x 150
6/2	2	3 x eating & spontaneous			2 x 150
7/2	2	2 x eating & spontaneous	Cranial osteo	Cranial osteo, relaxing.	2 x 150
8/2	2	3 x " "		Coffee and wine & peppermints taste awful	2 x 150
9/2	3	5			3x150
10/2	5	9 x cleaning teeth & face, eating & spontaneous	Eating very little	Tablets seem to have little effect	3 x 150
11/2	7	10 x as above		Did not go out into cold wind	3x150
12/2	7	4 x as above	Cancelled everything	4 tablets seem effective	4 x 150
13/2	7	1 x face	Lots of rest	Dont dare to go out, cold, very windy	4 x 150
14/2	0	0	Cranial osteo	Appetite generally reduced	4 x 150
15/2	0	0		Walk in Regents Park, slept afternoon	4 x 150
16/2	7	1 x breakfast		Slept during afternoon	4 x 150
17/2		0	Has it gone???	No breakfast. Nausious	4 x 150
18/2		0		Dropped one tablet	3 x 150
19/2	7 & 8	2 x brkfast & dinner	Definitely not gone!	back on full dose	4 x 150
20/2	7	1 x rinsing teeth am		Not eating breakfast. Slept afternoon	4 x 150
21/2	7	1 x spontaneous	Cleaned teeth OK	Not eating breakfast	" "
22/2	7	1 x spontaneous	Cleaned teeth OK	Slept afternoon	" "
23/2	0	0	Cleaned teeth OK		" "

Figure 4.7 Diary kept by patient of fourth episode of pain.

males. In a recent survey of UK general practitioner practices, it an incidence of 26.8 per 100 000 persons per year was estimated, but the disorder is often misdiagnosed, and in a similar study done in Holland, where neurologists validated the diagnosis, the incidence rate was 12.6 per 100 000 person years (confidence interval 10.5–15.1).

- The disease most frequently linked with TN is multiple sclerosis. Hypertension may be a risk factor, and tumours constitute a very small group of symptomatic cases. No genetic basis has been found, but there are reports of familial occurrence. Wu *et al.* (2015), in a population-based study in Taiwan, reports that TN was associated with increased depression, anxiety and sleep disturbance, but no other psychosis.

Aetiology and pathophysiology
- TN remains a disease of unknown aetiology and its pathophysiology is not completely understood (Devor *et al.*, 2002). A vascular compression of the trigeminal nerve at its root entry zone in the posterior fossa of the skull is

found in many patients. This causes demyelination and ephaptic transmissions, resulting in paroxysmal pain. Up to 20% of the population have neurovascular contact and yet only a small percentage develop TN. There is growing evidence that patients with TN have an abnormality of their sodium channels, which are important in nerve conduction, as well as a potential myelin defect, and central inhibitory pathways are abnormal.

Diagnosis
- The clinical features of TN have been described in a recent series of papers from the Danish Headache Centre (Maarbjerg *et al.*, 2014), but there are very few studies that have evaluated these over a longer period of time.
- More recently it has become increasingly clear that the classical description of TN as suggested in both the International Association for the Study of Pain and ICHD classifications is more complex (Headache Classification Committee of the International Headache Society (IHS), 2013).

2015 5th Episode	PAIN 0 - 10	DETAIL	ACTIVITY 0 - 10	SIDE EFFECTS 0 - 10	DOSAGE
28/3/15	5	1 x while eating	0 Ignored it		
29/3/	7	3 x spontaneous		1. Nose runny in morning	1 x 150gm
30/3	7	3 x eating & walking		1. Nose runny	1 x 150
31/3	7	4 x evoked & spontaneous	9 No aquarobics	4. drowsy	2 x 150
1/4	7	2 x on waking; 6x spontenous	Cranial osteopathy	Sleepy all day	2x150 & 1x300 @night
2	6	2 eating		Sleepy all day. no appetitie	" "
3	6	4 cleaning teeth & eating	10 Cancelled dinner with friends.	Nauseous, vomited in car	"
4	6	3 x waking & as above	Stayed home. No breakfast. Ate little	Nauseous morning. v. drowsy; nose still runny	" "
5	6	4 x waking, eating & talking	10 little food, no breakfast	" " " " "	" "
6			10 unable to eat	Very nauseous	
7	6	8 x cleaning teeth, eating, spontanious	10 Unable to eat	Vomited and nauseous	Reduced night to 150gm
8	5	4 x as above	Cranial osteopath	Sluggush & nauseous	3 x 150gm
9	4	2 x on getting up. Later in morning feel 75% better. Had lovely day out.	1 Lots of walking about	1st decent meal	3 x 150gm
10	10	Cleaned teeth - sensation of explosion in temple followed by pain paroxysm for 50 mins. countless shocks all day	10 Nothing, reading Cannot clean teeth or face.	Horrendous, only soup & of fruit juice via straw – too painful	2 x 150 + 300 at night
11	10	Woken at 5.50 by ½hr spasm, followed after ¼hr by another, & soon after yet another, each lasting ½hr. countless strong shocks throughout day, 50% are spontaneous	10 Still cannot clean teeth or face or hair. move slowly.	Bit of fruit smoothy & soup	3 x 150 + 300gm night
12	10	Woke at 8 to take med & another 25 min paroxysm of pain. leaves me trembling & exhaused – Carl too. Countless strong shocks. Another 25 min spasm at bedtime	10 Teeth & face still unwashed.Sitting in arm chair moving as little as possible. Not smiling or putting head down.	Unable to eat Yoghurt breakfast. Soup via straw, & smoothie.	

Figure 4.8 Diary kept by patient of fifth episode of pain.

- There are two conditions that have many similar characteristics to TN, short-lasting unilateral neuralgiform headache attacks with autonomics (SUNA), or short-lasting unilateral neuralgiform headache attacks with conjunctival injection and tearing (SUNCT). It is now being suggested that all these disorders may be part of a continuum of the same disorder, as autonomic features may be noted not only in these conditions but also with TN.
- Tölle *et al.* (2006), in their study of 89 European patients with TN, show the significant impact that this condition can have on activities of daily living as reported on the Brief Pain Inventory, a self-completed questionnaire. Using an extended Brief Pain Inventory Facial, neurosurgeons have been able to show how quality of life improves when patients are managed surgically. Phenotyping these patients at baseline is therefore crucial when assessing outcomes.

Management

- The wide range of treatments currently in use for TN is ample evidence that there is no simple answer to how TN should be managed. Trials in TN patients are difficult to conduct for a number of reasons, including; its relative rarity, its unknown aetiology, its natural history of spontaneous remission, its varying severity and the lack of objective diagnostic tests. The condition is in the first instance treated with anti-epileptic drugs, some of which have been evaluated in randomized controlled trials (Zakrzewska and Linskey, 2014).
- There is a wide range of surgical treatments (Zakrzewska and Linskey, 2014). Some are

destructive, mostly carried out at the level of the Gasserian ganglion under a short anaesthetic and result in pain relief for a few years but result in variable sensory loss. Microvascular decompression is a non-destructive procedure involving a major neurosurgical procedure linked with a 0.4% mortality rate. The procedure results in the longest pain-free interval. There are very few randomized controlled trials of surgery.

- Patient support groups have provided thousands of patients worldwide with access to improved quality data on which to make decisions about treatment and, more importantl, provide psychological support.

Diagnostic Criteria

ICHD 3rd edition (beta version) criteria for **Classic trigeminal neuralgia** (Headache Classification Committee of the International Headache Society (IHS), 2013).

A disorder characterized by recurrent unilateral brief electric-shock-like pains, abrupt in onset and termination, limited to the distribution of one or more divisions of the trigeminal nerve and triggered by innocuous stimuli. It may develop without apparent cause or be a result of another diagnosed disorder. There may or may not be, additionally, persistent background facial pain of moderate intensity.

TN developing without apparent cause other than neurovascular compression.

A. At least three attacks of unilateral facial pain fulfilling criteria B and C.

B. Occurring in one or more divisions of the trigeminal nerve, with no radiation beyond the trigeminal distribution.

C. Pain has at least three of the following four characteristics:

1. recurring in paroxysmal attacks lasting from a fraction of a second to 2 min;
2. severe intensity;
3. electric-shock-like, shooting, stabbing or sharp in quality;
4. precipitated by innocuous stimuli to the affected side of the face.

D. No clinically evident neurological deficit.

E. Not better accounted for by another ICHD-3 diagnosis.

Fundamental Points

- Correct diagnosis is essential, and this can only be achieved by listening carefully to the story. Owing to the severity of the attack, many will remember the circumstances surrounding their first attack. Clinical criteria:
  - **severity** – moderate to severe.
  - **duration and timing** – each episode comes and goes suddenly and lasts from seconds to 2 min; periods of remission vary from weeks to months or even years;
  - **character** – electric shock, sharp, shooting;
  - **location** – unilateral, within the trigeminal area both intraoral and extraoral, least likely only first division;
  - **factors affecting pain** – provoked by light touch activities, eating, brushing the teeth, washing the face, cold wind, vibrations;
  - **associated factors** – want to keep still; no gross neurological abnormalities.
- Dental causes must be excluded as it is easy to assume a dental cause and no irreversible procedures should be carried out if there is a lack of clinical signs.
- Carbamazepine or oxcarbazepine are anti-epileptics which should be used in the first instance and they are highly effective initially, but result in significant side effects.
- Patients should be referred early to specialists, and especially once the first-line drug becomes ineffective, for confirmation of diagnosis, imaging and either further medical management or surgery.
- Surgery is either destructive, providing a few years of pain relief with varying degrees of sensory loss, or attempts to decompress the trigeminal nerve, and so provide longer term relief without sensory loss.

Self-study Questions

1. What are the key features that distinguish TN from dental pain?

2. How would you manage the first episode of TN?

3. What key investigations does a TN patient need and why?

4. Why should patients be referred to specialist services?

5. Why would you consider surgery a better treatment option?

References

Devor M, Amir R, Rappaport ZH (2002) Pathophysiology of trigeminal neuralgia: the ignition hypothesis. *Clin J Pain* **18**:4–13.

Headache Classification Committee of the International Headache Society (IHS) (2013) The International Classification of Headache Disorders, 3rd edition (beta version). *Cephalalgia* **33**:629–808.

Maarbjerg S, Gozalov A, Olesen J, Bendtsen L (2014) Trigeminal neuralgia – a prospective systematic study of clinical characteristics in 158 patients. *Headache* **54**:1574–1582.

Rothman KJ, Monson RR (1973) Survival in trigeminal neuralgia. *J Chronic Dis* **26**:303–309.

Tölle T, Dukes E, Sadosky A (2006) Patient burden of trigeminal neuralgia: results from a cross-sectional survey of health state impairment and treatment patterns in six European countries. *Pain Pract* **6**:153–160.

Wu TH, Hu LY, Lu T, *et al.* (2015) Risk of psychiatric disorders following trigeminal neuralgia: a nationwide population-based retrospective cohort study. *J Headache Pain* **16**:64.

Zakrzewska JM, Linskey ME (2014) Trigeminal neuralgia. *BMJ* **348**:g474.

Answers to Self-study Questions

1. Pain is not confined to a tooth, begins at the start of eating rather than the end, very quick, very severe and does not respond to analgesics or any dental treatment.

2. Prescribe carbamazepine or oxcarbazepine initially in low doses and gradually increase to get good pain control. Provide information, contact with support group.

3. MRI to exclude multiple sclerosis or other lesions, such as a tumour or cyst.

4. To ensure correct diagnosis, use other drugs, obtain a neurosurgical opinion.

5. Surgery provides longer periods of pain relief with no drugs, and microvascular decompression tries to eliminate a major cause.

Case 4.3

Postherpetic Trigeminal Neuropathy

Gary M Heir

A. Demographic Data and Reason for Contact

- Hispanic male, 38 years old.
- Self-referred, due to pain of the right forehead and eye that he assumed was from an infection associated with a severely painful rash in the area of a previous trauma.

B. Symptom History

- The rash first appeared 2 months earlier and persisted for 3 weeks.
- The rash, which extended to the upper eyelid, was preceded by a tingling and burning sensation in the affected area. This was followed by the appearance of small, fluid filled blisters, which leaked a clear fluid.
- After the blisters had broken, crusted over and resolved, the skin was left scarred (Figure 4.9) and with burning pain in the distribution of the rash. Pain had persisted for 2 months at the time of the initial examination.
- The affected area was extremely sensitive to light touch. Even a non-noxious stimulus resulted in a report of significant stinging and burning pain.

C. Medical History

- No contributing medical history.
- The patient denies the use of alcohol, except socially, and does not smoke or use tobacco.
- A review of systems was negative.
- There was no report of allergies, illnesses, or hospitalization.
- The patient claimed he was in good health until an accident that occurred at work 11 months earlier. He incurred trauma to his right cheek.
- The patient has been edentulous in the maxillary arch for more than 10 years. All maxillary teeth were extracted secondary to dental caries and infection.

D. Psychosocial History

- The patient was born in Peru and has lived in the USA for 20 years.

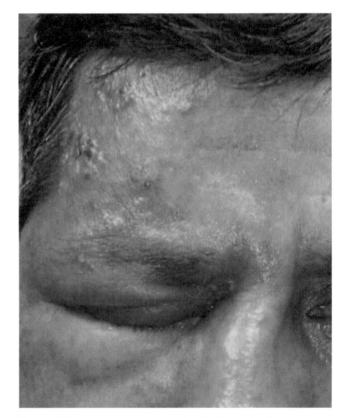

Figure 4.9 Appearance of patient at initial evaluation.

- Married, three children, age 6–10.
- Three siblings: an older brother, two sisters.
- Lower socio-economic status.
- The patient had normal scores for depression (PHQ-9), anxiety (GAD-7), physical symptoms (PHQ-15), and stress (PSS-10).
- He assumed a self-limiting infection.

E. Previous Consultations and Treatments

- Eleven months prior to the current complaint, the patient was working at the rear of a refuse collection vehicle. He explained he was struck across the right cheek by a cable bracing a utility pole. He did not see the cable and as the truck pulled ahead, he jumped from the truck striking his right cheek. This resulted in a nondisplaced zygomatic arch fracture and the loss of his maxillary denture. He was seen at a local emergency department, radiographs were taken, and no specific treatment offered, except palliative therapy for the pain and swelling of the right cheek. A new denture was fabricated.

- Thinking that the problem was secondary to the dental trauma, the patient consulted with the dentist who provided the new denture. He was offered a diagnosis of an allergic reaction and given a prescription of diphenhydramine. The rash began to fade, but at the same time the pain intensified. The patient was referred for an orofacial pain evaluation.

F. Extraoral Status

- The patient is approximately 172 cm in height.

Face

- The mandibular gait was somewhat guarded due to pain of the left temple and forehead.
- A bright red rash with the scars of numerous resolved vesicles was observed. The rash extended from the midline of the forehead across to the patient's hairline superiorly and laterally. It involved the entire upper eyelid. The remainder of the facial anatomy was within normal limits.
- With the exception of the rash, the patient's complexion was dark. Facial coloration and texture were otherwise uniform. Gross observation of facial movements was within normal limits.

Temporomandibular joint

- A palpatory examination of the TMJs found no tenderness laterally or posteriorly.
- Sounds consistent with soft crepitus emanated from the TMJs during function.

Masticatory muscles

- A palpatory examination of the masticatory musculature was performed as best as possible in the presence of the painful rash.
- Mild bilateral tenderness of the masseters and left temporalis muscles was detected without referral. The right temporalis could not be examined.
- No tender points reproduced familiar pain when palpated.

Jaw movements

- Maximum active opening was 42 mm measured interincisally.
- Bilateral movement was 8 mm to the left and 10 mm to the right.

- No deviations or deflections were noted other than a less than 2 mm deflection to the right at maximum opening.

Neck

- Cervical range of motion was normal; no movements evoked pain.
- No pain was elicited to palpation of the cervical and upper quarter musculature (trapezius, sternocleidomastoid, sub-occipital muscle groups).

G. Intraoral Status

Hard tissues

- The patient has a 1-year-old maxillary full denture that was provided. The denture is well made, well adapted, and functions properly.
- The edentulous maxillary ridge and mucosa are of normal appearance.
- The remaining mandibular dentition is intact with the exception of missing first and third molars.
- The patient is caries free with minimal posterior restorations.
- Anterior attrition of the mandibular incisors is noted, as is moderate gingival recession and inflammation.
- Hygiene is fair, with deposits of dental calculus and coffee stains noted.
- Missing mandibular molars are not replaced.

Soft tissues

- Normal appearance.

Occlusion

- Second molars have drifted mesially. The occlusion is stable.

H. Additional Examinations and Findings

- A cranial nerve examination found all cranial nerves intact. Note that the right occulomotor nerve could not be completely tested due to the closure of the right eye, and ophthalmic nerve could not be tested due to significant allodynia and hyperalgesia of the territory supplied by this nerve.

I. Diagnosis/Diagnoses

ICHD-3 beta

- Postherpetic trigeminal neuropathy (PHN) secondary to herpetic zoster of the ophthalmic division of the right trigeminal nerve.

J. Case Assessment

- This is a representative case of PHN after herpes zoster infection in the ophthalmic division of the right trigeminal nerve.

- If not for the classic presentation including the rash, a differential diagnosis might include trigeminal neuropathy.
- There was no history consistent with the current complaint as having any relationship to the accident of 1 year earlier.
- The presentation of the rash and associated symptoms is classic for herpetic zoster.
- No psychological factors were evident.

K. Evidence-based Treatment Plan including Aims

Aims

- Reduce pain.
- Prevent worsening of complaints.

Management

- The patient's initial presentation was approximately 1 or 2 months from the onset of an acute herpetic outbreak in the right ophthalmic division of the trigeminal nerve.
- The upper eyelid was closed, swollen, red, and crusty. It could not be opened. As there is a high risk of corneal scarring and loss of vision associated with ophthalmic herpetic zoster, the patient was urgently referred for an ophthalmologic evaluation on the same day as the initial evaluation. Antiviral ointments were prescribed.
- Systemic treatment included acyclovir 800 mg five times per day for 10 days.

L. Prognosis and Discussion

- Following the resolution of the initial outbreak, burning pain persisted for several months.
- At the time of the initial evaluation the patient's rash was present for over 1 week. Vesicles had begun to form scabs. Involvement of the upper eyelid increased the risk of corneal infection and scarring. Continuous burning pain in the area of the rash persisted for several months.
- A diagnosis of PHN is appropriate for an individual with pain that persists longer than 3 months after the resolution of confirmed herpetic zoster.
- Pain persists in the dermatomal distribution of the eruption, and is described in terms of burning and stinging. Pain is typically severe.
- After several months, pain slowly dissipated and, with the exception of facial scarring at the site of the rash, there were no sequelae. This favorable outcome is likely based on his young age and otherwise good health.

Background Information

Etiology and epidemiology

- PHN is more likely to occur in patients of greater than 60 years of age (Helgason et al., 2000).
- Most adults, especially those exposed to chickenpox as children, maintain the varicella virus in a dormant state in the dorsal root ganglia (DRG) of the sensory nervous system. Reactivation of the virus may occur in the presence of a compromised immune system. The dormant virus can reactivate in states of decreased immunosuppression, such as with aging. Exposure to the varicella virus, such as contact with a patient with chickenpox, is also a risk factor (Stankus et al., 2000).
- Up to 15% of patients who have suffered herpetic zoster will experience continued pain of postherpetic neuropathy.
- There is no gender specificity.
- Other risk factors for postherpetic neuropathy include the levels of intensity of pain associated with prodromal pain preceding the rash and the intensity of pain during the skin lesions. The more intense the prodromal pain, or pain during the outbreak of vesicles, the more likely painful postherpetic neuropathy will follow. Pain that persists for longer than 3 months is considered postherpetic neuropathy (Headache Classification Committee of the International Headache Society (IHS), 2013).
- Herpetic zoster of the ophthalmic division of the trigeminal nerves also poses a high risk factor for PHN and for ocular complications (Stankus et al., 2000).

Pathophysiology

- PHN is caused by reactivation of a dormant varicella zoster virus resulting in ectopic neuronal activity.
- The virus migrates toward the surface skin or mucosa along nerves associated with the DRG from where the virus has been reactivated.

- Neuronal injury of primary afferent neurons occurs during migration of the virus from the DRG to the skin or mucosa.
- The results of neuronal damage are:
  - sensory changes; allodynia and hyperalgesia;
  - central sensitization;
  - alteration of the pain inhibitory system.
  (Drummond, 2014)

Diagnostics

- The timing of the onset of the rash and observation associated with herpetic zoster, or obtaining a history of associated features, aid in the diagnostic process of postherpetic neuropathy.
- The vesicular outbreak is often preceded by prodromal symptoms of a tingling or burning sensation (Helgason *et al.*, 1996). This is due to the reactivation of the varicella virus as it travels along the affected nerve toward the skin or mucosa (Figure 4.10). This is followed by the appearance of multiple vesicles filled with clear fluid (Figure 4.11a). Vesicles eventually rupture and dry to form a scab during the healing process (Figure 4.11b). Scarring of the affected area may be apparent weeks later (Figure 4.11c). The affected area may exhibit sensory alterations, including hypoesthesia, allodynia, or hyperalgesia (Stankus *et al.*, 2000).

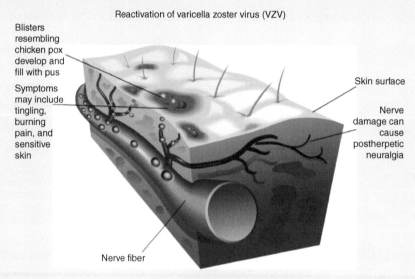

Reactivation of varicella zoster virus (VZV)

Blisters resembling chicken pox develop and fill with pus

Symptoms may include tingling, burning pain, and sensitive skin

Skin surface

Nerve damage can cause postherpetic neuralgia

Nerve fiber

Figure 4.10 Reactivation of varicella zoster virus. *Source:* courtesy Stephen Tyring, MD, Clinical Professor of Dermatology, University of Texas Health Science Center, Houston, TX.

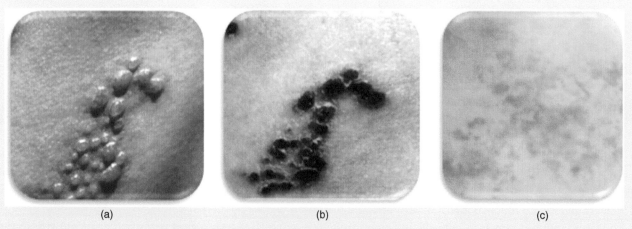

(a)　　　　　(b)　　　　　(c)

Figure 4.11 Vesicular outbreak of varicella zoster: (a) vesicles; (b) scab; (c) scarring. *Source:* courtesy Stephen Tyring, MD, Clinical Professor of Dermatology, University of Texas Health Science Center, Houston, TX.

Prognosis

- The prognosis for patients with PHN varies and is dependent upon the age of the patient (Gazewood and Meadows, 2003). One study included 2% of patients with PHN who were under age the age of 40, 21% who were aged 40–60, and 40% who were greater than 60 years old (Helgason et al., 1996, 2000). Pain was described as mild, moderate, or severe, with reports of the most severe complaints among those of greater than 60 years old. In the 60-year-old or older group, 18% reported continued mild pain at 3 months and 6% reported moderate to severe pain. At 1 year, 8% reported mild pain and 2% continued with moderate pain. Severe pain was not reported after 12 months (Helgason et al., 1996, 2000), although some had persistent mild discomfort. Only one patient in this study reported moderate pain after 7 years. The prognosis worsens with the age of the patient, and the probability of persistent PHN in the elderly is problematic. This is not only due to the loss of quality of life, but because of the side effects of the various medications used for management (Thyregod et al., 2007).

Diagnostic Criteria

ICHD 3rd edition (beta version) criteria for **Postherpetic trigeminal neuropathy** (Headache Classification Committee of the International Headache Society (IHS), 2013).

Unilateral head and/or facial pain persisting or recurring for at least 3 months in the distribution of one or more branches of the trigeminal nerve, with variable sensory changes, caused by herpes zoster.

A. Unilateral head and/or facial pain persisting or recurring for ≥3 months and fulfilling criterion C.
B. History of acute herpes zoster affecting a trigeminal nerve branch or branches.
C. Evidence of causation demonstrated by both of the following:
   1. pain developed in temporal relation to the acute Herpes zoster;
   2. pain is located in the distribution of the same trigeminal nerve branch or branches.
D. Not better accounted for by another ICHD-3 diagnosis.

Comment

Following acute herpes zoster, postherpetic neuralgia is more prevalent in the elderly. The first division of the trigeminal nerve is most commonly affected in PHN, but the second and third divisions can be involved also. Typically, the pain is burning and itching. Itching of affected areas may be very prominent and extremely bothersome. Sensory abnormalities and allodynia are usually present in the territory involved. Pale or light purple scars may be present as sequelae of the herpetic eruption.

Fundamental Points

Key points for diagnosis

- The observation or history of vesicles is key to the diagnosis of postherpetic neuropathy.
- An assessment must include a complete history and clinical evaluation.
  - This patient assumed an infection secondary to a prior trauma. Care was taken to obtain a detailed history and perform a thorough clinical evaluation. It was determined that the current complaint, nearly 1 year after the trauma, had no relationship. Further investigation found that the patient's youngest daughter had recently recovered from chickenpox, placing him at risk for varicella virus.
- Herpetic zoster may occur along any of the branches of the trigeminal nerve or along the course of any nerve in the body.
- Sensory alterations are common. Burning or stinging pain that persists for more than 3 months after the resolution of a confirmed herpetic zoster, and in the same territory as the eruption, is considered PHN.

Additional key points

- Unilaterality of the rash is characteristic of herpetic zoster.
- Vesicles may be found intraorally (Eisenberg, 1978), on the nasal mucosa, and in or around the ear.
- A differential diagnosis must begin with conditions requiring urgent attention. As seen in Figure 4.9, the patient suffered from a herpetic

outbreak in the right ophthalmic division of the trigeminal nerve. The eye is closed by swelling of the upper eyelid and is sealed by a dry, crusty material. Ophthalmic herpes zoster may result in corneal ulcerations. Urgent referral to an ophthalmologist was mandatory (Stankus *et al.*, 2000).

- Cutaneous scarring may be present.

Pharmacological treatment and prevention

- Medications that may shorten the course of herpetic zoster and prevent the formation of postherpetic neuropathy include antiviral medications such as acyclovir, valacyclovir, and famciclovir. These are most effective if administered within 72 h of the outbreak of the herpes zoster. These medications are often prescribed with steroids such as methylprednisone. While offering limited pain relief, they may reduce the incidence of PHN (Stankus *et al.*, 2000).

- Palliative treatment includes topical anesthetics via an adhesive patch, cream or spray, and systemic medications, including membrane stabilizer, anti-inflammatories, and analgesics. Systemic medications beginning with low-dose TCAs such as nortriptyline, antiseizure medications such as pregabalin, injections of steroids, and, in severe cases, opioids may be useful. (Lapolla *et al.*, 2011).

- The prevention for PHN is prevention of herpetic zoster. This may be accomplished by administration of a vaccine composed of attenuated chickenpox virus. However, data suggest it is only 50% effective.

Self-study Questions

1. How is postherpetic neuropathy diagnosed?
2. What are the common symptoms associated with postherpetic neuropathy?
3. Name three targets for treatment of postherpetic neuropathy and describe treatment.
4. What are the risk factors for PHN?
5. Is PHN preventable?

References

Drummond PD (2014) Neuronal changes resulting in up-regulation of alpha-1 adrenoceptors after peripheral nerve injury. *Neural Regen Res* **9**(14):1337–1340.

Eisenberg E (1978) Intraoral isolated herpes zoster. *Oral Surg Oral Med Oral Pathol* **45**(2):214–219.

Finnerup NB, Attal N, Haroutounian S, et al. (2015) Pharmacotherapy for neuropathic pain in adults: a systematic review and meta-analysis. *Lancet Neurol* **14**(2):162–173.

Gazewood JD, Meadows S (2003) What is the prognosis of postherpetic neuralgia? *J Fam Pract* **52**(6):485–497.

Headache Classification Committee of the International Headache Society (IHS) (2013) The International Classification of Headache Disorders, 3rd edition (beta version). *Cephalalgia* **33**(9):629–808.

Helgason S, Sigurdsson JA, Gudmundsson S (1996) The clinical course of herpes zoster: a prospective study in primary care. *Eur J Gen Pract* **2**:12–16.

Helgason S, Peturrson G, Gudmundsson S, Sigurdsson JA (2000) Prevalence of postherpetic neuralgia after a single episode of herpes zoster: prospective study with long term follow up. *BMJ* **321**:1–4.

Lapolla W, DiGiorgio C, Haitz K, et al. (2011) Incidence of postherpetic neuralgia after combination treatment with gabapentin and valacyclovir in patients with acute herpes zoster open-label. *JAMA Dermatol* **147**(8):901–907.

Oaklander AL (2008) Mechanisms of pain and itch caused by herpes zoster (shingles). *J Pain* **9**(1 Suppl 1):S10–S18.

Stankus SJ, Dlugopolski M, Packer E (2000) Management of herpes zoster (shingles) and postherpetic neuralgia. *Am Fam Physician* **61**(8):2437–2444.

Thyregod HG, Rowbotham MC, Peters M, et al. (2007) Natural history of pain following herpes zoster. *Pain* **128**(1–2):148–156.

Answers to Self-study Questions

1. Postherpetic neuropathy is diagnosed by the history. Postherpetic neuropathy is preceded by herpetic zoster, or a reactivation of the varicella zoster virus, commonly referred to as shingles. Therefore, the diagnosis of PHN requires a history consistent with an outbreak herpes zoster. The history is of significant importance in the diagnostic process. The patient will report:

   ○ An abnormal, unilateral tingling or burning sensation in the area of innervation of a specific nerve.
   ○ Within days of the abnormal sensation, an outbreak of small vesicles occurs if extraorally, or small ulcers intraorally. Vesicles occurring intraorally break down and ulcerate quickly (Eisenberg, 1978).
   ○ Vesicles rupture and leak a clear fluid. It is at this stage the virus may be easily transmitted to others.
   ○ The ruptured vesicles crust over and heal, often leaving a scar.

   The rash may persist for 7–10 days and the entire episode may average 4 weeks in duration. If pain persists for 3 months following an outbreak of herpetic zoster, it is considered postherpetic neuropathy. Its severity may depend on the intensity of prodromal pain and pain during the outbreak of vesicles.

2. Patients with PHN describe a variety of pain complaints ranging from moderate to severe. Severe pain is described as burning, sharp, electric-like and jabbing, or deep and aching. Patients suffering from PHN also report significant allodynia or pain to a nonpainful stimulus. These patients may report that even the light touch of loosely fit clothing may be intolerable. Less severe complaints include a numb, itchy, or pins-and-needles sensation.

3. Damage to the primary afferent receptors may occur at the site of herpetic vesicles. The inflammatory process reduces the firing threshold of these nociceptors, allowing the production of action potentials to non-noxious stimuli (allodynia). Sensitized receptors may remain in a hypersensitive state even after the inflammation has resolved. Affective treatment is via the use of topical anesthetics, specifically topical lidocaine patches applied to the painful areas.

Damage to the primary afferent neurons occurs as the reactivated virus travels along the nerve on its passage to the surface. Depending on the virulence, the result is neuronal damage, altering activity.

Ectopic discharge, ephaptic activity, and neuronal loss along with spontaneous C-nociceptor activity are likely (Oaklander, 2008). Treatment of this target involves membrane stabilization of primary afferent nociceptive neurons. First-line systemic medications useful in the management of PHN include serotonin–noradrenalin reuptake inhibitors (SNRIs) and TCAs (Finnerup et al., 2015). DRG cells infected by varicella virus acquire a sensitivity to noradrenaline by apparently upregulating alpha-1 adrenoceptors. They occur within the DRG and along the primary afferent neurons secondary to trauma; in this case, secondary to the passage of the varicella virus. This may explain the increased pain of PHN during times of increase noradrenaline (Drummond, 2014). Medications that can reduce the activity of alpha-1 adrenoceptors (agonists) include SNRIs and TCAs.

4. Up to 15% of patients who have suffered herpetic zoster will experience PHN. Risk factors include age greater than 60 years, a state of decreased immunosuppression, such as with aging, and exposure to the varicella virus, such as contact with a patient with chickenpox.

5. Yes. Vaccines are available to prevent herpes zoster. It is meant for individuals 60 years of age or older. It has an approximate 60% efficacy in preventing a recurrence of the virus and, therefore, is preventative for herpes zoster.

Case 4.4

Post-traumatic Trigeminal Neuropathy

Sowmya Ananthan, Junad Khan, Vincent B Ziccardi and Rafael Benoliel

A. Demographic Data and Reason for Contact

- Caucasian female, 59 years old.
- Pain and numbness in the lower right chin area for the past 6 months.

B. Symptom History

- The patient had an implant placed in area 46 around 6 months ago by her general dentist.
- The pain and sensory changes started right after the surgery.
- Initially, right after surgery, the pain was severe. Over time this became moderate to severe (6–7 on an NRS 0–10), located in the area of the right mental nerve, and did not spread significantly. The quality was described as burning and pain was present constantly, with some variations in severity through the day.
- Two weeks after initial placement, her general dentist, due to the pain and accompanying sensory changes, removed the implant.
- The symptoms did not subside on implant removal. One month after the initial injury, the general dentist referred the patient to an orofacial pain center.

C. Medical History

- Hypertension.
- Irritable bowel syndrome.
- Fibromyalgia.
- No known drug allergies.
- Current medications: Percocet® (combination of oxycodone 2.5 mg and acetaminophen 325 mg).

D. Psychosocial History

- Single.
- High school teacher.
- Pain is highly disabling, but moderately limiting (GCPS).
- Significant distress with moderate–severe symptoms of depression (PHQ-9), moderate anxiety (GAD-7), and moderate physical symptoms (PHQ-15).

E. Previous Consultations and Treatments

- The patient was evaluated at the orofacial pain center. Since the symptom history suggested trauma to the inferior alveolar nerve, CBCT was performed. This showed perforation of the roof of the inferior alveolar nerve canal in the area of tooth 46 (Figure 4.12).
- The patient was prescribed a course of steroids to reduce inflammation in the nerve vicinity. She was also given a referral to an oral surgeon to consult regarding nerve repair.
- After discussion of various options with the patient, the oral surgeon decided that the best course of action would be nerve decompression surgery.
- Nerve decompression surgery was performed, to relieve the inferior alveolar nerve in the area of injury, 3 months after the initial injury. Axoguard® was placed around the nerve. Axoguard is an extracellular matrix used to protect injured nerves and to reinforce

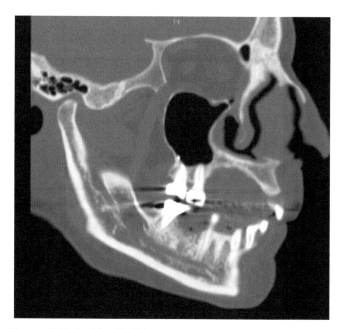

Figure 4.12 In this CBCT image, osteotomy site #46 shows breach of the roof of the inferior alveolar nerve canal.

nerve reconstruction, while preventing soft tissue attachments.

- Anesthesia in the initial area was relieved partially by the surgery by about 40%, and evolved into paresthesia, but the pain persisted.
- She was then referred back to the orofacial pain center for further management. On presentation after the surgery, she had both pain and sensory changes (paresthesia) in the right mental nerve distribution.

F. Extraoral exam
Face and neck

- No asymmetry.
- Skin color of affected area not different from surrounding noninjured area.
- No palpable lymph nodes.

Neurological findings

- Patient has an area of paresthesia (after the surgery) and allodynia (pain to light touch) extraorally in the right mental nerve territory in the mapped area (Figure 4.13).

Temporomandibular joint

- Moderate pain (not familiar) on palpation of the right TMJ.
- Opening click in right TMJ.
- Deviation to the right side with correction toward the midline.

Masticatory muscles

- Mild pain (not familiar) in the right superficial and deep masseter. No pain referral.

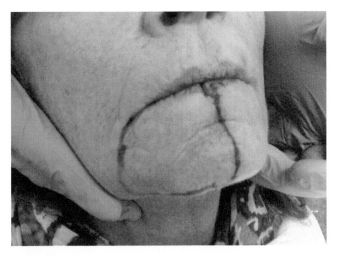

Figure 4.13 Mapped area of sensory changes extraorally at presentation at our center after the surgery.

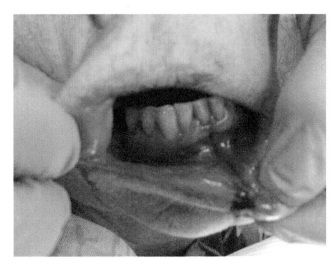

Figure 4.14 Mapped area of sensory changes intraorally.

G. Intraoral exam
Soft tissues

- Area of paresthesia and allodynia (pain to light touch) intraorally in the buccal gingiva from area 41 to 46 (Figure 4.14).
- There was no color change or swelling in the soft tissues of the injured area.
- The dorsum of the tongue was fissured.

Hard tissues

- Tooth 46 is missing. All other teeth in the mouth are present, with the exception of third molars.
- Teeth 34, 35, and 36 have crowns.
- Teeth 11, 12, 21, and 22 have veneers.
- Alveolar bone in the area of 46 has a bony depression, where the implant had been placed and removed.

H. Additional Examination and Findings
Neurosensory testing

- A cotton swab was first used to grossly delineate areas of pain and paresthesia. Within the delineated area, two additional tests were performed:
- (1) Mechanical test with Von Frey monofilaments:
  - Von Frey monofilaments are graded, calibrated nylon monofilaments, which are capable of delivering predetermined amounts of force.
  - There was hypoesthesia in the delineated area compared with the contralateral side.
- (2) Electrical test with Neurometer NervScan NS3000:
  - This device can deliver electrical stimuli at different frequencies, which are hypothesized to stimulate different nerve fibers.

Table 4.1 Detection thresholds of the affected (right) and unaffected dermatomes to electrical stimuli using the Neurometer

Frequency used	Right mental (mA)	Left mental (mA)	Ratio (right/left)
5 Hz (C fibers)	50	20	2.5
250 Hz (Aδ fibers)	90	30	3
2000 Hz (Aβ fibers)	380	220	1.7

mA: milliamperes.

- Expressing the electrical detection thresholds as the ratio between the injured and contralateral control side reduces any inconsistency with this method.
- This test showed hyposensitivity in the right mental nerve distribution compared with the contralateral side (Table 4.1).

I. Diagnosis

ICHD-3 beta

- Painful post-traumatic trigeminal neuropathy (PTTN).

J. Case Assessment

- The patient's symptoms and signs fit the diagnostic criteria for PTTN. She had unilateral facial pain located in the distribution of the right inferior alveolar nerve that developed immediately after the implant placement in the same distribution. She also had both a positive (allodynia) and a negative sign (hypoesthesia) of trigeminal nerve dysfunction.
- Localized sensory changes and persistent pain are indicative for PTTN. If left untreated, over time these changes may become persistent. It is important to evaluate these patients early (within days) after the initial injury to:
  - rapidly assess the degree of injury;
  - determine the possibility of nerve repair;
  - establish the early management strategy.
- Imaging is essential to determine the degree of nerve injury, the presence of a "compressing agent" (e.g., an implant), or any pathology (e.g., sequestrum).
- Neurosensory testing is also needed to localize and quantify nerve function.
- Discussion with the patient on management and prognosis.

K. Evidence-based Treatment Plan including Aims

Aims of treatment

- Reduce pain.
- Reduce extent (area) and severity of sensory changes.

Treatment plan

Pharmacologic management

- The patient was prescibed pregabalin 75 mg, three times a day, and duloxetine 20 mg, twice a day. At the same time she was titrated down from the oxycodone–paracetamol combination she was taking (Attal *et al.*, 2010; Finnerup *et al.*, 2015).

Psychosocial management

- The patient was referred for psychological counselling.

L. Prognosis and Discussion

- This case demonstrates how dental implant placement with nerve injury may result in neuropathic complications. In this case example, the patient had both sensory changes and persistent pain.
- Evidence suggests that patients who are female, with a history of painful dental procedures, high pain intensity around the area that is subsequently treated, and with comorbid pain conditions are more likely to suffer from PTTN following nerve injury. Two factors were present in this patient: female sex and fibromyalgia.
- Surgery improved the return of sensation, from complete anesthesia to paresthesia.
- The prognosis in this case is poor, as even after months of pharmacological management the overall pain relief was just under 30% (NRS ratings changed from 7/10 to 5/10).
- Surgery has mostly positive effects on sensory disturbances (Figure 4.15), but less effects on pain. Pharmacotherapy can help with pain management, but has minimal effects on sensory disturbances.

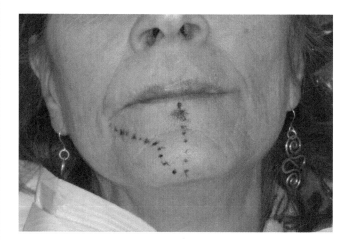

Figure 4.15 Mapped area of injury, 1 month after start of pharmacotherapy, showing shrinkage of the affected area.

Background Information

- Following dental implant surgery, up to 36% of patients may experience transient sensory changes, and up to ~7% of patients may have permanent sensory changes (unpublished systematic review in our center). The incidence of chronic pain is unclear.
- If surgery is considered, this should be made as early as possible and within the 3-month point if there is no, or minimal, return of sensation or in the presence of dysesthesia. The sensory outcomes are better if the repair is performed within 6 months of the initial injury (Nizam and Ziccardi, 2015).
- The mainstays of neuropathic pain management are the TCA and SNRI antidepressants, and the anti-epileptics. An evidence-based treatment algorithm for painful neuropathy is shown in Figure 4.16.

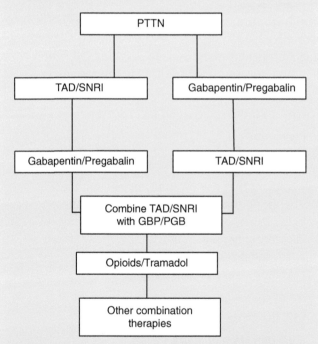

Figure 4.16 Evidence based management of painful neuropathies. Based on the patient's medical history and patient/physician preference either a TCA/SNRI antidepressant or pregabalin/gabapentin should be initiated. If these fail to offer sufficient relief the alternate drug should be tried, if the medical history permits. Further failure is an indication for a trial of both drugs at the same time. Failure of combination therapy may be an indication for opioid therapy or combined opioid–gabapentin therapy. In areas that are amenable, topical therapy may aid in pain management.

- PTTN can be associated with a significant psychosocial burden, where patients can display increased depression levels, pain catastrophizing, with lowered coping skills (Smith *et al.*, 2013).

Diagnostic Criteria

ICHD 3rd edition (beta version) criteria for **Post-traumatic trigeminal neuropathy** (Headache Classification Committee of the International Headache Society (IHS), 2013). Sensitivity and specificity have not been determined.

Unilateral facial or oral pain following trauma to the trigeminal nerve, with other symptoms and/or clinical signs of trigeminal nerve dysfunction.

Criteria

A. Unilateral facial and/or oral pain fulfilling criterion C.
B. History of an identifiable traumatic event (mechanical, chemical, thermal,or radiation exposure) to the trigeminal nerve, with clinically evident positive (hyperalgesia, allodynia) and/or negative (hypoesthesia, hypoalgesia) signs of trigeminal nerve dysfunction.
C. Evidence of causation demonstrated by both of the following:
1. Pain is located in the distribution of the same trigeminal nerve.
2. Pain has developed within 3–6 months of the traumatic event.
D. Not better accounted for by another ICHD-3 diagnosis.

Fundamental Points

Pharmacological treatment of post-traumatic trigeminal neuropathy

Tricyclic antidepressants

- Amitriptyline is approved by the US FDA for treatment of depression, but is the most validated TCA for neuropathic pain management. Off label, it has been used for the management of migraines, tension-type headache, irritable bowel syndrome, polyneuropathy, fibromyalgia, post-herpetic neuropathy, and myofascial pain.
- Amitriptyline may enhance descending inhibition via the inhibition of the reuptake of 5-HT

(serotonin) and noradrenaline, but also has opioid-enhancing properties and sodium, potassium, and calcium channel blocking properties. The analgesic effect is independent of the antidepressant actions and appears at lower doses.

- Recommended initial dose is 10 mg taken 1–2 h before bedtime. The dose may be increased if necessary at a rate of 10 mg a week to a maximum of 35–50 mg.
- Presence of cardiovascular disease requires medical consultation. When taken along with an SSRI, TCAs increase risk of upper gastrointestinal bleeding. Potential contraindications include urinary retention and narrow-angle glaucoma. Side effects include dry mouth, sedation, palpitations, nausea, sweating, and weight gain.

(Moore *et al.*, 2012)

Anti-epileptic drugs

- Anti-epileptic drugs are reasonably successful in the management of neuropathic pain.
- Gabapentin is FDA approved for treatment of seizures and postherpetic neuropathy. Off label uses include migraine management, diabetic neuropathy, trigeminal neuralgia, short-lasting neuralgiform headache attacks with conjunctival injection and tearing (SUNCT), and cluster headache.
- Pregabalin is FDA cleared for the treatment of partial seizures, diabetic neuropathy, postherpetic neuropathy, and pain from spinal cord injury.
- Anti-epileptic drugs suppress neuronal excitability via inhibition of glutamate neurotransmission, blockage of L-type calcium channel, blockage of voltage-gated sodium channels and enhanced GABAergic neurotransmission (enhanced GABA metabolism and release and GABA receptor activation).
- Recommended initial dose for gabapentin is 300 mg, increased by 300 mg daily over a period of 3 days. Maintenance doses of 900–2400 mg can be taken daily.
- Recommended initial dose for pregabalin is 50 mg three times/day or 75 mg two times/day. Maintenance dose is 75–150 mg daily.

- Precaution for gabapentin is the presence of renal problems. Side effects for gabapentin include dizziness, ataxia, and fatigue. Visual disturbances include tremor, weight gain, dyspepsia, amnesia, weakness, and paresthesia.
- Side effects of pregabalin include mild–moderate dizziness and somnolence, confusion, headache, amnesia, ataxia, and weakness. Constipation, dry mouth, and vomiting may also occur.

(Wiffen *et al.*, 2013)

Serotonin–noradrenaline reuptake inhibitors

- Duloxetine is a new-generation SNRI and is FDA approved for major depressive disorder, generalized anxiety disorder, fibromyalgia, chronic musculoskeletal pain, and painful diabetic neuropathy.
- It mainly inhibits the reuptake of serotonin and noradrenaline, but also shares some mode of action with the TCAs.
- Recommended initial dose is 20–40 mg increased to 60 mg daily.
- Contraindications include epilepsy, glaucoma, and hepatic impairment. Side effects: insomnia, headache, sleepiness, suicidal ideation.

(Lunn *et al.*, 2014)

Prevention

- Preoperative planning of safe implant placement (e.g., imaging – CBCT), determining length of implant that can be safely placed without violating the adjacent neural structures.
- Technical advances such as stops on the osteotomy drills to prevent overpenetration beyond planned depth.
- Postoperative analgesics and anti-inflammatories.

Patient assessment

Early detection of injury

- Reports suggest that cases identified and treated early have a better prognosis.
- Patients should be recalled soon after the surgery to assess any neurosensory complications from the surgery.
- Radiographic assessment should be routinely done after the implant placement surgery has been completed. This step will detect any neural impingement subsequent to surgery.

• Clinical assessment includes mapping of area of injury and neurological assessment. Simple chair-side neurological assessment can be done with standard dental instruments (e.g., probe, cotton wool). Difference in response to the stimuli between the injured and noninjured side should be quantified and documented.

Early management

• If the patient complains of neurosensory disturbances, they should be evaluated clinically and radiographically as detailed previously.

• If there is frank impingement on the nerve, the implant should be removed or shortened. The area should be debrided gently and sutured.

• The patient should be prescribed a course of steroids (such as prednisone 40–60 mg initially, then tapered over 7–10 days or dexamethasone 12 mg initially, then tapered over 7–10 days) to reduce inflammation. Preclinical evidence suggests that by inhibiting inflammation the incidence of neuropathy may be decreased.

• The patient should be referred to an oral surgeon with experience in microsurgery for assessment and to determine if the patient is suitable for nerve repair.

• If there is no neural impingement, the sensory disturbance could be the result of postsurgical inflammation surrounding the nerve. It is recommended to prescribe a course of steroids in this scenario and keep evaluating the patient closely.

Late management

• Pain management in established PTTN is very difficult.

• Late pharmacological management will follow the treatment algorithm described previously (Nizam and Ziccardi, 2015). The patient's medical background and preferences should be taken into consideration before prescribing any medications.

Self-study Questions

1. What important precautions should be taken after the implant surgery to minimize neurosensory complications?

2. What are some of the recommendations for early management of dental implant injuries?

3. How should the patient, who presents with neurosensory complications secondary to dental implant placement, be worked up?

4. What are the different types of medications that are available for "late" pharmacological management?

References

Attal N, Cruccu G, Baron R, et al. (2010) EFNS guidelines on the pharmacological treatment of neuropathic pain: 2010 revision. Eur J Neurol 17(9):1113-e88.

Finnerup NB, Attal N, Haroutounian S, et al. (2015) Pharmacotherapy for neuropathic pain in adults: a systematic review and meta-analysis. Lancet Neurol 14(2):162–173.

Headache Classification Committee of the International Headache Society (IHS) (2013) The International Classification of Headache Disorders, 3rd edition (beta version). Cephalalgia 33(9):629–808.

Lunn MP, Hughes RA, Wiffen PJ (2014) Duloxetine for treating painful neuropathy, chronic pain or fibromyalgia. Cochrane Database Syst Rev (1):CD007115.

Moore RA, Derry S, Aldington D, et al. (2012) Amitriptyline for neuropathic pain and fibromyalgia in adults. Cochrane Database Syst Rev (12):CD008242.

Nizam SA, II, Ziccardi VB (2015) Trigeminal nerve injuries: avoidance and management of iatrogenic injury. Oral Maxillofac Surg Clin North Am 27(3):411–424.

Smith JG, Elias LA, Yilmaz Z, et al. (2013) The psychosocial and affective burden of posttraumatic neuropathy following injuries to the trigeminal nerve. J Orofac Pain 27(4):293–303.

Wiffen PJ, Derry S, Moore RA, et al. (2013) Antiepileptic drugs for neuropathic pain and fibromyalgia – an overview of Cochrane reviews. Cochrane Database Syst Rev (11):CD010567.

Answers to Self-study Questions

1. After the final position of the implant is determined, a check X-ray should be taken to determine whether there is any neural impingement. The patient should be called the day of the surgery after the anesthesia should have worn off to ascertain if they are still having subjective signs of anesthesia. They should be prescribed postoperative analgesics and anti-inflammatories.

2. If the patient has subjective signs of persistent anesthesia they should be brought back immediately and a thorough clinical and radiographic exam should be conducted. If the implant is impinging on the nerve, the implant should be removed and the patient should be prescribed a course of steroids along with a referral to an oral surgeon with experience in microsurgery. If the implant is not in

violation of the neural structures, but the patient still is experiencing neurosensory disturbances, they should be prescribed steroids to reduce inflammation in the vicinity of the neural structures.

3. A thorough history should be obtained from the patient. A clinical exam should be performed, which should include mapping of the injured area and sensory testing.

4. For "late" pharmacological management, medications that can be used include TCAs, anti-epileptics, and SNRIs.

Case 4.5

Atypical Odontalgia/Persistent Dentoalveolar Pain

Maria Pigg and Lene Baad-Hansen

A. Demographic Data and Reason for Contact
- Female, 34 years old.
- Pain on right side of upper jaw and face.

B. Symptom History
- Dentoalveolar pain started 3 years ago in tooth 16, root-filled >10 years earlier.
- No known initiating event.
- Persistent, daily dentoalveolar pain, average intensity 6–8 (0–10 NRS). Occasionally increasing to 9–10 for 2–3 h.
- Dentoalveolar pain accompanied by a sensation of swelling and occasionally a "pins and needles" sensation in the area.
- No alleviating factors.
- Pain with average intensity 3–4 (NRS 0–10) and fatigue also frequently present in face/jaws.
- Chewing hard food aggravates the jaw pain.
- Patient suspects night bruxism, unconfirmed by partner.
- Clicking jaw joints (not painful), no locking.
- No associated autonomic symptoms.

C. Medical History
- Neck pain.
- Migraine without aura, occurring two or three times a year.
- No regular medications.

D. Psychosocial History
- Cohabiting with partner, no children, harmonious family relationships.
- Working full time, runs business and is also part-time employee (customer's service). Content with working situation but perceives it as stressful.
- Pain makes it difficult to concentrate.
- Increasingly avoids social activities because of weariness and low mood.
- Mild depression (PHQ-9), anxiety (GAD-7), and somatization (PHQ-15). Moderate stress (PSS-10) and severe catastrophizing (PCS).

E. Previous Consultations and Treatments
- Sudden onset 3 years ago of mild but increasing dentoalveolar pain in region 16.
- Pain was unexplained by clinical and radiographic findings according to dentist.
- Tooth 16 surgical endodontic retreatment by specialist in endodontics 4 months after pain onset. No explanatory findings during surgery. No change in pain post-surgery.
- Tooth 16 was extracted 5 months after endodontic surgery. Initial decrease in pain, but within 3–4 weeks the pain returned with intensity slowly increasing to present level.
- Referral to specialist in orofacial pain and TMD 2 years ago; received an occlusal appliance. Dentoalveolar pain was unchanged, but moderate improvement of jaw pain and fatigue.
- Referral to specialist in maxillofacial surgery 1.5 years ago; received MRI examination and arthroscopy of right-side TMJ; no conclusive findings.
- Paracetamol (acetaminophen) and diclofenac give only partial pain relief.

F. Extraoral Status
- TMJ: clicking right side, no associated pain.
- Masseter and temporalis muscles: localized familiar palpation pain bilaterally with no spreading or referral to tooth (Figure 4.17a).
- Jaw movement capacity: within normal limits.
- On maximum jaw opening, familiar pain in masseter muscle bilaterally.
- Neck: local palpation tenderness, no referral of pain to face or teeth, movement capacity within normal limits.
- Qualitative sensory examination of face: hypoesthesia to touch and cold in maxillary branch of trigeminal nerve (V:2), right side.
- Cranial nerve assessment: normal findings except for V:2 hypoesthesia.

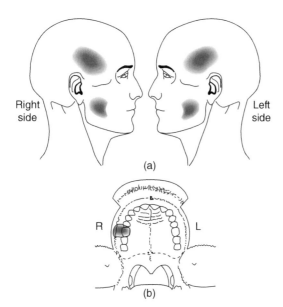

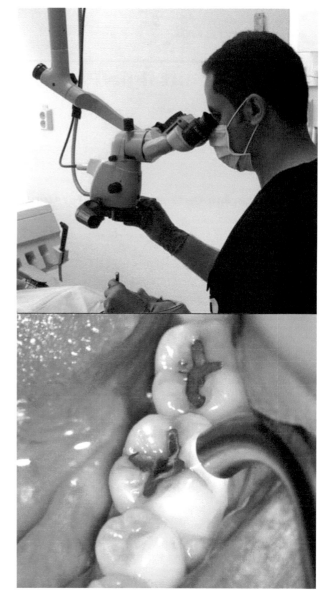

Figure 4.17 Anatomical drawing depicting pain locations (shaded areas): (a) face/jaw pain; (b) dentoalveolar pain.

G. Intraoral Status

- Tooth 16 missing.
- No caries, no periodontal disease, good oral hygiene.
- Soft tissues appear normal in the pain region, no swelling or redness.
- Dentoalveolar pain is localized to alveolar ridge and buccal area regio 16 (Figure 4.17b).
- Slight percussion tenderness upper molars bilaterally.
- Pulp vitality of teeth 15, 17, and 18 confirmed by electric pulp test.
- Microscope inspection with transillumination shows no tooth pathology (Figure 4.18).
- Radiographic examination shows no hard tissue pathology in the pain region (Figure 4.19).
- Occlusal contacts only on posterior teeth in intercuspal position.
- Dental wear according to age.
- Intraoral (region 16 with region 26 as control) qualitative sensory examination (QualST; see Figure 4.20 and Fundamental Points box) shows side differences: hypoesthesia to touch, hypoesthesia to cold, and hyperalgesia to pinprick, and repetitive pinprick stimulation increases pain from 4 to 7 (NRS 0–10); that is, sensory disturbances in the painful dentoalveolar region.

H. Additional Examinations and Findings

- Intraoral quantitative sensory testing (QST; see Fundamental Points box): confirmed sensory abnormalities in the pain region:
  - hypoesthesia to light mechanical stimulus (touch);

Figure 4.18 Operating microscope and enhanced light facilitates careful examination of teeth in the pain region.

  - hyperalgesia to cold and to heat;
  - mechanical pain (pinprick) threshold within the normal interval but considerably lower on the pain side.
- Diagnostic anesthesia: 40% pain reduction after infiltration injection with ropivacain; from initial 7 to 4 after 15 min and after 1 h and 5–6 after 6 h (NRS 0–10).

I. Diagnosis/Diagnoses
Other

- Atypical odontalgia (AO)/persistent dentoalveolar pain (PDAP) region 16.
- Myalgia neck muscles.

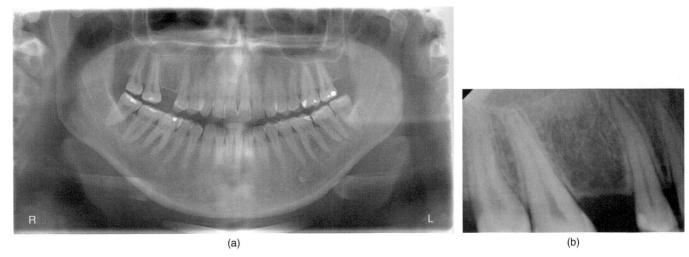

Figure 4.19 Pain is located to the right upper jaw, where tooth 16 was extracted after pain onset. Panoramic (a) and periapical (b) radiographs without signs of pathology.

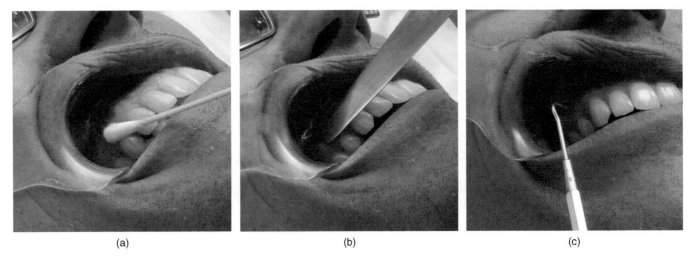

Figure 4.20 Example of intraoral qualitative sensory examination (QualST). Simple, easily available tools are used to compare the patient's perception of (a) touch, (b) cold, and (c) pinprick pain between pain site and corresponding contralateral gingival site.

ICHD-3 beta

• Persistent idiopathic facial pain.

DC/TMD

• Myalgia of masticatory muscles.
• Disc displacement with reduction right TMJ.

J. Case Assessment

• The dentoalveolar pain is suspected to be of neuropathic origin, although according to the patient's recollection no causative traumatic event in close timewise relationship with the pain could be clearly identified in the history. Central and/or peripheral mechanisms may be perpetuating the pain.
• Demonstration of sensory disturbances in the painful dentoalveolar region and V:2 extraorally.
• The sensory disturbances respect relevant neuroanatomical boundaries.
• Myalgia may be secondary to central sensitization.
• Disc displacement not bothersome to the patient
• Some degree of psychosocial distress.
• If bruxism is present, it may possibly contribute to myalgia and jaw fatigue, since this pain was reduced by occlusal appliance. Dentoalveolar pain, however,

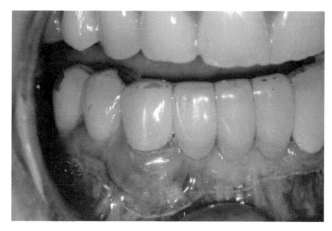

Figure 4.21 Soft splint with a reservoir in the pain region for deposition of lidocaine cream (in this example, a reservoir in region 43 is shown).

was not affected and therefore unlikely to be related to bruxism.

K. Evidence-based Treatment Plan including Aims

- Information about likely origin and causes of pain. Aim: educate the patient about the condition and reduce fear of malignant causes.
- Topical anesthesia (10% lidocaine cream deposited in soft splint with reservoir region 16; Figure 4.21). Aim: reduce peripheral sensory input from dentoalveolar pain area.
- Pharmacological treatment: pregabalin starting at 25 mg/day. Aim: reduce dentoalveolar pain and central sensitization.
- Psychological management based on CBT or acceptance and commitment therapy (ACT) principles. Aim: reduce affective/cognitive perpetuating factors.
- Jaw relaxation and exercises. Aim: reduce tension, fatigue, and pain in masticatory muscles.

L. Prognosis and Discussion

- After 3 months on pregabalin (daily dose stabilized to 2–3 × 50 mg) the pain was reduced to 1 in the mornings, increasing over the day to 4–5 (NRS 0–10).
- Patient also used soft splint with lidocaine cream regularly according to need, with good but temporary effect.
- Patient completed a CBT/ACT-based "pain school" program and learned strategies to function well despite ongoing pain.
- AO/PDAP is a chronic, often treatment-resistant, condition with no known cure.
- Treatment aims to reduce pain to a tolerable level.

- Multimodal management is an often recommended strategy (see Fundamental Points box), which was successful in this case.
- Prognosis is uncertain as to complete pain resolution.

Background information

- AO/PDAP has been estimated to occur in 1.4–5.5% of patients after endodontic treatment (Nixdorf *et al.*, 2010).
- AO/PDAP is often described as continuous and localized pain in one or more teeth or in the extraction region after tooth removal, in the absence of any dental cause (Woda *et al.*, 2005; Baad-Hansen, 2008). The pain is also usually described as continuous or present during most of the day, and non-paroxysmal in character.
- AO/PDAP may be considered a diagnosis of exclusion, which is unsatisfactory from a research perspective. The diagnosis has long been considered part of the group of idiopathic orofacial pain conditions (Woda *et al.*, 2005), but in recent decades there is increasing evidence supporting a neuropathic origin, including sensory disturbances and abnormal trigeminal reflexes (Forssell *et al.*, 2015). Hence, AO/PDAP may (at least in some cases) be of neuropathic origin due to damage to trigeminal afferent nerve fibers in association with, for example, endodontics, dentoalveolar surgery, or injection trauma/local anesthetic neurotoxicity.
- In cases where there is no clear evidence of nerve damage, AO/PDAP may be best grouped as "functional" pain (in terms of pathophysiological mechanism), with generalized hyperexcitability of the somatosensory system despite the absence of any demonstrable disease or nerve damage (Woolf *et al.*, 1998; Forssell *et al.*, 2015).

Diagnostic Criteria

ICHD 3rd edition (beta version) criteria for **Persistent idiopathic facial pain** persistent idiopathic facial pain (Headache Classification Committee of the International Headache Society (IHS), 2013: 781–782). Sensitivity and specificity have not been established.

Persistent facial and/or oral pain, with varying presentations but recurring daily for more than 2 h per day over more than 3 months, in the absence of clinical neurological deficit.

Criteria

A. Facial and/or oral pain fulfilling criteria B and C.
B. Recurring daily for >2 h per day for >3 months.
C. Pain has both of the following characteristics:
   1. poorly localized, and not following the distribution of a peripheral nerve;
   2. dull, aching, or nagging quality.
D. Clinical neurological examination is normal.
E. A dental cause has been excluded by appropriate investigations.
F. Not better accounted for by another ICHD-3 diagnosis.

Note: the term AO has been applied to a continuous pain in one or more teeth or in a tooth socket after extraction, in the absence of any usual dental cause. This is thought to be a subform of persistent idiopathic facial pain, although it is more localized, the mean age at onset is younger, and genders are more balanced. Based on the history of trauma, AO may also be a subform of painful PTTN. These subforms, if they exist, have not been sufficiently studied to propose diagnostic criteria.

DC/TMD criteria for **Myalgia**, see Case 3.3, and for **Disc displacement with reduction**, see Case 2.3 (Schiffman *et al.*, 2014).

Fundamental Points

Classification

• Persistent non-odontogenic dentoalveolar pain may currently be classified according to various classification systems from: the IHS, IASP, AAOP, and the RDC/TMD Consortium. For many years, AO has been the preferred term, with diagnostic criteria varying slightly between diagnostic systems. Without defining causative factors, the term PDAP has been suggested by some researchers (Nixdorf and Moana-Filho, 2011), whereas others prefer to include these patients in the painful PTTN category due to the evidence of involvement of neuropathic pain mechanisms in at least some of the patients (Benoliel *et al.*, 2012). Cases with sufficient

evidence of nerve damage obtained through patient history, somatosensory testing, and/or neurophysiological tests are probably most correctly labeled as painful PTTN (see Case 4.4).

Neurophysiological tests

• *Qualitative somatosensory testing (QualST)* can be done in a simple procedure. Testing may include perception of touch, cold, and pinprick pain in order to test different types of nerve fibers. Comparing the patient's pain site (gingival or mucosal) with the corresponding contralateral site may reveal side-to-side differences in perception indicating abnormal sensory function, possibly neuropathy (Figure 4.20).
• A more extensive examination, *quantitative somatosensory testing* (QST), measures sensory thresholds to different stimuli and responses to fixed-intensity stimuli (Rolke *et al.*, 2006). The comprehensive QST reveals sensory deficits in greater detail, comparing the patient's results with normative values (Baad-Hansen *et al.*, 2013).
• *Diagnostic anesthesia* examines if the pain is caused mainly by local, peripheral input or if central mechanisms contribute to pain maintenance. The effect on pain intensity by injection of a local anesthetic substance (local infiltration or regional nerve block) is assessed.
• Total pain relief may be interpreted as a local pain cause, possibly inflammatory pain.
• Incomplete or completely absent pain reduction may indicate central involvement; central sensitization mechanisms or referred pain from structures outside the anesthetized area.
• To exclude placebo effect and bias (influence of both patient's and dentist's expectations) on the outcome, diagnostic anesthesia can be executed in a two-appointment, randomized, double-blind, placebo-controlled procedure. In one appointment, active substance (local anesthetic compound) is injected, and in the other appointment an inactive substance (isotonic saline solution) is injected. The patient rates the pain intensity before and after injection. After the two appointments, the order is unveiled, and the effect of active substance and inactive substance can be evaluated independent of bias.

Management of atypical odontalgia/persistent dentoalveolar pain

- Management of chronic pain conditions in general is best performed in a multidisciplinary fashion. This is also true for chronic or persistent dentoalveolar pain. First, the patient with AO/PDAP should receive thorough education about the condition, as it is essential for the patient to understand and accept that there is no cure.
- Further invasive procedures such as endodontics or surgery (including explorative surgery) should be avoided unless there are clear signs of local pathology. Such unnecessary procedures are at risk of worsening the pain in such patients.
- Topical application of local anesthetics or capsaicin may be applied according to the patient's need (e.g., several times each day) using a soft reservoir splint (Figure 4.21). If the painful region cannot be targeted in this fashion, systemic pain management may be obtained using specific antidepressant (e.g., TCAs) or anti-epileptic (e.g., gabapentin, pregabalin) drugs, which is a strategy known to have some effect in neuropathic pain conditions.
- In addition to local or systemic pharmacologic treatment a CBT/ACT approach is often helpful, and hypnosis has also been shown to be effective in some patients.

Self-study Questions

1. What are the suggested pathophysiological mechanisms of AO/PDAP?

2. Describe how diagnostic anesthesia may help in the diagnosis and how it should best be performed?

3. How can AO/PDAP be managed?

4. What should be avoided when trying to manage AO/PDAP, and why?

References

Baad-Hansen L (2008) Atypical odontalgia – pathophysiology and clinical management. *J Oral Rehabil* **35**:1–11.

Baad-Hansen L, Pigg M, Elmasry Ivanovic S, *et al.* (2013) Intraoral somatosensory abnormalities in patients with atypical odontalgia – a controlled multicenter quantitative sensory testing study. *Pain* **154**(8):1287–1294.

Benoliel R, Kahn J, Eliav E (2012) Peripheral painful traumatic trigeminal neuropathies. *Oral Dis* **18**(4):317–332.

Forssell H, Jääskeläinen S, List T, *et al.* (2015) An update on pathophysiological mechanisms related to idiopathic oro-facial pain conditions with implications for management. *J Oral Rehabil* **42**(4):300–322.

Headache Classification Committee of the International Headache Society (IHS) (2013) The International Classification of Headache Disorders, 3rd edition (beta version). *Cephalalgia* **33**:629–808.

Nixdorf D, Moana-Filho E (2011) Persistent dento-alveolar pain disorder (PDAP): working towards a better understanding. *Rev Pain* **5**(4):18–27.

Nixdorf DR, Moana-Filho EJ, Law AS, *et al.* (2010) Frequency of nonodontogenic pain after endodontic therapy: a systematic review and meta-analysis. *J Endod* **36**(9):1494–1498.

Rolke R, Magerl W, Andrews Campbell K, *et al.* (2006) Quantitative sensory testing: a comprehensive protocol for clinical trials. *Eur J Pain* **10**:77–88.

Schiffman E, Ohrbach R, Truelove E, *et al.* (2014) Diagnostic Criteria for Temporomandibular Disorders (DC/TMD) for clinical and research applications: recommendations of the International RDC/TMD Consortium Network and Orofacial Pain Special Interest Group. *J Oral Facial Pain Headache* **28**(1):6–27.

Woda A, Tubert-Jeannin S, Bouhassira D, *et al.* (2005) Towards a new taxonomy of idiopathic orofacial pain. *Pain* **116**(3):396–406.

Woolf CJ, Bennett GJ, Doherty M, *et al.* (1998) Towards a mechanism-based classification of pain? *Pain* **77**(3):227–229.

Answers to Self-study Questions

1. Neuropathic pain origin is currently the most supported theory, more specifically traumatic or toxic damage to small peripheral sensory nerves with subsequent central sensitization. At times, a clear cause of neuropathy cannot be identified and the pain is then contributed to generalized hyperexcitability of the somatosensory system, "functional pain."

2. Diagnostic anesthesia may help differentiate between a local dental pain cause, with pain perpetuated by peripheral mechanisms (complete or substantial pain relief after injection) and pain that is partially or totally perpetuated by central mechanisms (incomplete or absent pain relief after injection). To avoid influence of bias, it should be done in a two-step, randomized, double-blinded, placebo-controlled procedure.

3. Pain in AO/PDAP, like many severe chronic pain states, is often best managed with a multimodal approach. Sensory, emotional, and behavioral aspects of the pain experience should be evaluated and targeted. This can include information about origin and reasons for pain, medications, and

psychological interventions. Pain reduction and rehabilitation are the main goals.

4. Further invasive treatment of the painful tooth, including explorative surgery, should be avoided since it is generally ineffective for pain relief and risks making the pain worse. For diagnostic purposes, noninvasive methods should be selected. In general, teeth in the pain area should be assessed with caution, and irreversible treatments (root canal treatment, extraction) avoided unless there is very clear pathology.

Case 4.6

Clinical Case: Burning Mouth Syndrome

Jean-Paul Goulet and Christine Nadeau

A. Demographic Data and Reason for Contact

- Caucasian woman, 42 years old.
- Chief complaint of "persistent burning mouth sensation and metallic taste."

B. Symptom History

- Reports a sudden onset of burning sensation on the tip of the tongue about 1 year ago.
- Intermittent metallic taste first noticed 4 months ago.
- Location of the burning sensation on the dorsum and lateral borders of the tongue, palate, and inside both cheeks.
- Burning always affects the tongue but is "on" and "off" at other sites.
- Reports daily burning with no recall of symptom-free days over the past few months.
- Burning starts soon after awakening and persists all day.
- Increases as the day goes by, reaching a peak by the end of the afternoon.
- Denies interfering with falling asleep and sleeps through the night without a problem.
- Intensity varies between 2 and 6 on 0–10 pain rating scale.
- Denies any triggering and aggravating factors, including the consumption of pine nuts.
- Burning disappears with food intake/chewing but returns immediately afterward.
- Denies dry mouth sensation and any skin, eye, or genital symptoms.

C. Medical History

- Hospitalized for delivery and 10 years ago for a tonsillectomy.
- Sees her family physician once a year, and her last medical check-up was normal.
- Does not report any medical problem, and review of systems not contributory.
- No current medication and denies intake of vitamins, over-the-counter products, and natural products.

- No known allergies to any medication or foods.
- Visits her dentist once a year for routine care.

D. Psychosocial History

- Married with two children, aged 14 and 11 years old.
- Works as a full-time reception clerk in a medical clinic.
- Exercises once or twice a week.
- Maintains an active lifestyle and social activities with friends and colleagues.
- Both parents and family siblings alive and in good health.
- Drinks two to four glasses of wine per week;, no other alcohol consumption.
- No history of smoking or drug abuse.
- Keeps on doing regular activities, but the burning sensation affects her quality of life.
- Burning-related unpleasantness rated 5 on a 0–10 rating scale.
- Shows no distress or anxious feeling.
- Defines herself as a happy and active person.

E. Previous Consultation and Treatments

- Saw her dentist for a clinical examination: Within normal limits.
- Dentist prescribed a symptomatic treatment with chlorhexidine gluconate mouth rinse twice a day for 2 weeks; did not notice any improvement.

F. Extraoral Status

- Inspection of the head, face and neck: within normal limits, no evidence of pallor, redness, swelling, or any other contributory physical manifestations.
- Palpation of major salivary glands, jaw muscles, TMJ, lymph nodes, and neck: within normal limits, no evidence of lumps, tenderness, or other contributory physical signs.
- No evidence of jaw tremor, facial tic, or mannerism.
- Exposed extremities including nails: within normal limits.

G. Intraoral Status

- Fully dentate except for upper and lower third molars.
- Oral mucosa well lubricated with clear and watery saliva.
- Inspection and palpation of labial, vestibular, buccal, palatal, and floor of the mouth mucosa: no evidence of lesion and absence of allodynia, hypo-/hyperesthesia, and hyperalgesia.
- Inspection of oropharynx: negative for lesions, redness, and impaired motor function.
- Inspection and palpation of tongue: within normal limits with no evidence of superficial or deep lesions and absence of allodynia, hypo-/hyperesthesia, and hyperalgesia (Figure 4.22).
- Gingival, periodontal, dental, and occlusion status: within normal limits.
- Stimulation of the major salivary glands: patent ducts with normal saliva leakage.

H. Additional Examinations and Findings

- Ordering complementary tests and referring for a consult depends on the degree of certainty for identifying burning mouth syndrome (BMS) by the ICHD-3 criteria and exclusion based on the history, review of system, and clinical examination.
- Chair-side assessment of the resting whole salivary flow rate: within normal limits with a flow rate of 0.4 mL/min (low normal rate value: 0.1 mL/min).

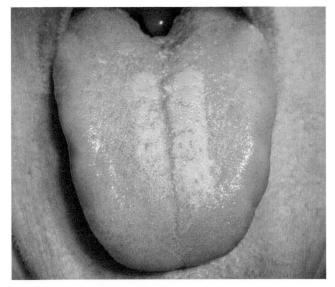

Figure 4.22 Except for the coated tongue, the clinical examination is within normal limit for this 42-year-old female patient complaining of burning sensations.

- Laboratory tests ordered for uncovering systemic factors: all results within normal limits.
- PHQ-4: normal with a score of 0 (scale 0–12).
- No evidence of local pathology, systemic, and psychological factors combined with the ICHD-3 criteria support a diagnosis of BMS.

I. Diagnosis/Diagnoses

ICHD-3 beta

- BMS.

J. Case Assessment

- The ICHD-3 criteria define BMS on two aspects: one describing the clinical presentation and the other identifying the condition by the exclusion of local, systemic, or psychological pathologies.
- Overt clinical manifestations attributed to local factors and/or systemic conditions that may cause burning sensations preclude a diagnosis of BMS.
- In this case, the age and sex of the patient fall into the population mostly affected by BMS (please refer to Background Information box).
- The fact that the patient has daily burning mouth symptoms and denies any aggravation following food intake helped to rule out burning sensation caused by consumption/usage of certain foods or products: intermittent burning and dysguesia associated pine nut syndrome (Chinese *Pinus armandii*), allergic reaction to sorbic acid, cinnamon, nicotinic acid, propylene glycol, and benzoic acid.
- The possibility of a subclinical systemic condition or psychological etiology needs consideration before a final diagnosis of BMS is made.

K. Evidence-based Treatment Plan including Aims

- The overall treatment aims for any patients with BMS are: (1) reassure and inform about the condition; (2) relieve symptoms; and (3) give psychological and social support as needed.
- This lady, in otherwise good health, was bothered by the burning sensations but there was no sign of distress or anxiety related to her condition.
- Explanations were given regarding the occurrence of burning mouth sensations despite the normal appearance of intraoral tissues and the lack of local or systemic disorder. The same was done for the metallic taste.
- Any concern about mouth cancer wase addressed and clarified with the patient.

- She was informed that there was no treatment cure for BMS and the duration of the syndrome is highly variable and unpredictable.
- She was warned to pay attention to and avoid any traumatic habits she might have that can make symptoms worse.
- The treatment options were presented with emphasis on goals, benefits, disadvantages, duration of drug therapy, and follow-up.
- She agreed to do a topical treatment three times a day (t.i.d.) after each meal for 1 month with clonazepam. She was instructed to suck a tablet containing 1 mg of clonazepam while retaining the saliva in her mouth near the pain site for 5 min without swallowing and then expectorate.
- At 1-month follow-up visit, she reported improvement with the topical treatment modality. Recommendation was made to continue current medication regimen, monitor progression and side effects, and resume regular follow-up.
- In the case of no improvement with the recommended topical treatment, an alternative option included switching to systemic clonazepam 0.5 mg at bedtime (h.s.), monitor side effects, and continue regular follow-up.

L.   Prognosis and Discussion

- The clinical and laboratory findings, as well as the psychosocial assessment, leave no doubt as to the idiopathic nature of the burning mouth symptoms in this case.
- A diagnosis of BMS is most likely when the ICHD-3 criteria are fulfilled, laboratory findings are within normal limits, food intake eliminate the burning sensation, resting whole salivary flow is within normal limits, the score on the PHQ-4 that screens for anxiety and depression is below 3 or the score for the GAD-7 (anxiety) and PHQ-9 (depression) are each below 5.
- As no factors can predict how long the burning sensation will last, the patient was informed that remission occurs in approximately 50–60% of patients after a few months or years and that the symptoms can persist to some degree even with pharmacologic treatment.
- When no improvement is reported at follow-up with the selected drug treatment, another medication may be tried after discussion with the patient.
- CBT can be used alone and in combination with pharmacological therapy to improve treatment response.

Background Information

Clinical presentation

- BMS is a chronic pain disorder characterized by burning sensation of the oral mucosa occurring in the absence of local, systemic, and psychological causes, often accompanied by subjective symptoms of mouth dryness and metallic taste.
- It is a distinctive nosological entity with poorly understood pathophysiology.
- Location of the burning is usually bilateral and independent of a nervous pathway.
- In most cases BMS starts on the tip of the tongue and may extend to the lateral border and other intraoral sites, most notably the palate and labial mucosa, but rarely to extraoral sites.
- The burning varies in intensity with no paroxysm and the patient may report an absence of burning on awakening that escalates throughout the day with peaking intensity in late afternoon/early evening.
- Sleep disturbance is infrequent.
- Many patients report disappearance of the burning with food intake or chewing but it resumes afterward and not infrequently the same happens with the metallic taste.

(Gurvits and Tan, 2013; Zakrzewska and Buchanan, 2016)

Terminology, prevalence, and incidence

- Former terms used to designate BMS in the literature are glossopyrosis, glossodynia, sore tongue, stomatodynia, stomatopyrosis, oral dysesthesia, and sore mouth.
- More recently BMS has also been called "burning mouth disorder" and "complex oral sensitivity disorder."
- To emphasize its idiopathic nature BMS is also referred to as "primary or essential BMS."
- Burning sensation that results from local, systemic, or psychological condition as confirmed by clinical examination and additional investigations is designated "burning mouth symptom" or "secondary BMS."
- Prevalence data on BMS varies widely across studies, and this is mainly explained by the fact that most studies are based on self-report without physical examination; only a paucity of studies were conducted on a representative

sample of the population, and different diagnostic criteria have been used.

- Cross-sectional population-based epidemiologic surveys indicate that 0.2–4% of adults report burning sensation not associated with oral lesions.
- BMS rarely occurs before the age of 30 and is more frequent amongst the elderly, with up to 90% of patients being peri- and postmenopausal women.
- The incidence rate of BMS adjusted for age and sex in a North American Caucasian population has been estimated at 11.4 per 100 000 person-years.

(Gurvits and Tan, 2013)

Etiology and pathophysiology

- The etiology of BMS remains unknown, and no causal relationship has been shown between depression and/or anxiety and BMS, although these patients are liable to anxiety and depressive state.
- Oral dryness is frequently reported by BMS patients; however, measurement of the whole resting salivary flow rate shows values above what seems critical for inducing burning sensation (0.1mL/min).
- Current evidence on pathophysiology favors a neuropathic background, but what the trigger is for the proposed mechanisms remains an unanswered question.
- Findings from psychophysical, electrophysiological, immunohistochemical, neuropathologic, and functional brain imaging studies indicate a complex pathophysiology involving heterogeneous neurological pathways at different level of the nervous system with the potential contribution of local environmental factors.
- The pathophysiological processes currently proposed for BMS are the following:
  - Damage to the taste system carried by the facial (chorda tympani), glossopharyngeal, and vagus nerves leads to the loss of tonic inhibition of the trigeminal nerve and simultaneous dysfunction of the sensory components.
  - Axonal degeneration in the epithelial and sub-papillary nerve fibers, which is

responsible for a trigeminal small-fibers sensory neuropathy and dysfunction of the trigeminal pain pathway.
  - Impairment of the central pain modulation pathway resulting from a presynaptic dysfunction of the nigrostriatal dopaminergic system.
  - Drastic and concomitant changes in sources of steroids known to play a role in neuroregeneration and protection in the peripheral and central nervous system cause neurodegeneration and dysfunction of the trigeminal pain processes.

(Eliav et al., 2007; Woda et al., 2009; Jääskeläinen, 2012)

Diagnostic Criteria

ICHD-3 beta criteria for **Burning mouth syndrome** (Headache Classification Committee of the International Headache Society (IHS), 2013:781–782). Sensitivity and specificity have not been established.

An intraoral burning or dysesthetic sensation, recurring daily for more than 2 h per day over more than 3 months, without clinically evident causative lesions.

Criteria

A. Oral pain fulfilling criteria B and C.
B. Recurring daily for >2 h per day for >3 months.
C. Pain has both of the following characteristics:
   1. burning quality;
   2. felt superficially in the oral mucosa.
D. Oral mucosa is of normal appearance, and clinical examination, including sensory testing, is normal.
E. Not better accounted for by another ICHD-3 diagnosis.

Fundamental Points

Diagnostics

- A detailed symptom history is important and should cover every aspect of the burning sensations (onset, site, intensity, duration, pain-free period, aggravating and alleviating factors), associated symptoms, treatment history, impact on function and well-being, coping capacity, elements suggestive of anxiety, depression, hypochondria, and catastrophizing (e.g., cancerophobia).

- Self-administered questionnaires considered helpful for assessing psychosocial factors include: GCPS, PHQ-9 for depression, GAD-7 for anxiety (or PHQ-4 screening tool), and PHQ-15 for nonspecific physical symptoms (Kroenke et al., 2010).
- To date, there are no universally accepted diagnostic criteria, laboratory tests, imaging studies, or other modalities that confirm the diagnosis of BMS. A diagnosis based on the International Headache Society criteria indicates that BMS represents an idiopathic pain condition and that any local, systemic, or psychological causes have been excluded (Gurvits and Tan, 2013).
- All aspects of the current medical status are not always completely covered by a self-administered medical questionnaire, and a comprehensive review of systems is required.
- A careful review of the patient's medication list is imperative, with special attention to antihypertensive agents such as angiotensin-converting enzyme inhibitors, antiretrovirals, antidepressants, anxiolytics and anticonvulsants.

Physical examination
- To avoid overlooking potential causes of burning mouth and associated symptoms the physical examination goes beyond the affected area and includes a thorough visual inspection and palpation of extraoral and intraoral structures looking for any clinical manifestations of local pathology or systemic disorder that could explain the patient's symptoms.
- Somatic signs to look for are pallor, redness, erosion, ulcer, swelling, lump, network of interlacing white lines (lichenoid lesions), white plaque, desquamation, atrophy of lingual papillae, and lack of saliva.
- Consider doing an abbreviated cranial nerve examination in the presence of sensory deficit or any other neurological signs.
- Additional chair-side tests to consider include assessment of whole resting salivary flow rate

and assessment of taste sensation (sweet, salty, bitter, and sour).
- Laboratory tests to consider for assessing systemic factors include: complete and differential blood counts; sedimentation rate; serum iron, ferritin, transferrin, vitamin B12, folic acid, zinc; blood sugar level; thyroid function; immunoserology for *Helicobacter pylori*, rheumatoid factor, antinuclear antibodies, anti-anti-Sjögren's syndrome A and B.

Potential causes of burning mouth symptoms to exclude
- Local causes of burning mouth symptoms to exclude:
  - mechanical trauma of any types, including tongue thrusting, lip or cheek biting, lip licking;
  - allergic contact reaction to dental material, oral care products, foods;
  - infection (Figure 4.23);
  - oral manifestation of a mucodermatosis;
  - hyposalivation secondary to drug intake, head and neck radiotherapy, or other salivary dysfunction;
  - food consumption such as Chinese pine nut (*Pinus armandii*).
- Systemic causes to exclude:
  - hematologic disorders – anemia

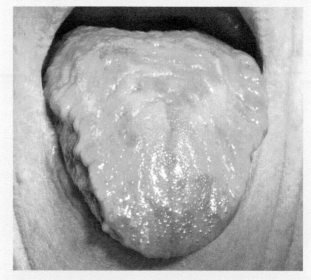

Figure 4.23 A 52-year-old female known to have a fissured geographic and tongue (benign migratory glossitis) for many years presenting with burning sensations caused by a candida infection.

- vitamins or nutritional deficiencies – B complex, folate, iron, zinc;
- endocrine disorders – diabetes, hypothyroidism, hormonal deficiencies;
- gastrointestinal disorders – gastroesophageal reflux;
- autoimmune disorders – Sjögren syndrome;
- adverse effect from medication.
- Psychologic conditions to exclude:
  - depression;
  - anxiety;
  - other psychiatric/mental disorders.

(Patton *et al.*, 2007)

Treatment options for burning mouth syndrome

- Reassure patients, stress that this is a real pain and that it is probably a form of neuropathic pain.
- Therapy should be tried at least for 1 month if no adverse effect before considering another treatment modality.
- Tailored CBT is recommended for patients showing maladaptive coping or are interpersonally distressed or dysfunctional.
- Refer patients for standardized taste testing when taste dysfunction is suspected.
- There is no specific treatment for the metallic taste reported by BMS patients and it usually improves in parallel with the burning.
- In the presence of patients refusing drug therapy or if not an option due to medical condition, self-treatment based on anecdotal reports worth trying include:
  - tabasco rinse (one or two drops per 15 mL of water) rinse/spit after each meal;
  - over-the-counter topical anesthetic, oral spray and gel.
- Therapies tested in double-blind randomized controlled trials with placebo showing efficacy for managing BMS symptoms:
  - topical (let it dissolve, retain saliva 5 min without swallowing and expectorate)
  - clonazepam troche or tablet (1.0 mg, after each meal).
  - Systemic
    - clonazepam (0.5 mg h.s.)
    - alpha lipoic acid (200 mg t.i.d.)
    - alpha lipoic acid (600 mg/day) + gabapentin (300 mg/day)
    - capsaicin (0.25% capsules t.i.d.)
  - nonmedicinal
    - CBT
    - low-level laser therapy
    - Catuama® herbal compound (310 mg twice a day)
- Therapies reported effective for managing BMS symptoms based on expert report and clinical practice but not yet tested in double-blind randomized controlled trials with placebo:
  - Topical
    - capcaisin cream (0.025%)
  - systemic
    - amitriptyline (10–50 mg h.s.)
    - nortriptyline (10–30 mg h.s.)
    - pregabalin (50–150 mg/day)
    - amisulpride (50 mg/day)
    - paroxetine (20 mg/day)
    - sertraline (50 mg/day)
    - duloxetine (30–60 mg/day).

(Patton *et al.*, 2007; Zakrzewska and Buchanan, 2016)

Self-study Questions

1. During the case history, aside from the clinical features of the burning sensation, what important aspects must be covered?

2. What history and clinical features best describe BMS?

3. How do we define BMS and what are the relevant diagnostic criteria?

4. What is known about the prevalence of BMS and the populations at risk?

5. What local factors and systemic conditions must be ruled out before considering a diagnosis of BMS?

6. What is known about the pathophysiology of BMS?

7. When managing patients with BMS, what important aspects must be covered and discussed?

8. What are the treatment modalities for BMS?

References

Eliav E, Kamran B, Schaham R, *et al.* (2007) Evidence of chorda tympani dysfunction in patients with burning mouth syndrome. *J Am Dent Assoc* **138**(5):628–633.

Gurvits GE, Tan A (2013) Burning mouth syndrome. *World J Gastroenterol* **19**(5):665–672.

Headache Classification Committee of the International Headache Society (IHS) 2013. The international Classification of Headache disorders, 3rd edition (beta version). *Cephalalgia* **33**:629–808.

Jääskeläinen SK (2012) Pathophysiology of primary burning mouth syndrome. *Clin Neurophysiol* **123**(1):71–77.

Kroenke K, Spitzer RL, Williams JB, Löwe B (2010) The patient health questionnaire somatic, anxiety, and depressive symptom scales: a systematic review. *Gen Hosp Psychiatry* **32**(4):345–359.

Patton LL, Siegel MA, Benoliel R, De Laat A (2007) Management of burning mouth syndrome: systematic review and management recommendations. *Oral Surg Oral Med Oral Pathol Oral Radiol Endod* **103**(Suppl):S39.e1–S39.e13.

Woda A, Dao T, Gremeau-Richard C (2009) Steroid dysregulation and stomatodynia (burning mouth syndrome). *J Orofac Pain* **23**(3):202–210.

Zakrzewska J, Buchanan JA (2016) Burning mouth syndrome. *BMJ Clin Evid* Jan 7; pii: 1301.

Answers to Self-study Questions

1. Patient's medical status, list of medications, detailed review of systems for hematologic, endocrine, gastrointestinal, renal, hepatic, autoimmune, and psychiatric disorders; patient well-being, fear of cancer, anxiety, depression, and coping ability (see Fundamental Points box).

2. History of the chief complaint of BMS is characterized by a continuous burning sensation of the mucosa of the mouth, typically involving the tongue with or without extension to the lips and oral mucosa. The burning sensation is usually bilateral. Most patients will be symptom free upon waking up but will report a continuous burning sensation that gradually increases throughout the day and disappears with food intake or chewing. Clinical features will be unremarkable, with no evidence of any local causes or oral manifestations of systemic diseases/disorders. In addition to the burning sensation, patients may report dryness of the mouth and a metallic taste.

3. BMS is defined by recurring symptoms of oral burning in the absence of tissue abnormalities, laboratory findings for systemic diseases, and psychological disorders. No laboratory tests, imaging studies, or other modalities can confirm the diagnosis of BMS. Despite no universally accepted diagnostic criteria, the International Headache Society (Headache Classification Committee of the International Headache Society (IHS), 2013:781–782) defines BMS according to the following set of empirically derived criteria:

A. Oral pain fulfilling criteria B and C.
B. Pain recurring daily for >2 h/day for >3 months.
C. Pain has both of the following characteristics:
   1. burning quality;
   2. felt superficially in the oral mucosa.
D. Oral mucosa is of normal appearance, with a normal clinical examination including sensory testing.
E. Not better accounted for by another ICHD-3 diagnosis (see Background Information box)

4. BMS is more prevalent in women in the age range corresponding to the peri-/postmenopausal time period. BMS occurs rarely before the age of 30. Prevalence data vary widely across studies because of methodological and case definition issues. Cross-sectional population-based epidemiologic surveys indicate that 0.2–4% of adults report a burning sensation unassociated with oral lesions which could represent cases of BMS (see Background Information box).

5. Local factors to be ruled out include: (a) mechanical trauma of any type resulting from oral habits and parafunctions; (b) soft tissue lesions resulting from infection, contact allergic reactions, or mucodermatosis; and (c) a lack of saliva.

   Systemic conditions/diseases that may cause oral burning include: (a) hematologic (anemia); (b) endocrine (diabetes, thyroid dysfunction); (c) gastrointestinal (gastroesophageal reflux disease); (d) autoimmune (Sjögren syndrome); and (e) psychiatric disorders. Vitamin and nutritional deficiencies as well as adverse effects from medications may be involved. Therefore, a complete medical history and detailed review of systems are warranted to assess a complaint of burning mouth sensation (see Fundamental Points box).

6. To date, the cause of BMS is unknown. Current studies suggest complex mechanisms leading to a dysfunction of the trigeminal pain pathway. The pathophysiology of BMS falls under two main theories: an imbalance between the gustatory and sensory systems and trigeminal sensory neuropathy in the peripheral and/or central nervous system resulting from one or more processes such as small-fiber axonal degeneration, dysfunction of the dopaminergic system, and loss of protective neurosteroids (see Background Information box).

7. The patient must be informed that we do not yet fully understand the cause of the burning sensation and accompanied symptoms, nor can we predict how

long it will last. Clinicians must also address the patient's well-being and coping ability. Although available treatments focus on alleviating symptoms, there is no cure for BMS. Patients must be reassured and informed on the absence of cancer.

8. Various treatment modalities include topical, systemic, and cognitive behavioral treatments. A stepwise approach is usually deemed appropriate, starting with one topical treatment; if no improvement is reported, a systemic treatment is then envisaged. Topical or systemic clonazepam represents the first-line drug to use. A single or combined treatment option may be necessary in order to alleviate the burning sensations and improve patient well-being (see Fundamental Points box).

C: Dental Pain and Tooth Wear

Case 4.7

Pain Due to Pulpitis

Natasha M Flake

A. Demographic Data and Reason for Contact

- Female, 32 years old.
- Reports on an emergency basis with pain in the maxillary left posterior.

B. Symptom History

- Sensitivity to cold for a few weeks and spontaneous pain the past 2 days. The sensitivity to cold is a sharp, shooting pain, which lasts minutes after the cold has been removed from the tooth. The spontaneous pain is a throbbing sensation. The pain woke her up last night. The spontaneous pain varies in intensity from 3 to 6 (NRS 0–10), but the pain to cold is 9 (NRS 0–10). At its worst, the pain radiates in the maxillary left quadrant and toward her temple and ear, making it feel like the whole left side of her head hurts, but the patient can point to the tooth that she believes is the source of her pain. She has been taking over-the-counter acetaminophen for the past day, under the instruction of her obstetrician. The acetaminophen helps, but does not eliminate the pain.

C. Medical History

- Pregnant, 25 weeks.
- History of hypothyroidism.
- Penicillin allergy.
- Blood pressure 132/82 mmHg.
- Pulse 54 bpm.
- Temperature 37.1 °C.
- Medications:
  - levothyroxine, 123 µg/day
  - ferrous sulfate, 325 mg/day
  - prenatal vitamin.

D. Psychosocial History

- Married.
- Employed as a research technician.
- History of sporadic dental care. Usually only sees a dentist when in pain.
- No psychological assessment done.

E. Previous Consultations and Treatments

- None related to the present chief complaint.

F. Extraoral Status

- The extraoral exam is within normal limits. No asymmetries, swellings, erythema, or other abnormalities of the TMJ and muscles are noted.

G. Intraoral Status

Soft tissues

- No swelling, no sinus tract stoma, no exudate evident.

Hard tissues and dentition

- Tooth 24 has a do composite restoration; 25 has an mod composite restoration; 26 has mo and o amalgam restorations; and 27 is a virgin tooth. The margins of all restorations are intact. No recurrent caries is noted.

H. Additional Examinations and Findings

- Diagnostic test results show that tooth 26 has a hypersensitive and lingering response to cold and is sensitive to percussion (Table 4.2).
- Radiographic examination showed that all restorations appear to have intact margins. No caries is noted. The lamina dura appears intact and the periodontal ligament space of normal width for teeth 24–27 (Figure 4.24). There is moderate horizontal bone loss on 26d.

I. Diagnosis/Diagnoses

Other

- Symptomatic irreversible pulpitis tooth 26.
- Symptomatic apical periodontitis tooth 26.

J. Case Assessment

- The source of the patient's pain in this case is inflammation of the pulp of the maxillary left first molar. The etiology of the pulpal inflammation is bacteria, likely due to a history of dental caries.

Table 4.2 Diagnostic test results

Tooth	Percussion	Palpation	Cold	EPT	Mobility	Probing depth (mm)			
						b	l	m	d
24	WNL	WNL	WNL	24	0	2	3	3	4
25	WNL	WNL	WNL	27	0	2	2	4	3
26	+	WNL	+L	32	0	3	3	4	6
27	WNL	WNL	WNL	20	0	3	2	4	4

Endodontic diagnostic test results are listed for the teeth in the maxillary left posterior. Tooth 26 is sensitive to percussion with respect to the adjacent teeth and has an exaggerated and lingering response to the cold test. EPT, electric pulp test (0–80); b, buccal; l, lingual; m, mesial; d, distal; WNL, within normal limits; +, hypersensitive; +L, hypersensitive and lingering.

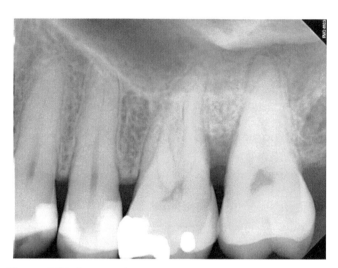

Figure 4.24 Preoperative radiograph of teeth 24–26.

Bacteria may also induce an inflammatory response in the pulp due to a crack or leaking restoration in the tooth.

- The patient's history, signs, and symptoms are a classic example of pain due to symptomatic irreversible pulpitis.
- The diagnoses in this case were made based on the patient's reported history of pain and the diagnostic test results. The patient's history of pain, presence of spontaneous pain, and intense and lingering sensitivity to cold are all suggestive of a pulpal diagnosis of symptomatic irreversible pulpitis. This pulpal diagnosis was confirmed clinically by the hypersensitive and lingering response to the cold test. The periapical diagnosis of symptomatic apical periodontitis was made due to the presence of percussion sensitivity on the tooth. All diagnostic test results were assessed in relation to the adjacent teeth in the quadrant.
- The differential diagnosis could include reversible pulpitis or a non-odontogenic toothache. However, the patient's history of pain, spontaneous pain, and

lingering pain to cold clearly suggest a diagnosis of symptomatic irreversible pulpitis. In this case, the inflammation of the pulp has spread beyond the pulp and has begun to affect the periapical tissues, resulting in sensitivity to percussion.

K. Evidence-based Treatment Plan including Aims

- Treatment options for tooth 26 include: (1) nonsurgical root canal therapy, followed by a definitive build-up restoration and crown; (2) extraction, and (3) do nothing.
- The aim of the treatment is to remove the inflamed tooth pulp to eliminate the source of the patient's pain. This can be accomplished through endodontic therapy or extraction of the tooth. After the inflamed tooth pulp is removed, the inflammation of the periapical tissues should resolve. If the patient elects to maintain the tooth through endodontic therapy, the tooth must be properly restored after root canal therapy. A crown restoration is recommended in order to prevent fracture of the tooth or recontamination of the root canal system through coronal leakage, and to provide long-term function for the patient.
- Emergency treatment plan: pulpectomy (Figure 4.25).
- Definitive treatment plan: nonsurgical root canal therapy.
- Restorative treatment plan: build-up and crown.

L. Prognosis and Discussion

- The prognosis is favorable. When the inflamed tooth pulp is removed, the patient's pain will resolve. If proper endodontic therapy and restoration are provided (Figure 4.26) there should be no further bacterial contamination of the root canal system. This will prevent the development of apical periodontitis, and the tooth should provide long-term function for the patient (Figure 4.27).

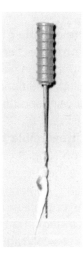

Figure 4.25 Extirpated tooth pulp.

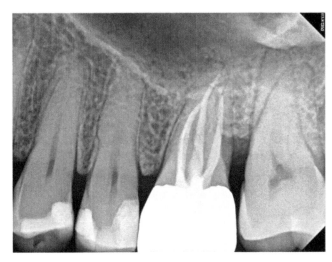

Figure 4.27 The 1 year follow-up radiograph.

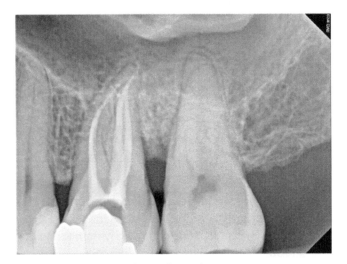

Figure 4.26 Postoperative radiograph.

emergency patients was removal of the dental pulp (23% of patients) (Portman-Lewis, 2007). According to a survey of dentists in the USA in 2005–2006, over 22 million endodontic procedures including over 15 million root canals were performed annually by private practitioners in the USA (American Dental Association (ADA), 2007).

- Removal of the inflamed pulp tissue by a pulpectomy in cases of irreversible pulpitis provides significant pain relief (Menhinick *et al.*, 2004). Removal of the pulp will eliminate the temperature sensitivity on the treated tooth. When inflammation of the pulp spreads from the coronal aspect of the tooth apically, the periapical tissues also become inflamed. The patient may then become sensitive to biting or chewing, and the clinician can reproduce this as percussion sensitivity during diagnostic testing. A pulpectomy will also help alleviate percussion sensitivity, although percussion sensitivity may take more time to completely resolve than temperature sensitivity.

Background Information

- Nine percent of adult patients who visited a general dentist reported having pain related to the teeth and surrounding tissues within the past year (Horst *et al.*, 2015). This dentoalveolar pain was the most frequently reported type of orofacial pain, and was reported more often by patients who did not receive regular dental care and those seeking treatment in community-based public health clinics (Horst *et al.*, 2015). In a study of after-hours calls for a group of dentists over a 5-year period, 52% of calls recorded were related to acute pulpitis or apical periodontitis (Portman-Lewis, 2007). The most common treatment provided for these

Diagnostic Criteria

American Association of Endodontists (AAE) consensus conference for diagnosis of **Symptomatic irreversible pulpitis** (American Association of Endodontists (AAE), 2009).

Symptomatic irreversible pulpitis is based on subjective and objective findings that the vital inflamed pulp is incapable of healing and that root canal treatment is indicated. Characteristics may include sharp pain upon thermal stimulus, lingering pain (often 30 s or longer after stimulus removal), spontaneity (unprovoked pain), and referred pain. Sometimes the pain may be accentuated by postural changes, such as lying down or bending over, and over-the-counter analgesics are typically ineffective. Common etiologies may include deep caries, extensive restorations, or fractures exposing the pulpal tissues. Teeth with symptomatic irreversible pulpitis may be difficult to diagnose because the inflammation has not yet reached the periapical tissues, thus resulting in no pain or discomfort to percussion. In such cases, dental history and thermal testing are the primary tools for assessing pulpal status.

For **Symptomatic apical periodontiti**s, see Case 4.8.

Fundamental points

Endondontic diagnostics

- All endodontic examinations should results in two diagnoses: a pulpal and a periapical diagnosis to describe the status of both the dental pulp and the periapical tissues. Historically, many different terms have been used to describe pulpal and periapical conditions, with some terms being based on clinical characteristics and some on histological characteristics. The following are the recommended diagnostic terms adopted by the American Association of Endodontists (AAE) (2009, 2015).

Pulpal diagnoses

- **Normal pulp.** A clinical diagnostic category in which the pulp is symptom free and normally responsive to pulp testing.
- **Reversible pulpitis.** A clinical diagnosis based on subjective and objective findings indicating that the inflammation should resolve and the pulp return to normal.

- **Symptomatic irreversible pulpitis.** A clinical diagnosis based on subjective and objective findings indicating that the vital inflamed pulp is incapable of healing. Additional descriptors: lingering thermal pain, spontaneous pain, referred pain.
- **Asymptomatic irreversible pulpitis.** A clinical diagnosis based on subjective and objective findings indicating that the vital inflamed pulp is incapable of healing. Additional descriptors: no clinical symptoms but inflammation produced by caries, caries excavation, trauma.
- **Pulp necrosis.** A clinical diagnostic category indicating death of the dental pulp. The pulp is usually nonresponsive to pulp testing.
- **Previously treated.** A clinical diagnostic category indicating that the tooth has been endodontically treated and the canals are obturated with various filling materials other than intracanal medicaments.
- **Previously initiated therapy.** A clinical diagnostic category indicating that the tooth has been previously treated by partial endodontic therapy (e.g., pulpotomy, pulpectomy).

Apical diagnoses

- **Normal apical tissues.** Teeth with normal periradicular tissues that are not sensitive to percussion or palpation testing. The lamina dura surrounding the root is intact, and the periodontal ligament space is uniform.
- **Symptomatic apical periodontitis.** Inflammation, usually of the apical periodontium, producing clinical symptoms including a painful response to biting and/or percussion or palpation. It might or might not be associated with an apical radiolucent area.
- **Asymptomatic apical periodontitis.** Inflammation and destruction of apical periodontium that is of pulpal origin, appears as an apical radiolucent area, and does not produce clinical symptoms.
- **Acute apical abscess.** An inflammatory reaction to pulpal infection and necrosis characterized by rapid onset, spontaneous pain, tenderness of the tooth to pressure, pus formation, and swelling of associated tissues.
- **Chronic apical abscess.** An inflammatory reaction to pulpal infection and necrosis

characterized by gradual onset, little or no discomfort, and the intermittent discharge of pus through an associated sinus tract.

- **Condensing osteitis.** Diffuse radiopaque lesion representing a localized bony reaction to a low-grade inflammatory stimulus, usually seen at apex of tooth.

Assessing the status of the pulp

- The most common diagnostic tests used to assess the status of the dental pulp in clinical practice are the cold test and the EPT. These tests are referred to as pulp sensibility tests, as they assess the ability of the pulp to detect stimuli applied to the tooth. The cold test is thought to stimulate fluid movement within dentinal tubules, which then stimulates neurons within the pulp. The cold test is most commonly performed using a refrigerant (1,1,1,2-tetrafluorethane) sprayed onto a cotton pellet and applied to the tooth (Figure 4.28). The patient is asked to indicate if they feel the cold, the intensity of the sensation, and whether or not the sensation lingers after the cold is removed (compared with control teeth). The EPT uses an electrical current to stimulate neurons in the dental pulp. The patient states only whether or not they feel the stimulus. The EPT is useful in determining the presence of functional neurons in the pulp (i.e., pulp vitality); the cold test is useful in determining both pulp vitality and the health status of the pulp (i.e., differentiating between normal pulp, reversible pulpitis, and irreversible pulpitis). Diagnostic test results must always be interpreted with respect to control teeth. Control teeth typically are the adjacent teeth, but may be contralateral teeth in some cases. Caution must be used in interpreting cold test and EPT results in immature teeth with open apices and in teeth that have been traumatized, as false negatives may be obtained in these cases.

- Additional pulp tests that may be used in clinical practice include the heat test and the test cavity. The heat test is used when the patient's chief complaint is sensitivity to heat, and the test cavity is used only when all other diagnostic tests yield equivocal results. Pulse oximetry and laser Doppler flowmetry may also be used to assess the status of the pulp. These tests detect blood flow within the tooth, but are not commonly available in clinical practice.

- The validity of pulp testing has been assessed, and although the tests are generally quite accurate in the clinical setting, they are not perfect. Weisleder *et al.* (2009) pulp tested teeth and compared the results with direct inspection of the pulp upon initiating endodontic therapy (a tooth was considered vital if blood was present in the canal upon access). Ninety-seven percent of teeth that responded to cold and EPT contained vital pulps; 90% of teeth that failed to respond to cold or EPT contained necrotic pulps (Weisleder *et al.*, 2009). In another study, Chen and Abbott (2011) found EPT to be 98% accurate, while spray refrigerant was 91% accurate in assessing the pulp vitality. Use of more than one pulp test should provide the most reliable test results, and use of more than one test is especially indicated in cases that are diagnostic challenges. In addition, pulp test

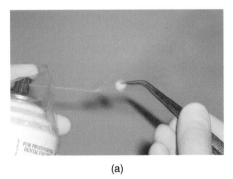
(a)

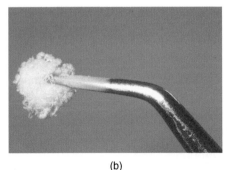
(b)

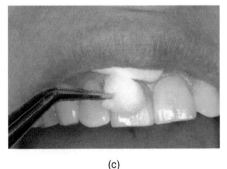
(c)

Figure 4.28 Cold testing. (a) Spraying refrigerant onto a #2 cotton pellet held by a cotton plier. (b) Cold cotton pellet ready for cold testing. (c) Placing cold cotton pellet on the facial surface of the tooth to be tested.

results should always be interpreted in conjunction with radiographic and clinical exam as well as the patient's reported history.

Assessing the status of the periapical tissues

• The status of the periapical tissues is commonly assessed using percussion, palpation, mobility, and periodontal probing. Percussion is performed by gently tapping on the tooth. Percussion is typically performed apically, but may also be performed in a lateral direction. Sensitivity to percussion indicates inflammation of the periapical tissues. Palpation is performed by feeling the attached gingiva and the alveolar mucosa on both the buccal and lingual aspects of the area of interest. Sensitivity to palpation indicates that inflammation has spread to include the periosteum surrounding the affected tooth. Mobility assesses the periodontal support of the tooth, and may be useful in assessing the periodontal prognosis and treatment planning. Assessing mobility is also a critical part of the exam following dental trauma. Periodontal probing is important for both diagnosis and assessing prognosis. Probing assesses the periodontal status of the tooth and may help differentiate between periodontal lesions, endodontic lesions, and perio-endo lesions. An isolated deep probing may suggest the presence of a sinus tract draining through the gingival sulcus or the presence of a longitudinal fracture. As with pulp tests, it is imperative to interpret all test results in comparison with control teeth and in conjunction with radiographic and clinical exam.

Self-study Questions

1. What treatment is indicated to provide pain relief for a patient who presents with symptomatic irreversible pulpitis?

2. What pulpal diagnosis terms are recommended by the American Association of Endodontists?

3. What periapical diagnostic terms are recommended by the American Association of Endodontists?

4. What two diagnostic tests are most commonly used in dental practice to assess the status of the dental pulp?

5. What diagnostic tests are commonly used in clinical practice to assess the status of the periapical tissues, and what do abnormal results to these tests suggest?

Acknowledgments

I thank Dr Randy Ball and Dr David Pitts for use of images.

References

American Association of Endodontists (AAE) (2015) *Glossary of endodontic terms*. http://www.nxtbook.com/nxtbooks/aae/endodonticglossary2015/ (accessed November 14, 2016).

American Association of Endodontists (AAE) (2009) AAE Consensus Conference Recommended Diagnostic Terminology. *J Endod* **35**(12):1634.

American Dental Association (ADA) (2007) 2005–06 Survey of Dental Services Rendered. http://ebusiness.ada.org/productcatalog/product.aspx?ID=1428 (accessed November 21, 2016)).

Chen E, Abbott PV (2011) Evaluation of accuracy, reliability, and repeatability of five dental pulp tests. *J Endod* **37**(12):1619–1623.

Horst OV, Cunha-Cruz J, Zhou L, et al. (2015) Prevalence of pain in the orofacial regions in patients visiting general dentists in the Northwest Practice-based REsearch Collaborative in Evidence-based DENTistry research network. *J Am Dent Assoc* **146**(10):721–728.e3.

Portman-Lewis S (2007) An analysis of the out-of-hours demand and treatment provided by a general dental practice rota over a five-year period. *Prim Dent Care* **14**(3): 98–104.

Menhinick KA, Gutmann JL, Regan JD, et al. (2004) The efficacy of pain control following nonsurgical root canal treatment using ibuprofen or a combination of ibuprofen and acetaminophen in a randomized, double-blind, placebo-controlled study. *Int Endod J* **37**(8):531–541.

Weisleder R, Yamauchi S, Caplan DJ, et al. (2009) The validity of pulp testing: a clinical study. *J Am Dent Assoc* **140**(8):1013–1017.

Answers to Self-study Questions

1. In a patient with symptomatic irreversible pulpitis, pain relief is provided by removing the inflamed dental pulp. This may be accomplished through endodontic therapy (a pulpectomy as an emergency treatment or root canal therapy) or extraction.

2. The recommended pulpal diagnosis terms are normal pulp, reversible pulpitis, symptomatic irreversible pulpitis, asymptomatic irreversible pulpitis, pulp necrosis, previously treated, and previously initiated therapy.

3. The recommended periapical diagnosis terms are normal periapical tissues, symptomatic apical periodontitis, asymptomatic apical periodontitis, acute apical abscess, chronic apical abscess, and condensing osteitis.

4. The cold test and the EPT are the most common diagnostic tests used in clinical practice to assess the status of the dental pulp.

5. Percussion and palpation are commonly used to assess the status of the periapical tissues.

Sensitivity to percussion suggests that the periapical tissues are inflamed. Sensitivity to palpation indicates that the periapical tissues are inflamed and that the inflammation has spread to affect the periosteum. Mobility and periodontal probing are also be used to assess the periapical tissues and provide information about the periodontal support for the tooth. Probing is particularly useful in assessing longitudinal fractures and sinus tracts that drain through the sulcus.

Case 4.8

Pain Due to Apical Periodontitis

Natasha M Flake

A. Demographic Data and Reason for Contact
- Male, 49 years old.
- Reports with pain in the mandibular right posterior.

B. Symptom History
- Sensitivity to chewing on the mandibular right side for about 1 month, which has been getting progressively worse. The sensitivity is a dull ache, but getting more intense over time. He now avoids chewing on the right side. In the past few days the pain intensity has been between 4 at rest and 7 when chewing on the right side (NRS 0–10). The pain is localized to the mandibular right quadrant, and the patient can point to the tooth that he believes is the source of his pain. The patient says the mandibular right first molar (tooth 46) is sore when he presses on it with his tongue. He reports no sensitivity to hot or cold. The patient has been taking over-the-counter ibuprofen for the past few days, which helps the pain.

C. Medical History
- Stage I hypertension, controlled with medication.
- Blood pressure 130/74 mmHg.
- Pulse 62 bpm.
- Temperature 36.9 °C.
- Medications: hydrochlorothiazide, 25 mg/day.

D. Psychosocial History
- Married.
- Employed as an information technology specialist.
- History of regular dental care.
- No psychological assessment done.

E. Previous Consultations and Treatments
- None related to the present chief complaint. The restoration on tooth 46 was completed approximately 1.5 years ago.

F. Extraoral Status
- The extraoral exam is within normal limits. No asymmetries, swellings, erythema, or other abnormalities of the TMJ or muscles are noted.

G. Intraoral Status
Soft tissues
- No swelling, no sinus tract stoma, no exudate evident.

Hard tissues and dentition
- Tooth 45 has a do amalgam restoration; 46 has a dol amalgam restoration; 47 has a mo amalgam restoration. The margins of all restorations are intact. No recurrent caries is noted.

H. Additional Examinations and Findings
- Diagnostic test results show that tooth 46 is hypersensitive to percussion and does not respond to cold or the EPT (Table 4.3).
- Radiographic examination shows that all restorations appear to have intact margins (Figure 4.29). No caries is noted. The lamina dura appears intact and the periodontal ligament of normal width for tooth 47. There is a loss of the lamina dura and a diffuse periapical radiolucency around the mesial and distal roots of tooth 46, approximately 10 mm × 20 mm (height × width). Crestal bone height is within normal limits.

I. Diagnosis/Diagnoses
Other
- Pulp necrosis tooth 46.
- Symptomatic apical periodontitis tooth 46.

J. Case Assessment
- The source of the patient's pain in this case is inflammation of the periapical tissues of the mandibular right first molar. The etiology of the patient's problem is bacteria. The pulp has undergone necrosis, and the periapical tissues are inflamed as result of bacteria, necrotic tissue, and inflammatory mediators in the root canal system. Bacteria likely entered the pulp due to a history of dental caries, but a crack or leaking restoration are other possible etiologic factors.

Table 4.3 Diagnostic test results

	Percussion	Palpation	Cold	EPT	Mobility	Probing depth (mm)			
						b	l	m	d
45	WNL	WNL	WNL	27	0	2	2	3	3
46	+	WNL	NR	NR/80	0	2	2	3	4
47	WNL	WNL	WNL	20	0	2	2	4	4

Endodontic diagnostic test results are listed for the teeth in the mandibular right posterior. Tooth 46 is sensitive to percussion with respect to the adjacent teeth and does not respond to cold or electric pulp test (EPT; 0–80); b, buccal; l, lingual; m, mesial; d, distal; WNL, within normal limits; +, hypersensitive; NR, no response.

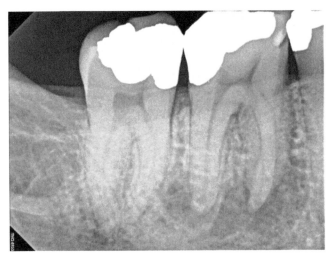

Figure 4.29 Preoperative radiograph.

- The patient's history, signs, and symptoms are a classic example of pain due to symptomatic apical periodontitis. The differential diagnosis could include an acute apical abscess, chronic apical abscess, or pain of non-odontogenic origin. However, the clinical exam does not indicate evidence of pus formation, and the radiographic findings indicate the presence of apical periodontitis due to endodontic origin.
- The diagnoses in this case were made based on the patient's reported history of pain, the diagnostic test results, and the radiographic findings. The patient's history of sensitivity to chewing is suggestive of a periapical diagnosis of symptomatic apical periodontitis. This periapical diagnosis was confirmed clinically by the sensitivity to percussion. The presence of periapical radiolucencies on the radiograph further indicate the presence of apical periodontitis. The pulpal diagnosis of pulp necrosis was made based on the lack of response to the cold test and EPT. All diagnostic test results were assessed in relation to the adjacent teeth in the quadrant.

K. Evidence-based Treatment Plan including Aims

- Treatment options for tooth 46 include: (1) nonsurgical root canal therapy, followed by a definitive build-up restoration and crown, (2) extraction, and (3) do nothing.
- The aim of the treatment is to eliminate the bacteria, necrotic tissue, and inflammatory mediators in the root canal system to eliminate the source of the patient's pain. This can be accomplished through endodontic therapy or extraction of the tooth. After the bacteria, necrotic tissue, and inflammatory mediators are removed, the inflammation of the periapical tissues should resolve.
- Endodontic treatment plan: nonsurgical root canal therapy (Figure 4.30).
- If the patient elects to maintain the tooth through endodontic therapy, the tooth must be properly restored after root canal therapy. A crown restoration is recommended in order to prevent fracture of the tooth or recontamination of the root canal system

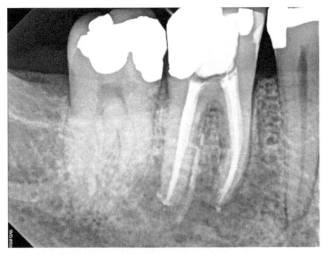

Figure 4.30 Postoperative radiograph.

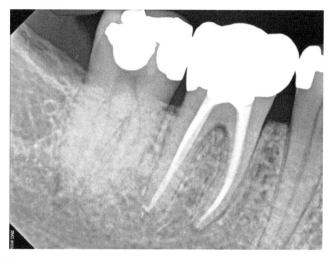

Figure 4.31 The 1 year follow-up radiograph.

through coronal leakage, and to provide long-term function for the patient.

- Restorative treatment plan: build-up and crown.

L. Prognosis and Discussion

- The prognosis is favorable. After the root canal system is cleaned and disinfected, periapical inflammation and the patient's pain should resolve. If proper endodontic therapy and restoration are provided, there should be no further bacterial contamination. The apical periodontitis will heal, and the tooth will provide long-term function for the patient. Resolution of apical periodontitis is evidenced by resolution of the patient's symptoms in the short term, and radiographic evidence of healing in the long term (Figure 4.31).

Background Information

- Apical periodontitis is inflammation of the tissues surrounding the apex of a tooth. Asymptomatic apical periodontitis is defined as inflammation and destruction of the apical periodontium that is of pulpal origin, appears as an apical radiolucent area, and does not produce clinical symptoms (American Association of Endodontists (AAE), 2015).
- Symptomatic apical periodontitis is defined as inflammation usually of the apical periodontium, producing clinical symptoms including a painful response to biting and/or percussion or palpation. It might or might not be associated with an apical radiolucent area (American Association of Endodontists (AAE), 2015).

- Apical periodontitis is a common condition in the adult population. For research purposes, the prevalence of apical periodontitis is typically measured by detecting the presence of radiographic changes. In a sample of over 5000 adults in Finland, the prevalence of apical periodontitis as detected on panoramic radiographs was 27% of subjects. The prevalence was greatest on teeth with inadequate root canal fillings, and apical periodontitis was more prevalent in males versus females (Huumonen *et al.*, 2016).

Diagnostic Criteria

American Association of Endodontists (AAE) (2009) consensus conference for diagnosis of **symptomatic apical periodontitis**.

Symptomatic apical periodontitis represents inflammation, usually of the apical periodontium, producing clinical symptoms involving a painful response to biting and/or percussion or palpation. This may or may not be accompanied by radiographic changes (i.e., depending upon the stage of the disease, there may be normal width of the periodontal ligament or there may be a periapical radiolucency). Severe pain to percussion and/or palpation is highly indicative of a degenerating pulp and root canal treatment is needed.

Fundamental Points

Outcomes of endodontic treatment

- Research investigating the outcomes of endodontic therapy vary widely in their protocols and outcome measures reported. Some studies report "success" and others report "survival" of the treated tooth. These outcomes may be defined differently in different studies, but success is the more stringent outcome measure and usually accounts for radiographic healing in addition to the tooth being present and symptom free in the mouth. In a prospective study, Ng *et al.* (2011a,2011b) investigated both periapical health and tooth survival following nonsurgical root canal therapy. An 83% success rate was found, with success defined as the absence of apical periodontitis assessed both clinically and radiographically at least 2 years after treatment (Ng *et al.*, 2011a). Of teeth with a recall of at least 4 years, the survival rate was over 95%, which meant the tooth was still present and potentially functional in the mouth (Ng *et al.*, 2011b). Furthermore, in a systematic review of the literature, Ng *et al.* (2010) found that tooth survival ranged between 86 and 93% over 2–10 years following root canal therapy.

Factors affecting prognosis of endodontic treatment

- Research into endodontic outcomes has attempted to identify factors that are associated with success or failure of root canal treatment. With dozens of published studies, two factors repeatedly have been shown to have an effect on treatment outcome: (1) the presence of a preoperative periapical radiolucency; and (2) definitive restoration of the tooth.

- Classic and contemporary literature show that teeth with preoperative periapical radiolucencies have a poorer prognosis than teeth without preoperative periapical radiolucencies. Teeth with a periapical radiolucency are thought to be infected; whereas teeth without a periapical radiolucency may or may not be infected. Thus, teeth with a periapical radiolucency are more difficult to disinfect than teeth with intact periapical tissues. In a systematic review and meta-analysis of the literature, Ng *et al.* (2008) found 49 studies published between 1922 and 2002 that investigated the effect of periapical status on treatment outcome following root canal therapy. The preoperative absence of a periapical radiolucency significantly improved the outcome of root canal treatment. Additional studies published since 2002 have corroborated these results. In a prospective study of factors affecting the outcomes of nonsurgical root canal treatment, the absence of a periapical lesion (or, if present, the smaller its size) significantly increased the probability of apical healing (Ng *et al.*, 2011a).

- Research also highlights the importance of a definitive coronal restoration in the long-term prognosis of endodontically treated teeth. In a systematic review, the presence of a crown restoration was the factor that most

impacted tooth survival 2–10 years after root canal therapy (Ng *et al.*, 2010). In a prospective study of the factors affecting the outcomes of nonsurgical root canal treatment, the presence of a satisfactory coronal restoration significantly affected both periapical healing and tooth survival after root canal therapy (Ng *et al.*, 2011a,b). Furthermore, in a large study of an insurance database of over 1.4 million teeth treated with root canal therapy, 97% of teeth were retained in the mouth 8 years after the initial root canal therapy. Of the 3% of teeth that required additional treatment (retreatment, apical surgery, or extraction), 85% had no full coronal restoration (Salehrabi and Rotstein, 2004).

One- versus two-visit endodontic treatment

- The number of visits in which root canal treatment should be completed has been greatly debated. Consensus exists that a tooth with a vital pulp may have root canal therapy completed in one visit, time permitting, because the canals are not infected. Consensus also exists that root canal therapy should not be completed in one visit when the patient has swelling or the canal cannot be dried due to blood or exudate seepage from the periapical tissues. In these cases, the clinician should wait until the swelling has resolved and the canal can be dried completely prior to obturation.

- Disagreement exists on whether necrotic teeth with asymptomatic apical periodontitis, symptomatic apical periodontitis, or a chronic apical abscess should be treated with single- or multiple-visit root canal therapy. The rationale for completing treatment in two visits is that the intracanal medicament placed between visits facilitates disinfection of the root canal system. Despite the sound scientific rationale for completing root canal therapy of necrotic teeth in two visits using an intracanal medicament, there is a lack of clinical outcomes data to support the idea that two-visit treatment results in a better prognosis. Systematic reviews of the available literature have found no significant effect of the number of treatment visits on radiographic success of root canal therapy (Ng *et al.*, 2008; Su *et al.*, 2011). However, it is important to note that these studies are limited in power.

Self-study Questions

1. What is the difference between success and survival of an endodontically treated tooth?

2. What two factors have consistently been shown to have an effect on outcome of endodontic treatment?

3. What is the rationale for providing root canal therapy in two visits versus one visit?

4. What are the differences in outcomes for root canal therapy provided in one visit versus two visits?

Acknowledgments

I thank Dr Randy Ball for use of images.

References

American Association of Endodontists (AAE) (2009) AAE Consensus Conference Recommended Diagnostic Terminology. *J Endod* **35**(12):1634.

American Association of Endodontists (AAE) (2015) *Glossary of endodontic terms.* http://www.nxtbook.com/nxtbooks/aae/endodonticglossary2015/ (accessed November 14, 2016).

Huumonen S, Suominen AL, Vehkalahti MM (2016) Prevalence of apical periodontitis in root filled teeth: findings from a nationwide survey in Finland. *Int Endod J* in press. doi: 10.1111/iej.12625.

Ng YL, Mann V, Rahbaran S, *et al.* (2008) Outcome of primary root canal treatment: systematic review of the literature – Part 2. Influence of clinical factors. *Int Endod J* **41**(1):6–31.

Ng YL, Mann V, Gulabivala K (2010) Tooth survival following non-surgical root canal treatment: a systematic review of the literature. *Int Endod J* **43**(3):171–189.

Ng YL, Mann V, Gulabivala K (2011a) A prospective study of the factors affecting outcomes of nonsurgical root canal treatment: part 1: periapical health. *Int Endod J* **44**(7):583–609.

Ng YL, Mann V, Gulabivala K (2011b) A prospective study of the factors affecting outcomes of non-surgical root canal treatment: part 2: tooth survival. *Int Endod J* **44**(7):610–625.

Salehrabi R, Rotstein I (2004) Endodontic treatment outcomes in a large patient population in the USA: an epidemiological study. *J Endod* **30**(12):846–850.

Su Y, Wang C, Ye L (2011) Healing rate and post-obturation pain of single- versus multiple-visit endodontic treatment for infected root canals: a systematic review. *J Endod* **37**(2):125–132.

Answers to Self-study Questions

1. Endodontic success is defined as the treated tooth having no signs or symptoms of endodontic pathosis, as well as complete radiographic healing of any periapical lesion. Survival is a less stringent outcome and refers to the tooth being present in the mouth.

2. The presence of a preoperative periapical radiolucency and definitive restoration of the tooth have an effect on outcome of endodontic treatment. Teeth without a preoperative periapical radiolucency and teeth that have been satisfactorily restored have better outcomes than teeth with a preoperative periapical radiolucency and those without a satisfactory definitive restoration.

3. The rationale for providing root canal therapy in two visits versus one is that placement of an intracanal medicament between visits facilitates disinfection of the root canal system.

4. The available literature has found no significant difference in outcomes between root canal therapy performed in one visit versus two visits.

Case 4.9

Pain Due to Traumatic Occlusion

Natasha M Flake

A. Demographic Data and Reason for Contact
- Male, 53 years old.
- Reports with pain in the maxillary anterior teeth.

B. Symptom History
- Patient reports with a chief complaint of "My front tooth is sensitive and I feel like it is loose." Patient reports pain in his maxillary anterior teeth, specifically the maxillary right central incisor (tooth 11). The pain varies in intensity from 1 to 3 (NRS 0–10). The pain is intermittent; the tooth will hurt for several days and then the pain will subside for several days. Sometimes the pain radiates up to his forehead. The pain is increased by pressure and cold.

C. Medical History
- Blood pressure: 140/82 mmHg.
- Pulse: 62 bpm.
- No medications.

D. Psychosocial History
- Single.
- Employed as a carpenter.
- History of sporadic dental care; has not seen a dentist in 3 years.
- No psychological assessment done.

E. Previous Consultations and Treatments
- None related to the present chief complaint.

F. Extraoral status
- The extraoral exam is within normal limits. No asymmetries, swellings, erythema, or other abnormalities of the TMJ and muscles are noted.

G. Intraoral Status
Soft tissues
- No swelling, no sinus tract stoma, no exudate evident.

Hard tissues and dentition
- Teeth 12–22 and 32–42 are intact and have no noted caries or restorations. Tooth 41 is facially positioned and in end-to-end occlusion with tooth 11. Occlusal registration shows a supra-occlusal contact in intercuspal position. Calculus is present on the lingual aspect of the mandibular anterior teeth.

H. Additional Examinations and Findings
- Diagnostic test results are as follows (Table 4.4).
- Radiographic examination showed mild to moderate horizontal bone loss in the maxillary and mandibular anterior. The lamina dura appears intact and the periodontal ligament of normal width for the maxillary (Figure 4.32a) and mandibular incisors (Figure 4.32b). No caries was noted.

I. Diagnosis/Diagnoses
Other
- Traumatic occlusion tooth 11.

J. Case Assessment
- The working diagnosis in this case is traumatic occlusion, and the source of the patient's pain is inflammation of the pulp and periapical tissues due to chronic occlusal trauma. The differential diagnosis for the pulp and periapical tissues includes reversible pulpitis, symptomatic irreversible pulpitis, and symptomatic apical periodontitis.
- The absence of any caries, restoration, crack, or known history of trauma to the tooth renders pathosis of endodontic origin an unlikely cause of the patient's pain.
- In the absence of tooth pathology, the plan is to address the occlusion and monitor for resolution of symptoms, rather than perform root canal therapy.
- The diagnosis in this case was made based on the patient's reported history of pain, the clinical and radiographic exam, and the diagnostic test results. The clinical exam and examination of the occlusion were critical in making the diagnosis.

Table 4.4 Diagnostic test results

Tooth	Percussion	Palpation	Cold	EPT	Mobility	Probing depth (mm)			
						b	l	m	d
12	WNL	WNL	WNL	27	1	3	2	4	4
11	+	WNL	+L	32	1	3	2	4	4
21	WNL	WNL	WNL	20	1	3	2	4	4
22	WNL	WNL	WNL	42	1	2	2	4	4
32	WNL	WNL	WNL	25	1	2	2	3	3
31	WNL	WNL	WNL	50	1	2	3	3	4
41	WNL	WNL	WNL	40	1	2	2	4	4
42	WNL	WNL	WNL	39	1	2	2	4	3

Endodontic diagnostic test results are listed for the maxillary and mandibular incisors. Tooth 11 is sensitive to percussion with respect to the adjacent teeth and has an exaggerated and lingering response to the cold test. EPT, electric pulp test (0–80); b, buccal; l, lingual; m, mesial; d, distal; WNL, within normal limits; +, hypersensitive; +L, hypersensitive and lingering.

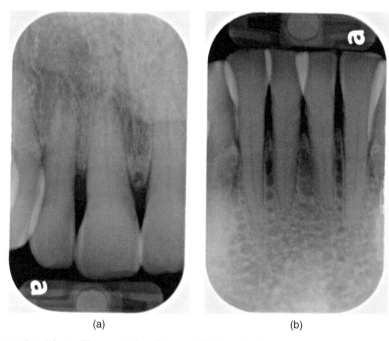

(a)　　　　　　　　　　(b)

Figure 4.32 Periapical radiographs: (a) maxillary anterior; (b) mandibular anterior.

K. Evidence-based Treatment Plan including Aims

- Treatment options for tooth 11 include (1) occlusal adjustment and monitor for resolution of symptoms, (2) root canal therapy, (3) extraction, and (4) do nothing.
- The treatment plan is to perform an occlusal adjustment on tooth 41, which occludes end to end with tooth 11. The aim is to remove the source of the pulpal and periapical inflammation, thereby eliminating the patient's pain. The patient will be monitored for resolution of symptoms after the occlusal adjustment. If symptoms do not resolve, the patient will be reevaluated for the need for endodontic therapy or other treatment.

L. Prognosis and Discussion

- The prognosis is favorable. However, if the occlusal adjustment does not relieve the symptoms, then root canal therapy or other treatment may be indicated.
- In the case presented, occlusal adjustment was performed on tooth 41, which occluded end to end with tooth 11. The next day, the patient reported his symptoms had resolved. The tooth was not endodontically treated. Had root canal therapy been performed instead of the occlusal adjustment, it is likely that the treatment would have alleviated the patient's sensitivity to cold, but not all of his symptoms, as the tooth would still have been in traumatic occlusion.

Background Information

- The American Academy of Periodontology (AAP, 2012) defines occlusal trauma as injury resulting in tissue changes within the attachment apparatus due to physiologic or parafunctional forces which may exceed its adaptive capacity. Primary occlusal trauma is injury resulting in tissue changes from excessive occlusal forces applied to a tooth or teeth with normal support. Secondary occlusal trauma is injury resulting in tissue changes from normal or excessive occlusal forces applied to a tooth or teeth with reduced support. Traumatic occlusion is occlusion that produces such trauma.

- The relationship between traumatic occlusion and dental pain symptoms is recognized by clinicians, but there is little available literature to describe this clinical phenomenon. The majority of what is known about pain due to traumatic occlusion is based on clinical observations and small case reports. There is no known published data on the incidence or prevalence of pain due to traumatic occlusion, and no known published controlled clinical studies on treatment. Thus, there is a great need for clinical research on pain due to traumatic occlusion.

- Painful symptoms associated with traumatic occlusion have been described as including temperature sensitivity, pressure sensitivity, and spontaneous pain. These symptoms reflect pulpal and periapical inflammation, and therefore may mimic pain of endodontic origin. However, endodontic therapy is not indicated in these cases, if the traumatic occlusion is addressed and symptoms resolve. Treatment of traumatic occlusion may include an occlusal splint and/or occlusal adjustment, in addition to other therapies. Root canal therapy is only indicated in cases where the dental pulp has become irreversibly inflamed or necrotic.

Diagnostic Criteria

There are no criteria for **Traumatic occlusion** so the diagnosis is solely based on the patient's reported history of pain, the clinical and radiographic exam, and the diagnostic test results. Absence of caries, restoration, crack, or known history of trauma to the tooth renders pathology of endodontic origin an unlikely cause of the patient's pain. The clinical exam and examination of the occlusion are critical in making the diagnosis.

Fundamental Points

Literature in humans

- There is a lack of data available on traumatic occlusion as an etiology of dental pain, and the clinical literature includes a few case reports. Cooke (1982) reported a case of reversible pulpitis in the maxillary anterior teeth due to protrusive bruxism. After the patient was treated with a night guard, the symptoms resolved, and the teeth responded within normal limits to all tests upon reevaluation after 1 year. Yu (2004) reported two cases of traumatic occlusion playing a role in the initiation and progression of pulp and periapical inflammation. Symptoms did not resolve after endodontic therapy, and traumatic occlusion was identified as the etiology of the patients' pain. Symptoms resolved after occlusal adjustment was performed, and occlusal splints were recommended.

- Caviedes-Bucheli *et al.* (2011) investigated the effect of experimentally induced occlusal trauma on substance P (SP) expression in healthy human pulp and periodontal ligament. Human subjects whose treatment plan included premolar extractions were studied. Occlusal trauma was induced by having subjects chewing on gum for 30 min with an interference placed on an occlusal surface. Teeth were then extracted and levels of SP were measured in the pulp and periodontal ligament. After occlusal trauma, there was a 45% increase of SP in the pulp and a 120% increase in the periodontal ligament compared with contralateral control teeth. In a review, Caviedes-Bucheli *et al.* (2016) concluded that human dental pulp responds to occlusal trauma with a neurogenic inflammatory response. This inflammatory response leads to angiogenesis, which is needed to produce mineralized tissue formation as a defense mechanism.

Mechanisms of pain due to traumatic occlusion: animal studies

- Although little data exist on pain due to traumatic occlusion in human populations, studies using animal models provide some insight into mechanisms that may underlie such pain.
- In a classic study using a rat model, pins were placed in maxillary molars to produce sustained forces on the opposing teeth. Effects of the traumatic occlusion on the periodontium were seen in a matter of days, but after months effects were also seen in the pulp. The pulp contained increased numbers of macrophages and lymphocytes, as well as formation of reparative dentin (Cooper *et al.*, 1971).
- In another study in rats, blood flow to the pulp and periodontal ligament was measured during experimental traumatic occlusion in the maxillary and mandibular molars (Kvinnsland *et al.*, 1992). An increase in blood flow in the pulp and periodontal ligament was observed on teeth with traumatic occlusion compared with the contralateral side. In addition, over time an increase in blood flow on both sides was observed compared with control animals. Thus, unilateral occlusal trauma induced increased blood flow on both the affected tooth and the contralateral side.
- Also using a rat model, traumatic occlusion was induced by adding 1 mm of composite to the occlusal surface of the maxillary first molar (Kvinnsland and Heyeraas, 1992). An increase in the density of nerve fibers containing SP and calcitonin gene-related peptide was seen in the gingiva, periodontal ligament, and the pulp. Axonal proliferation also occurred. The changes were greatest in the pulp.
- Collectively, these results suggest that traumatic occlusal forces may induce changes in neuropeptides, nerve morphology, and blood flow in the pulp and periodontium that could lead to clinical symptoms.

Self-study Questions

1. What is the difference between primary occlusal trauma and secondary occlusal trauma?
2. Traumatic occlusion might present as what painful symptoms in a patient?
3. In case reports of patients who have presented with pain due to traumatic occlusion, what treatments have helped to alleviate the patients' pain?
4. Based on data from animal studies, what mechanisms may underlie pain due to traumatic occlusion?

Bibliography

AAP (2012) *Glossary of periodontal terms*. http://members.perio.org/libraries/glossary (accessed November 16, 2016).

Caviedes-Bucheli J, Azuero-Holguin MM, Correa-Ortiz JA, *et al.* (2011) Effect of experimentally induced occlusal trauma on substance P expression in human dental pulp and periodontal ligament. *J Endod* **37**(5):627–630.

Caviedes-Bucheli J, Gomez-Sosa JF, Azuero-Holguin MM, *et al.* (2016) Angiogenic mechanisms of human dental pulp and their relationship with substance P expression in response to occlusal trauma. *Int Endod J*. doi: 10.1111/iej.12627.

Cooke HG (1982) Reversible pulpitis with etiology of bruxism. *J Endod* **8**(6):280–281.

Cooper MB, Landay MA, Seltzer S (1971) The effects of excessive occlusal force on the pulp. II. Heavier and longer term forces. *J Periodontol* **42**(6):353–359.

Kvinnsland I, Heyeraas KJ (1992) Effect of traumatic occlusion on CGRP and SP immunoreactive nerve fibre morphology in rat molar pulp and periodontium. *Histochemistry* **97**(2):111–120.

Kvinnsland S, Kristiansen AB, Kvinnsland I, Heyeraas KJ (1992) Effect of experimental traumatic occlusion on periodontal and pulpal blood flow. *Acta Odontol Scand* **50**(4):211–219.

Yu CY (2004) Role of occlusion in endodontic management: report of two cases. *Aust Endod J* **30**(3):110–115.

Answers to Self-study Questions

1. Primary occlusal trauma is injury resulting in tissue changes from excessive occlusal forces applied to a tooth or teeth with normal support. Secondary occlusal trauma is injury resulting in tissue changes from normal or excessive occlusal forces applied to a tooth or teeth with reduced support.
2. Traumatic occlusion might present as temperature sensitivity, pressure sensitivity, and/or spontaneous pain.
3. In patients with pain due to traumatic occlusion, night guards, occlusal adjustments, and occlusal splints have helped to alleviate the patients' pain.
4. Mechanisms that may contribute to pain due to traumatic occlusion include increased numbers of immune cells in the pulp, increased blood flow to the pulp and periodontal ligament, increased neuropeptides in the pulp and periodontal ligament, and axonal proliferation.

Case 4.10

Extreme Tooth Wear

Peter Wetselaar

A. Demographic Data and Reasons for Contact

- Male, 44 years old, concerned about excessive tooth wear.

B. Symptom History

- Patient has been concerned because of his worn teeth for some time. After looking at a 20-year-old photograph of himself smiling he noticed that the teeth had changed a lot. Recently, he decided to contact his dentist about this.
- Reported no problems with dry mouth.

C. Medical History

- Healthy, but at times problems with heartburn; no diagnosis.

D. Psychosocial History

- Engineer, not married, no children.
- Describes himself as a calm person, but with high current stress level due to demanding work load. No depression according to PHQ-9 and no anxiety according to GAD-7. No physical symptoms according to PHQ-15. Severe stress according to PSS-10. Poor sleep quality (PSQI).
- Nonsmoker, moderate alcohol consumption.

E. Previous Consultations and Treatments

- No orthodontic treatment; teeth 14 and 24 are missing due to hypodontia. Wisdom teeth were extracted. Over several decades, some direct fillings were made, resulting in 11 fillings and one endodontic treatment in tooth 46 at the age of 36. On tooth 46 a crown was made. In the last couple of years there was an acceleration of complaints, resulting in endodontic treatments in teeth 16 and 13. In teeth 16 and 46 the endodontic treatment was revisited; in tooth 16, apical surgery was performed. An endodontic treatment was started in tooth 36. The crown on tooth 46 was fractured. Because of the accumulation of complaints, the patient asked for a referral.

F. Extraoral Status

- No asymmetries, swelling, redness, or other specific findings, but bilateral masseter muscle hypertrophy.
- DC/TMD examination shows normal findings for jaw movement capacity, movement pain, joint sound, and TMJ and muscle palpation (Schiffman et al., 2014).
- Qualitative somatosensory testing: no abnormalities were found (Baad-Hansen et al., 2013).

G. Intraoral Status

Soft tissues

- Bilateral tongue scalloping and mucosal ridging.
- The gingiva around teeth 36 and 46 was swollen and red.

Hard tissues and dentition

- Full dentition with the exception of wisdom teeth.
- Tooth wear examination revealed severe tooth wear with occlusal cupping, cratering, rounding of cusps, wear on non-occluding surfaces, raised restorations, broad concavities within smooth surface enamel, convex areas flatten, or concavities (Figures 4.33 and 4.34).
- The (avital) teeth 16, 13, 46, and 36 did not respond to the sensitive endodontic tests. The majority of the other (vital) teeth had a prolonged reaction time. Teeth 36 and 46 were painful on percussion, palpation of the apical region; in particular, the bite test with a Fractfinder or the Tooth Slooth was painful, and showed deep pockets. It was concluded that both teeth 36 and 46 were cracked, resulting in this deep pocketing, and therefore re-endodontic treatment and saving these two teeth was no longer possible.

Occlusion

- There was a normal occlusion (Angle class I, both frontal and posterior). Concerning the articulation patterns, the right (Figure 4.33b) and left (Figure 4.33c) lateral movements showed group guidance; in protrusion, frontal guidance existed.

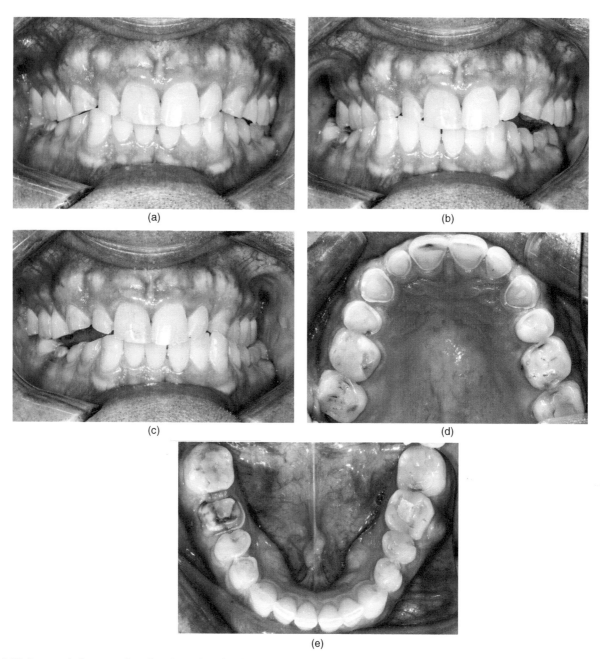

Figure 4.33 Intraoral photographs of patient showing intercuspal position (a), tooth contacts during right (b) and left (c) lateral excursion as well as maxillary (d) and mandibular (e) occlusal surfaces. Severe wear is noted.

Saliva

- Evaluation of the salivary parameters, like the salivary flow, buffer capacity, and pH, revealed normal values.

H. Additional Examination and Findings

- Panoramic imaging showed three endodontically treated teeth and periapical radiolucent areas for 36 and 46 (Figure 4.35).
- Additional questionnaires regarding oral hygiene products, food diary, reflux, xerostomia. These showed an acidic diet, use of hard toothbrush in combination with abrasive toothpaste, possible reflux, but no xerostomia.
- Patient was referred to a gastroenterologist.

I. Diagnosis/Diagnoses
Other

- Tooth wear.
- Probable bruxism.
- Asymptomatic apical periodontitis.

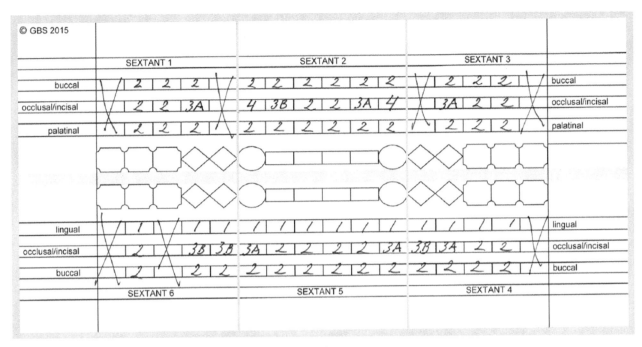

Figure 4.34 Completed chart of tooth wear from clinical examination.

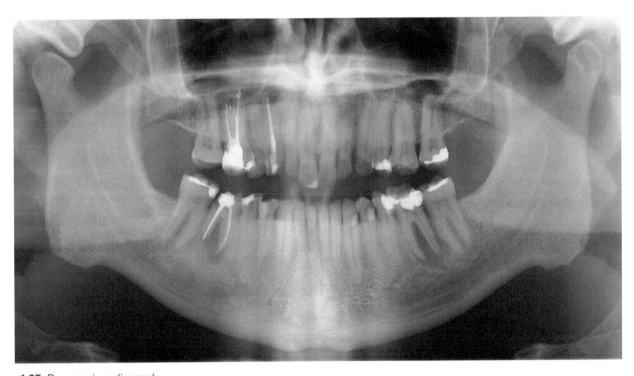

Figure 4.35 Panoramic radiograph.

J. Case Assessment

- The findings from the tooth wear evaluation system (TWES), Tables 4.5, 4.6, 4.7, and 4.8, were in line with the oral history taking and the answers to the questionnaires (OBCL, oral hygiene products, food diary, xerostomia).

- Both the oral history taking and the questionnaires revealed that awake and sleep bruxism were present. The intraoral findings of the soft tissues also supported bruxism. Based on this information, and the clinical examination, a diagnosis of probable bruxism was made (Lobbezoo *et al.*, 2013).

Table 4.5 TWES: overview of modules

Diagnostic modules

Basis diagnostic (general practitioner)
Module Qualification
Module Quantification, screening module *or*
Module Quantification, clinical crown length module Recording
 of tooth wear (intraoral photographs, dental casts)

Extended diagnostic (referral clinic)
Module Quantification, finer-grained occlusal/incisal and
 non-occlusal/non-incisal
Module Oral history, questionnaires
Module Salivary analysis

Treatment/management modules
Module Complaints of the patient versus reasons for the
 clinician to start treatment/management
Module Start of treatment/management
Module Level of difficulty

- Concerning the dental hard tissues, it was found that, beside chemical tooth wear, mechanical tooth wear was also present. For the diagnosis of bruxism, the clinical findings: "enamel and dentin wear at the same rate" and "matching wear on occluding surfaces or corresponding features at the antagonistic teeth" were present. This can be the reason for the clinical signs of attrition (see earlier).

- Knowledge about the use of oral hygiene products of the patients is important, because these products can be abrasive. The patient is using an abrasive dentifrice and a hard toothbrush; this can be part of the reason for the clinical signs of abrasion (see earlier).

- The food diary revealed an acidic diet; this can be the reason for the clinical signs of erosion (see earlier). The reflux questionnaire revealed that the patient sometimes experienced complaints that could fit with gastroesophageal reflux disease, like heartburn and regurgitation. This also can be the reason for the clinical signs of erosion (see earlier), especially the clinical finding "preservation of enamel cuff in gingival crevice." Also, during the oral history taking, the patient reported that sometimes he suffers from heartburn and regurgitation.

- The module "Quantification" of the TWES (Table 4.7) showed that the patient could be classified as having both localized extreme (sextant 2) and generalized severe (sextants 1, 3, 4, 5, and 6) tooth wear. Concerning the origin of the tooth wear, this case was classified as tooth wear with a mixed origin: mechanical/intrinsic (attrition), mechanical/extrinsic (abrasion), chemical/intrinsic (erosion), and chemical/extrinsic (erosion). The origin was based on

Table 4.6 TWES: module "Qualification"

Clinical signs of erosion
1. Occlusal "cupping," incisal "grooving," "cratering,"[a] rounding of cusps and grooves[b]
2. Wear on non-occluding surfaces[a]
3. "Raised" restorations[a,b]
4. Broad concavities within smooth surface enamel,[a] convex areas flatten, or concavities become present, width exceeds depth[b]
5. Increased incisal translucency[a]
6. Clean, nontarnished appearance of amalgams[a]
7. Preservation of enamel "cuff" in gingival crevice[a,b]
8. No plaque, discoloration, or tartar[b]
9. Hypersensitivity[a]
10. Smooth silky-shining, silky-glazed appearance, sometimes dull surface[b]

Clinical signs of attrition
1. Shiny facets,[a] flat and glossy[b]
2. Enamel and dentin wear at the same rate[a]
3. Matching wear on occluding surfaces,[a] corresponding features at the antagonistic teeth[b]
4. Possible fracture of cusps or restorations[a]
5. Impressions in cheek, tongue, and/or lip

Clinical signs of abrasion
1. Usually located at cervical areas of teeth[a]
2. Lesions are more wide than deep[a]
3. Premolars and cuspids are commonly affected[a]

[a] According to Gandara and Truelove (1999).
[b] According to Ganss and Lussi (2014).

Table 4.7 TWES: module "Quantification"

Eight-point ordinal scale for occlusal and incisal grading
For each tooth the grade is determined
0 = no (visible) wear
1a = (within the enamel) minimal wear of cusps or incisal tips
1b = (within the enamel) facets parallel to the normal planes of contour
1c = (within the enamel) noticeable flattening of cusps or incisal edges
2 = wear with dentin exposure and loss of clinical crown height $\leq 1/3$
3a = wear with dentin exposure and loss of clinical crown height 1/3–1/2
3b = wear with dentin exposure and loss of clinical crown height 1/2–2/3
4 = wear with dentin exposure and loss of clinical crown height of $\geq 2/3$

Three-point ordinal scale for non-occlusal/non-incisal grading
For each tooth the grade is determined, both buccal/labial as palatinal/lingual
0 = no (visible) wear
1 = wear confined to the enamel
2 = wear into the dentin

Source: Wetselaar *et al.* (2009).

the qualification, the oral history taking, and some questionnaires.

K. Evidence-based Treatment Plan including Aims

- The first aim was to eliminate infections in 36 and 46.
- Teeth 36 and 46 were surgically removed.
- The second aim was to determine if the patient had any gastrointestinal condition that could be part of the etiology of the tooth wear. The patient was therefore referred to a gastroenterologist, who diagnosed gastroesophageal reflux disease. Medication with a proton pump inhibitor was prescribed.
- The third aim was to prevent pain/sensitivity, restore esthetics, and prevent further loss of hard dental tissues and breaking of restorations. Restorative treatment was started according to a so-called dynamic treatment plan. This means to start only with the necessary steps, and if possible use reversible techniques. All existing restorations were removed before restoring all teeth with direct composite restorations.

L. Prognosis and Discussion

- There is evidence that a restorative treatment plan with direct composite material has a good prognosis (Milosevic and Burnside, 2015). The biggest

advantage of this kind of treatment is to avoid further loss of dental hard tissues by using a nonpreparation or minimal invasive restoration technique. When doing so, the dental clinician can monitor the patient and see if other diagnostic steps or treatments are necessary. Common complications are wear or breaking of the restorations. To avoid these complications, a protective stabilization splint can be made. In this case this was not done, because it was thought that the chemical wear was of greater importance than the mechanical wear. Although the patient used medication for the gastroesophageal reflux disease, it is nevertheless known that (a part of) the reflux can remain. If so, the splint may retain gastric acidic content that may cause an adverse effect.
- When using indirect techniques, preparation of the teeth is necessary; more dental tissue is sacrificed. There is a higher risk for endodontic treatment, and, for example, when bruxism exists, a higher risk of breaking of these indirect restoration, and even worse of the roots themselves. If that were the case, more teeth would have been lost. Making three-unit-bridges to close the existing diastema is a possibility; in this case no improvement in esthetics or masticatory function will be achieved; again, a greater risk of these roots should be the case. Placement of dental implants on the location of teeth 36 and 46 is a better option than the three-unit-bridges. There is no higher risk for complications of the adjacent teeth, but again no gain in esthetics or masticatory function will be achieved.

Background Information

Qualification (intraoral examination)

- Tooth wear is a multifactorial condition, leading to the loss of dental hard tissues; namely, enamel and dentin.

   Three subtypes of tooth wear can be present: erosion, attrition, and abrasion. The following signs of erosion (chemical wear) may occur: occlusal cupping, cratering, rounding of cusps, wear on non-occluding surfaces, raised restorations, broad concavities within smooth surface enamel, convex areas flatten, or concavities become present, width exceeds depth, preservation of enamel "cuff" in gingival crevice, and a smooth silky-shining, silky-glazed appearance, and sometimes a dull surface. Signs of attrition (mechanical wear) may

Table 4.8 TWES: module "Start of treatment/management"

Primary criterion	Treatment/management	Secondary criterion
I The amount of tooth surface loss	Wear within the enamel: counselling/monitoring Wear with dentin exposure: counselling/monitoring grade 0, 1, 2 Wear with dentin exposure and loss of clinical crown height: restorative treatment advised grade 3, 4	1. *Speed of the tooth wear process* Slow process: counselling/monitoring Fast process: restorative treatment advised
II Which surfaces are affected	Non-occlusal/non-incisal wear (no potential loss of clinical crown length; no disturbance of occlusion/articulation: counselling/monitoring Occlusal/incisal wear, and wear of the palatinal surfaces of sextant 2 (disturbance of occlusion/articulation): restorative treatment advised	2. *Age of the patient* The younger the patient, the sooner restorative treatment is advised 3. *Etiological factors* The more factors are present and the more difficult these are to eliminate, the sooner restorative treatment is advised
III The number of teeth that are affected	Limited number of teeth/sextants show wear (localized wear, 1 or 2 sextants): counselling/monitoring Increasing number of teeth/sextants show wear (generalized wear, 3 to 6 sextants): restorative treatment advised	

be shiny facets, flat and glossy on the incisal surfaces of the incisors, enamel and dentin wear at the same rate, matching wear on occluding surfaces or corresponding features at the antagonistic teeth. Signs of abrasion are usually located on cervical areas of teeth, lesions being of greater width than depth, and commonly affects premolars and cuspids (Gandara and Truelove, 1999; Ganss and Lussi, 2014).

Quantification (intraoral examination)
The severity of the tooth wear may be quantified using the TWES module Quantification into finer-grained occlusal/incisal and finer-grained non-occlusal/non-incisal. The grading scales that are used are an eight-point ordinal scale for the occlusal/incisal surfaces and a three-point ordinal scale for the non-occlusal/non-incisal surfaces (Wetselaar *et al.*, 2009).

Classification
- Filling in the module Quantification, finer-grained occlusal/incisal and non-occlusal/non-incisal, it was revealed that this patient could be classified

concerning the distribution and severity as: localized extreme (sextant 2) and generalized severe (sextants 1, 3, 4, 5, and 6) tooth wear. Concerning the origin of the tooth wear, this case was classified as tooth wear with a mixed origin: mechanical/intrinsic (attrition), mechanical/extrinsic (abrasion), chemical/intrinsic (erosion), and chemical/extrinsic (erosion). The origin was based on the qualification, the oral history taking, and some questionnaires.

Diagnostic Criteria
TWES criteria for **Tooth wear** (Wetselaar and Lobbezoo, 2016). Sensitivity and specificity have not been established.
    The TWES includes tools to assess:

1. Distribution of wear
        localized (1–2 sextants);
        generalized (3–6 sextants).
2. Severity of wear
        mild (wear within the enamel; occlusal/incisal and/or non-occlusal/non-incisal);

moderate (wear with dentin exposure; occlusal/incisal and/or non-occlusal/non-incisal);

severe (wear with dentin exposure and loss of clinical crown height <2/3 occlusal/incisal; regardless of the non-occlusal/non-incisal wear)

extreme (wear with dentin exposure and loss of clinical crown height ≥2/3 occlusal/incisal, regardless of the non-occlusal/non-incisal wear).

3. Origin

mechanical/intrinsic (attrition);

mechanical/extrinsic (abrasion);

chemical/intrinsic (erosion);

chemical/extrinsic (erosion).

Proposed criteria for **Sleep or awake bruxism** (Lobbezoo *et al.*, 2013). Sensitivity and specificity have not been established. The diagnosis is based on patient report, clinical examination, and polysomography.

- Possible sleep or awake bruxism
  - Self-report of sleep or awake bruxism (questionnaires or patient interview).
- Probable sleep or awake bruxism.
  - Self-report plus clinical examination.
- Definite sleep or awake bruxism.
  - Self-report, a clinical examination and a polysomnographic recording.

Fundamental Points

Tooth wear evaluation system

- Because of its multifactorial etiology, tooth wear can manifest itself in many different representations, and therefore it can be difficult to diagnose and manage the condition. A systematic approach is a *sine qua non*, to improve the diagnosis and management of this condition.
- In the TWES, all the necessary tools for a clinical guideline are present in different modules. This allows the dental clinician, in a general practitioner setting as well as in a referral practice setting, to perform a state-of-the-art diagnostic process.
- Since the TWES is a modular system, the dental clinician can select the proper modules for each individual patient. It is divided into several Diagnostic modules and Treatment/management modules (Tables 4.5, 4.6, 4.7, and 4.8).

Self-study Questions

1. How is qualification of tooth wear possible?
2. How is quantification of tooth wear possible?
3. How can one unravel the etiology of tooth wear?
4. Based on which findings can one decide which kind of treatment one should start?
5. Based on which findings can one judge if to perform a restorative treatment by oneself or to refer to a dental clinician specialized in restorative treatment of tooth wear patients.

References

Baad-Hansen L, Pigg M, Ivanovic SE, *et al.* (2013) Chairside intraoral qualitative somatosensory testing: reliability and comparison between patients with atypical odontalgia and healthy controls. *J Orofac Pain* **27**:165–170.

Gandara BK, Truelove EL (1999) Diagnosis and management of dental erosion. *J Contemp Dent Pract* **1**:16–23.

Ganss C, Lussi A (2014) Diagnosis of erosive tooth wear. *Monogr Oral Sci* **25**:22–31.

Lobbezoo F, Ahlberg J, Glaros AG, *et al.* (2013) Bruxism defined and graded: an international consensus. *J Oral Rehabil* **40**:2–4.

Milosevic A, Burnside G (2016) The survival of direct composite restorations in the management of severe tooth wear including attrition and erosion: a prospective 8-year study. *J Dent* **44**:13–19.

Schiffman E, Ohrbach R, Truelove E, *et al.* (2014) Diagnostic Criteria for Temporomandibular Disorders (DC/TMD) for clinical and research applications: recommendations of the International RDC/TMD Consortium Network and Orofacial Pain Special Interest Group. *J Oral Facial Pain Headache* **28**(1):6–27.

Wetselaar P, Lobbezoo F (2016) The tooth wear evaluation system (TWES): a modular clinical guideline for the diagnosis and management planning of worn dentitions. *J Oral Rehabil* **43**:69–80.

Wetselaar P, Lobbezoo F, Koutris M, *et al.* (2009) Reliability of an occlusal and non-occlusal tooth wear grading system: clinical use versus dental cast assessment. *Int J Prosthodont* **22**:388–390.

Answers to Self-study Questions

1. Qualification of tooth wear can be accomplished by the use of clinical signs of mechanical and chemical wear. It is the first step for the dental clinician to map the tooth wear.

2. Quantification of tooth wear is possible with one of the many existing grading scales. This grading is necessary to assess the severity of the tooth wear, to classify the tooth wear, and to decide which kind of treatment is necessary (management/restorative treatment).

3. To unravel the etiology of the tooth wear, necessary steps are (1) qualification, (2) structured oral history; and (3) proper questionnaires.

4. A helpful tool is the module "Start of treatment/management" of the TWES.

5. This is possible with the lists of "General complicating factors" and "Specific complicating factors," as described in the module "Level of difficulty" of the TWES.

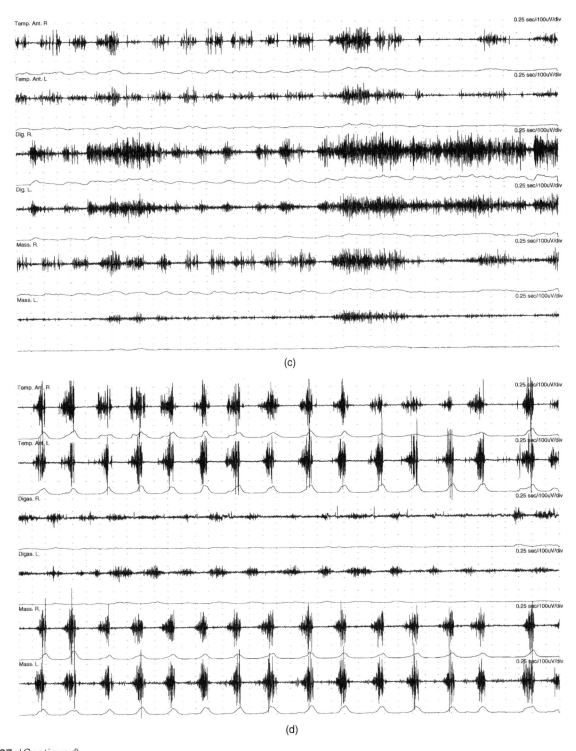

Figure 4.37 (*Continued*)

for facial pain was seldom. The maximal active jaw mobility increased from 52 mm to 58 mm and the blockages of the jaw during mastication decreased.
- There was a great need for oral rehabilitation and general dental treatment; however, treatment may be difficult to manage in these cases because of the dystonic activity (especially tooth preparations, dental impressions, etc.) and of the costs of extensive dental reconstructions (e.g., the patient's financial condition, insurance). Protection of the teeth with splints is seldom used, as the dystonic movements are usually only present during wakefulness.

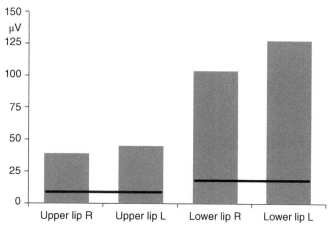

Figure 4.38 High dystonic activity in the lips during resting posture in the case patient. The gray columns represent the average levels of the mean rectified voltages recorded with bipolar surface electrodes over the superior orbicularis (Upper lip R and L) and the inferior orbicularis oris muscles (Lower lip R and L) (Bakke *et al.*, 2013). The black lines indicate the mean plus two standard deviations of corresponding reference values from surface EMG in healthy subjects (Electromyography Laboratory, Clinical Oral Physiology).

Background Information

Definition of dystonia

- Dystonia is a movement disorder characterized by sustained or intermittent muscle contractions causing abnormal, often repetitive, movements, postures, or both. Dystonic movements are typically patterned, twisting, and may be tremulous. Dystonia is often initiated or worsened by voluntary action and associated with overflow muscle activation (Albanese *et al.*, 2013).

Characteristics of oromandibular dystonia

- OMD is a rare focal neurological disorder localized to the lower part of the face and jaws and affecting less than 30 per 100 000 persons.
- Onset is often in the sixth decade of life and more common in women than in men.
- OMD is caused by functional changes in brain areas that contribute to control and performance of conscious and unconscious movements; it may be inherited or acquired, but in most cases OMD is idiopathic.
- OMD is characterized by jaw movements and deviations, restless tongue, and facial grimacing caused by the masticatory, facial, pharyngeal, lingual, and/or lip muscles; consequently,

chewing, swallowing, and speech may be hampered.
- OMD is usually associated with a feeling that the face and jaws are never at rest as well as fatigue in affected muscles, but rarely with pain.
- OMD may look similar to sleep bruxism, but it is present when the patient is awake and usually ceases during sleep.
- OMD is incapacitating as it may affect facial expression, resulting in social isolation and lack of acceptance from those around him.
- OMD may cause severe attrition of the teeth and problems with prosthetic reconstructions and dentures.
- OMD may be misdiagnosed as TMDs, dental problems, or as psychiatric manifestations.
- In most countries, specialists in neurology have the responsibility for the final decision on the diagnosis as well as the treatment of OMD, but dentists should be able to recognize the condition and refer to the proper specialists.
- Presently, there is no general agreement about a precise definition of OMD and the difference between OMD and dyskinesia; however, dyskinesia is in contrast to dystonia most often described as a side effect of medication.
- OMD has currently no cure, but there are treatment options to manage symptoms, such as peroral medication with clonazepam, intramuscular injections with BoNT and in special cases deep brain stimulation with implanted electrodes.

(Bakke *et al.*, 2007, 2013; Balasubramaniam and Ram, 2008)

Diagnostic Criteria

Expanded DC/TMD criteria for **Oromandibular dystonia** (Peck *et al.*, 2014). *Sensitivity and specificity have not been established.*

Excessive, involuntary, and sustained muscle contractions that may involve the face, lips, tongue, and/or jaw.

History. Positive for both of the following:
1. Neurological diagnosis of OMD.
AND
2a. Arthralgia that worsens with episodes of dystonia.

OR

2b. Myalgia that worsens with episodes of dystonia.

Examination. Positive for all of the following:

1. Sensory and/or motor nerve conduction deficit. AND

2. Central and/or peripheral myopathic disease. AND

3. Dystonia confirmed by intramuscular EMG. AND

4a. Arthralgia.

OR

4b. Myalgia.

Note: The pain is not better accounted for by another pain diagnosis.

DC/TMD criteria for **Arthralgia**, see Case 2.1, and for **Myalgia**, see Case 3.3 (Schiffman *et al.*, 2014).

Fundamental Points

- BoNT is a neurotoxin produced by the anaerobic bacterium *Clostridium botulinum*.
- BoNT can be injected to achieve therapeutic benefit across a large range of clinical conditions (e.g., dystonia, spasticity, drooling).
- Evidence-based reviews have evaluated BoNT to be possibly effective for OMD.
- BoNT binds to the nerve terminals and inhibits the release of acetylcholine and this chemo-denervation reduces muscle contractions.
- EMG is essential for precise identification of the muscles involved, for accurate and safe delivery, and for satisfactory therapeutic effect of BoNT in small muscle groups.
- Depending on the anatomic region, misplacement of BoNT during injection may lead to significant but temporary discomfort.
- The latency for the effect is just over 1 week, and BoNT is most effective within the first 1.5 months.
- The neuromuscular transmission regenerates slowly; the effect ceases and normal muscle function is restored after 3–6 months.
- BoNT treatments are typically repeated three or four times per year.

(Møller *et al.*, 2003, 2007; Hallett *et al.*, 2013)

Self-study Questions

1. Which relevant history and clinical observations may indicate the diagnosis of OMD?

2. How do you reach the diagnosis?

3. What is the cure for OMD?

References

Albanese A, Kallash B, Bressman SB, *et al.* (2013) Phenomenology and classification of dystonia: a consensus update. *Mov Disord* **28**(7);863–873.

Bakke M, Larsen BM, Dalager T, Møller E (2013) Oromandibular dystonia – functional and clinical characteristics: a report on 21 cases. *Oral Surg Oral Med Oral Pathol Oral Radiol* **115**(1):e21–e26.

Bakke M, Møller E, Thomsen CE, *et al.* (2007) Chewing in patients with severe neurological impairment. *Arch Oral Biol* **52**(4):399–403.

Balasubramaniam R, Ram S (2008) Orofacial movement disorders. *Oral Maxillofac Surg Clin North Am* **20**(2):273–285.

Conte A, Berardelli I, Ferrazzano G, *et al.* (2016) Non-motor symptoms in patients with adult-onset focal dystonia: sensory and psychiatric disturbances. *Parkinsonism Relat Disord* **22**(Suppl 1):S111–S114.

Hallett M, Albanese A, Dressler D, *et al.* (2013) Evidence-based review and assessment of botulinum neurotoxin for the treatment of movement disorders. *Toxicon* **67**:94–114.

Møller E, Bakke M, Dalager T, Werdelin LM (2007) Oromandibular dystonia involving the lateral pterygoid muscles: four cases with different complexity. *Mov Disord* **22**(6):785–790.

Møller E, Werdelin LM, Bakke M, *et al.* (2003) Treatment of perioral dystonia with botulinum toxin in 4 cases of Meige's syndrome. *Oral Surg Oral Med Oral Pathol Oral Radiol Endod* **96**(5):544–549.

Peck CC, Goulet JP, Lobbezoo F, *et al.* (2014) Expanding the taxonomy of the diagnostic criteria for temporomandibular disorders. *J Oral Rehabil* **41**(1):2–23.

Schiffman E, Ohrbach R, Truelove E, *et al.* (2014) Diagnostic Criteria for Temporomandibular Disorders (DC/TMD) for clinical and research applications: recommendations of the International RDC/TMD Consortium Network and Orofacial Pain Special Interest Group. *J Oral Facial Pain Headache* **28**(1):6–27.

Answers to Self-study Questions

1. Information about tiredness, twitches of the face, involuntary movements of the jaw during wakefulness, severe dental attrition.

2. The diagnosis is reached by a neurological examination supplemented by EMG.

3. There is no cure for OMD, but the condition is often alleviated by daily intake of peroral medication and/or repeated injections of BoNT.

Index

Printed and bound by CPI Group (UK) Ltd, Croydon, CR0 4YY
24/05/2022
03125561-0001